'In the transition from recommendation to
to help them make relevant and meaningful ⌐⌐⌐ ⌐
have pulled together fantastic systems-orientated therapeu⌐⌐⌐   t
will complement or independently propel individuals towards their g⌐⌐⌐ ⌐f
nutrition-orientated optimal health.

Practitioners of functional medicine and others will cherish this book, as it
solves the question: so what CAN I eat, and how do I make it tasty, healthy and
family friendly?'

> *— Michael Ash BSc, DO, ND, F.DipION, osteopath, naturopath, nutritional*
> *therapist and managing director of Integrated Health Consultancy Ltd*

'Integrating nutrition science with Functional Medicine through an evidence-
based approach, this highly practical book is an excellent resource for any
nutrition-oriented healthcare practitioner helping individuals make dietary
changes to support their health. Combining simple advice with delicious,
nutritious recipes suitable for all, it's certainly a book to reach for in the kitchen
on a daily basis.'

> *— Jane Nodder, senior lecturer, clinic tutor and nutritional therapist*

'All the foods we consume affect our function in a positive or negative way. This
health-promoting recipe book will be an invaluable tool for health practitioners
and their patients to identify foods that have a positive function. It is full of
delicious recipes which specifically target the nutritional imbalances associated
with key body systems that are the underlying cause of many health conditions.
This functional approach to eating and lifestyle deals with the root cause of
disease, not just the symptoms.'

> *— Ken Eddie, managing director of Nutri, leaders in the field of Functional Medicine*
> *education*

'This is a cookbook that has just been waiting to happen. A great practitioner
companion to *Biochemical Imbalances in Disease*. The well-referenced text helps
practitioners to readily justify nutrition recommendations for their clients in an
evidence-informed manner, and guide them towards reading specific chapters
and key recipes to support their personalised plan. The brilliance of a functional
nutrition cookbook is that as new data emerges it is relatively straightforward to
update text and revise recipes in a highly relevant and practical way. Personalised
healthcare is here to stay and this cookbook will likely be the first of many that
truly attempts to address the importance of diets for the individual rather than
the population.'

> *— Kate Neil MSc (Nutritional Medicine) MBANT NTCC CNHC Registered*
> *Practitioner, managing director and Head of Quality Assurance, Centre for Nutrition*
> *Education and Lifestyle Management*

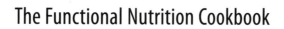

The Functional Nutrition Cookbook

by the same author

Biochemical Imbalances in Disease
A Practitioner's Handbook
Edited by Lorraine Nicolle and Ann Woodriff Beirne
Foreword by David S. Jones M.D.
ISBN 978 1 84819 033 7
eISBN 978 0 85701 028 5

of related interest

Make Yourself Better
A Practical Guide to Restoring Your Body's Wellbeing through Ancient Medicine
Philip Weeks
ISBN 978 1 84819 012 2
eISBN 978 0 85701 077 3

Breaking Free from Persistent Fatigue
Lucie Montpetit
ISBN 978 1 84819 101 3
eISBN 978 0 85701 081 0

THE
FUNCTIONAL
NUTRITION
COOKBOOK

ADDRESSING BIOCHEMICAL
IMBALANCES THROUGH DIET

LORRAINE NICOLLE AND CHRISTINE BAILEY

FOREWORD BY THE INSTITUTE FOR FUNCTIONAL MEDICINE

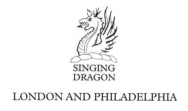

SINGING
DRAGON

LONDON AND PHILADELPHIA

First published in 2013
by Singing Dragon
an imprint of Jessica Kingsley Publishers
73 Collier Street
London N1 9BE, UK
and
400 Market Street, Suite 400
Philadelphia, PA 19106, USA

www.singingdragon.com

Library of Congress Cataloging in Publication Data
Nicolle, Lorraine.
   The functional nutrition cookbook : addressing biochemical imbalances through diet / Lorraine Nicolle and Christine Bailey ; foreword by the Institute for Functional Medicine.
      p. cm.
   Includes bibliographical references and index.
   ISBN 978-1-84819-079-5 (alk. paper)
   1. Nutrition. 2. Nutrient interactions. I. Bailey, Christine, 1970- II. Institute for Functional Medicine. III. Title.
   QP141.N497 2012
   612.3--dc23

                                                          2012012755

British Library Cataloguing in Publication Data
A CIP catalogue record for this book is available from the British Library

ISBN 978 1 84819 079 5
eISBN 978 0 85701 052 0

Printed and bound in Great Britain by Bell and Bain Ltd, Glasgow

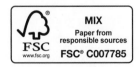

Contents

Contents

Foreword

Nutrition is coming to the fore as a major modifiable determinant of chronic disease, with scientific evidence increasingly supporting the view that alterations in diet have strong effects, both positive and negative, on health throughout life. Most importantly, dietary adjustments may not only influence present health, but may determine whether or not an individual will develop such diseases as cancer, cardiovascular disease and diabetes much later in life.[1]

It is a special pleasure for faculty and staff at The Institute for Functional Medicine to introduce this book on functional nutrition cooking for healthcare practitioners and their patients. In this age of highly processed, nutrient-poor food driving a devastating epidemic of chronic disease in both developed and developing nations, the need for a different approach to selecting, preparing and eating 'our daily bread' is urgent. By now, most people in the relatively affluent countries of the world are familiar with the push to eat less fat, less sugar and more fresh food. Unfortunately, changing eating behaviours is far more complex – and far more difficult – than that.

Dietary choice is a complicated amalgam of culture, availability, marketing, taste preferences, stress, knowledge, habit, relationships and economics (not to mention allergies, intolerances and other health factors). Access to healthy food can be compromised by commercial food practices, inadequate government regulation, the location and inventory of neighbourhood food stores, lack of time to shop and prepare food, and limited finances. While public health officials speak with great urgency about the need to change food production and dietary practices, commercial growers continue their heavy use of toxic pesticides and herbicides and genetic alteration of the food supply, while food manufacturers continue to rely heavily on additives, excessive salt, fat, and sugar, harmful processing, and sophisticated and pervasive marketing strategies to keep us buying the very foods that are making us sick.

Hence, even a quick glance at the issue tells us that helping people adopt healthier diets is not simply a matter of individual self-discipline or knowledge. We need to educate policymakers as well as individuals about why specific changes are important, what the health consequences of not making those changes are likely to be, and exactly how to make step-by-step improvements that will shift our trajectory towards health and away from illness. Physicians and other health practitioners must become ardent advocates for these changes, helping young people avoid or significantly postpone serious disease and assisting older people to halt or reverse the many chronic conditions that are so intimately related to diet: not just heart disease, diabetes and cancer, but arthritis, allergies and autoimmune diseases as well.

The Functional Nutrition Cookbook just made that job a lot easier. Organised by physiological processes (e.g. detoxification, glucose/insulin regulation, immune regulation and half a dozen others), the book provides relatively detailed explanations of how food impairs (or enhances) each of the core functional systems of the body (references are provided at the ends of chapters). This will be familiar territory for clinicians with solid nutrition training and those who have learned a great deal about functional medicine, but it may well represent considerable new information for those without that background.

Meal plans for each chapter are followed by recipes for suggested dishes. The recipes include a per-serving analysis of the basic nutritional components of each dish (protein, fat, carbohydrate and calories). Accommodations are frequently recommended for vegan, vegetarian and gluten-free eating. A very useful set of general guidelines (e.g. how/when to eat; basic stocks, sauces and dressings) is included in the first chapter ('Why and How to Use this Book').

The technical explanations of various physiological processes are likely to be challenging for the average patient, and the meal plans and recipes involve a sea change from the way most people eat. Therefore, just handing (or recommending) the book to patients may not be the most effective way to use it. Practitioners who become familiar with the book's contents and who can speak from firsthand experience about incorporating this approach to food into their own lives will be well equipped to suggest appropriate chapters based on the needs of each individual patient.

The final chapter, 'Healthy Ageing', discusses several basic mechanisms of age-related changes in gene expression that lead to cellular damage and organ dysfunction. For example, an association between hyperinsulinemia and telomere shortening (and between insulin sensitivity and longevity) serves to reinforce the material in the glucose/insulin chapter about the importance of maintaining normal blood sugar regulation. The authors conclude with a brief exploration of the dietary habits of long-lived populations, followed by some general guidelines about which foods to eat regularly and which to avoid, as well as some lifestyle recommendations for healthy living and ageing.

Overall, this dietary manual (it really is much more than a cookbook) provides a very thorough examination of the kinds of changes in food choice and preparation that will be required to regain some mastery over the health of our populations. We highly recommend it and wish you a safe and happy journey to a long and vibrant life.

The Institute for Functional Medicine
505 S. 336th, Suite 500
Federal Way, WA 98003
functionalmedicine.org

References

1. World Health Organization (2003) 'Diet, Nutrition, and the Prevention of Chronic Diseases.' *WHO Technical Report, Series 619*. Geneva: WHO. Available at http://whqlibdoc.who.int/trs/who_trs_916.pdf, accessed on 25 July 2012.

1

Why and How to Use this Book

> Throughout your life the most profound influences on your health, vitality and function are not the doctors you have visited, surgery, or other therapies you have undertaken. The most profound influences are the cumulative effects of the decisions you make about your diet and lifestyle on the expression of your genes.[1]

This quotation, by the nutritional biochemist Dr Jeffrey Bland, succinctly captures our reasons for writing *The Functional Nutrition Cookbook*. For, if our state of health is the lifelong culmination of the interactions between our genes and our lifestyle, we are all invested with the capability to alter our current state of wellbeing and our likely risk of developing degenerative diseases.

Systems versus symptoms

In this and the following chapters you will find eating guidelines, meal plans and recipes to give you some ideas for designing and implementing the *dietary* changes that will bring you the most benefit.

The recommendations are not organised according to disease states or symptoms. Rather, they are categorised according to specific physiological processes of the human body. This is because chronic diseases are almost always 'preceded by a lengthy period of declining function in one or more [such]…body systems'.[2] (Indeed, such a decline in function generally exists long before any signs or symptoms manifest.)

The body systems taking centre stage in this book are:

- gastro-intestinal function

- detoxification processes

- cell membrane function and the balance of fatty acid metabolites

- blood glucose and insulin control

- thyroid and adrenal function

- sex hormone balance

- immune tolerance and the control of inflammation

- antioxidant processes

- brain chemistry.

We believe that rather than simply treating clinical symptoms, these are more valuably used as indicators of underlying functional problems within such body systems. The consequent diet and lifestyle recommendations are therefore designed to provide support to the systems that appear imbalanced.

The benefit of this deep approach is not only the management of symptoms but also a new-found feeling of vitality and the potential prevention of long-term chronic conditions, such as cancer, cardiovascular disease, diabetes, autoimmunity and mental health problems.

A personalised approach

With the exception of identical twins, we are each endowed with a unique set of genes. We also each have a life history like no one else's. As we progress through this unique story (that is, as we age), our experiences trigger changes in the way our genes are expressed (see the section on 'epigenetic changes' in Chapter 11). In biochemical terms, then, each of us is truly *individual*.

Thus, while there are certain dietary modifications that are likely to benefit everyone (such as avoiding *trans*-fats, for example), the one-size-fits-all 'healthy diet' does not exist. Rather, the diet of most benefit to your health will be one that is specifically designed to meet your individual biochemical needs. This practice is known as personalised nutrition and it is different from standard nutrition advice, such as the 'five-a-day' mantra, which aims to achieve incremental improvements in the health of the wider population.

Most countries have in place, for example, a system of 'recommended daily allowances' (RDAs) for nutrients, and these may be useful for benchmarking the basic nutritional status of populations. However, it's now thought that up to a third of all genetic variations between individuals affect the ways in which vitamins and minerals bind to their receptors in order to make everyday biological processes happen.[3] This means that if you have one of these genetic variations, you are likely to need far higher than average levels of certain micronutrients in order to function normally. Thus these standard nutrition recommendations do not, and cannot, take account of biochemical individuality.

Moreover, the more progressive nutrition scientists point out that because these RDA-type systems were originally designed to help prevent the classic deficiency diseases (such as scurvy, caused by vitamin C deficiency, and rickets, caused by lack of vitamin D), they are too low to be used as targets for peak health. This is because they do not take into account the insidious consequences of long-term, milder insufficiencies.[4] Such insufficiencies may go unnoticed for decades, all the while disrupting physiological systems, damaging cells and eventually leading to premature ageing and age-related diseases.[3, 4, 5, 6]

Thus optimal (and personalised) intakes of all nutrients are crucial throughout life, and this can only be achieved through a personalised dietary and lifestyle plan.

A model for organising these principles

This type of personalised, systems-oriented approach to dietary intervention is based on an evidence-based model of chronic healthcare known as 'functional medicine' (FM). Started in the 1990 by Dr Jeffrey Bland, FM is now practised by a growing number of US medical doctors and is included in an increasing number of academic healthcare programmes.

FM's starting point is to consider not what disease the patient has but what type of individual has the disease. You can read more about functional medicine at the Institute for Functional Medicine's website.[7]

All roads lead to and from inflammation

When aiming to improve the functioning of physiological systems, it's important to be mindful that they don't operate in isolation. Rather, they are inextricably linked to each other through a complex web of interactions. Hence, the dietary and lifestyle recommendations in each of this book's chapters, while focused on one body system, will also likely influence others. So you'll see that we will often cross-refer you to advice on the pages of other chapters.

This is never more the case than in addressing problems with the body's ability to regulate inflammation. Long-term, low-grade inflammation is at the route of all chronic, degenerative illness. But in order to address the inflammation, you often need to rebalance other body processes.

For example, poor blood glucose control leads to glycation (see Chapter 11), which leads to oxidation (see Chapter 9), causing inflammation. A microflora imbalance in the gastro-intestinal tract (see Chapter 2) leads to compromised detoxification processes (see Chapter 3), which causes an increased oxidative load (see Chapter 9) and then inflammation. Poor methylation (see Chapter 7) leads to high blood levels of the transient amino acid homocysteine. This damages cells in the walls of the blood vessels, leading to inflammation.

There are various natural interventions that can reduce the symptoms of inflammation (curcumin, from the turmeric spice, being one such example). A truly effective approach to long-term health, however, will complement any such intervention with a strategy to identify and address the underlying causes of the inflammation (see Chapter 8).

Nutrition as part of the overall picture of health

It's also worth remembering that dietary interventions will have limited effects unless they are also accompanied by improvements to other aspects of your life; hence, we have included some lifestyle recommendations in each of the chapters. Researchers studying communities throughout the world with higher than average proportions of long-lived, healthy inhabitants, sometimes referred to as 'Blue Zones', propose the following overall approach to a longer, healthier life:[8]

- Build more natural physical movement into every day (e.g. by rejecting some of the time-saving electronic equipment that has 'simplified' your life).

- Live with a sense of purpose.

- Adopt daily stress-management behaviours.

- Eat only until you are 80 per cent full. This will stop you from overeating and help to optimise digestive function and weight management. Reduce the size of your plates. Don't eat in front of the television – focus on your meal.

- Use plants as the basis of your diet. The majority of your calories should come from vegetables, nuts and seeds.

- Have a sense of spiritual belonging, whether this is through a religious faith or through accessing the spiritual qualities of art and/or nature.

- Spend regular, quality time with your children, your partner and other loved ones.

- Be part of a supportive community of friends, colleagues, acquaintances and/or neighbours.

In addition, many long-lived communities regularly drink a little antioxidant-rich red wine (with friends and food). Outside these communities, however, there is a high prevelance of addictions and chronic diseases, such as cancer, and we therefore advocate assessing the benefits of alcohol consumption on an individual basis.

An evidence-based approach

A personalised, systems-oriented approach may be a departure from conventional nutritional practice but it is no less evidence-informed. Every chapter in this book carries a list of references to medical lectures and scientific papers, the vast majority from well-established peer-reviewed journals. The summaries of these are freely available from the US National Institutes of Health database, Pubmed.[9]

Evidence presented includes randomised controlled trials of human subjects, population-based studies, animal studies and laboratory work. While some of the research findings may be viewed as 'preliminary', they have been included because the consequent recommendations for dietary and lifestyle changes are unlikely to carry negative side effects.

Putting this approach into practice

How do you identify the body systems that need the most support, in your particular case? Ideally, it's best to work with a healthcare practitioner using personalised nutrition. He or she will take a detailed case history and may recommend some laboratory testing. This process helps to identify the underlying physiological processes that are flagging (and contributing to symptoms). Each of these body processes has the potential to be altered so as to improve the function of your cells and organs.

Once the order for supporting the body systems has been prioritised, you and your practitioner can design your individual health plan, based on the ideas and recipes in the relevant chapters of this book.

A final note before we begin

While this book is written for nutrition-oriented healthcare practitioners to use in clinic, appropriate chapters can also be recommended to patients, as a support to their personalised healthcare plans.

The book is designed to be read as a stand-alone resource. However, practitioners may prefer to use it as a companion to the personalised nutrition textbook *Biochemical Imbalances in Disease*.[10] Where appropriate, we have referenced and directed you to the relevant sections of this textbook for further information.

Be aware that these meal plans and recipes are not designed to be exhaustive or prescriptive, but as bases to be adapted to your individual needs. While we have included a range of recipes in each chapter, some are interchangeable, so please look through all the recipes in the book and adapt the meal plans accordingly. Please also note that the advice is not meant as an alternative to seeing your doctor, nor should it be viewed as a diagnosis of any condition. You should visit your doctor if you or your practitioner suspect that you may have a medical condition or if you have undiagnosed symptoms. Moreover, you should not discontinue, nor alter the dosage of, any medication without the knowledge of your doctor.

Some general dietary guidelines

- Start each day with a cup of warm water. You can add lemon juice or fresh ginger (steep the root) if desired. Some people find this helps to stimulate the digestive tract and the bowel.

- Eat three meals a day, at regular times, and always have breakfast (by 10am).

- Snacks are optional. Do not eat them unless you are genuinely too hungry to wait until the next meal. You can also skip a snack in order to use it as a dessert. We have included snacks for the benefit of individuals with large appetites, who are doing more physical activity and/or who are vulnerable to hypoglycaemic states between meals. If you are not affected by these issues, it may be appropriate to do without snacks. This will give your digestive system a rest.

- Never eat to the extent that you feel stuffed – always stop eating before you feel full (see the 80% rule above).

- Don't overdo the calories. The UK Government recommends 2,500 calories per day for men, and 2,000 for women. However, the amount needed by an individual will vary and is also influenced by activity levels.

- Eat fruits and/or vegetables at every meal, making each plate as colourful as possible, so that you are taking in a broad range of beneficial phytonutrients (see Chapter 9). Some of these should be raw every day – in the form of salads, green juices and smoothies, vegetable crudités and/or marinated vegetables, for example.

- Vegetables should comprise a half to two-thirds of your plate at lunch and dinner, with the remaining third protein. Starches (grains and potatoes) are optional – if you want to include them, use small portions only.

- Eat lean protein with every meal and snack. A portion of protein in a meal should measure approximately the size of the palm of your hand. If you are a vegan, combining grains with beans, pulses, nuts or seeds will provide good-quality protein.

- Include raw nuts and seeds daily, or you could use nut butters and cold-pressed seed oils instead.

- Eat a variety of whole, natural, unprocessed foods and try not to eat the same food every day. This ensures a wide range of nutrients and reduces the chance of developing food addictions and sensitivities. Try to prepare meals from scratch, using simple whole foods and nutritious ingredients.

- Eat organic food wherever possible, to minimise your exposure to antibiotics, growth promoters, pesticides, fertilisers and other chemical residues. Know the provenance of your meat and check that it is free-range and grass-fed.

- Avoid genetically modified foods.

- Replace all white starches (bread, bagels, rice, pasta) with wholemeal varieties.

- Aim to eat most of your food raw, baked, boiled, steamed, steam-fried or cooked in a slow-cooker. Lower-temperature cooking preserves the food's health-giving nutrients. Browning food creates potentially damaging molecules, some of which are known carcinogens (such as polycyclic aromatic hydrocarbons). Microwaving is a relatively novel cooking method. The evidence for its effects on food quality appears somewhat contradictory and thus minimal usage only is recommended.

- Eat primarily fresh or frozen foods, although tinned beans and pulses can be used if they are free of added salt and sugar.

- Avoid commercially processed foods as much as possible. Get used to reading labels and don't buy foods with added colourings, preservatives or sweeteners.

- Don't add polyunsaturated oils (vegetable, seed and corn oils) to foods for cooking, as they degrade when heated and produce 'free radicals' that damage cells. Saturated fats, such as butter, lard and coconut oil, are stable at high temperatures and can therefore be used for cooking. Coconut oil is the healthiest of these three and that is why we have used it in our recipes. However, it is more expensive than some other oils. You can use olive oil for cooking at lower temperatures. The polyunsaturated oils can be poured over-cooked or raw food or used in dressings; keep them in the fridge because they go rancid quickly.

- Chew all food thoroughly. Chewing triggers the rest of the digestive process.

- Do not eat when stressed, overly tired or upset, as these factors impair digestion.

- Eat slowly and enjoy your food, sharing it with friends and family whenever possible.

- Drink 1.5 litres/3 pints of water a day (more with physical activity). This includes soups and broths, herbal teas and vegetable smoothies. A water filter is useful to reduce unwanted chemicals and toxic metals. If you are caffeine-sensitive, limit your intake of coffee and black tea. (Caffeine tolerance varies considerably between individuals, so you should discuss this with your nutrition practitioner.)

- If you have a particularly large appetite, have some extra vegetables on the side. Use one of the vegetable dishes outlined in this book, or simply chop, steam and dress any available vegetables with a mixture of cold-pressed olive or flax oil and cider vinegar or lemon juice, adding chopped herbs, garlic and/or tamari (wheat-free) soy sauce if desired.

- Stick to these guidelines as much as you can – but don't become obsessive.

Notes about the meal plans and recipes

- Many of the lunches are portable: soups can be carried around in a flask and salads can be taken in plastic pots.

- Many of the dishes can be made in large quantities and frozen in individual portions. Each recipe has a nutritional analysis per serving (including any dressings or sauces, unless specified or listed as 'optional').

- The inclusion in the recipes of xylitol and other natural sugars is optional and is primarily for the benefit of readers who are gradually moving from a high-sugar to a low-sugar diet. If you do not need the sweetness, it is best to reduce or omit these sugars, to avoid encouraging a desire for sweet-tasting foods. (Also note that dogs should not be given access to xylitol, as they are unable to metabolise it.)

Basic recipes

Here are some basic recipes, many of which form part of the meal plans in the following chapters.

Stocks

Fish Stock

250g/9oz fish trimmings (you can include heads, bones and skin of most types of fish, but avoid salmon, red mullet and oily fish)
1 large leek, chopped
1 fennel bulb
1 large carrot, chopped
1 celery stick, including the leafy top, sliced
Handful of parsley, including the stalks

Rinse the fish bones and trimmings of any blood.

Place the vegetables in a large pan or stockpot.

Roughly chop the parsley, including the stems, and add to the stockpot.

Add the fish trimmings to the stockpot.

Pour in enough cold water to cover the fish and vegetables (about 1 litre/2 pints).

Bring to the boil, then simmer. Remove the scum that forms on the surface with a spoon and discard. Simmer, covered, for about 25 minutes, skimming as necessary.

Strain, discarding the fish trimmings and the vegetables.

Cool and store in the fridge for up to 3 days or freeze for up to 1 month.

Vegetable Stock

1 leek, diced
1 carrot, diced
1 small bulb fennel, diced
2 garlic cloves, peeled
1 head of broccoli
2 sticks celery, diced
Handful of spinach leaves
Potato peelings (optional)

Chop up all the vegetables.

Place in a pan and add enough cold water to cover the vegetables generously.

Bring to the boil, cover and simmer for 20–30 minutes.

Strain the liquid and drink the broth or use as a stock.

Cool and store in the fridge for up to 3 days or freeze for up to 1 month.

Chicken Stock

1 organic chicken or 3–4lbs chicken parts with bones
1 onion, coarsely chopped
3 carrots, chopped
2 celery sticks, chopped
2–3 courgettes (zucchini), sliced into 5cm/2in rounds
2 garlic cloves

Place the chicken in a large stockpot and add enough water to cover the chicken. Add the rest of the ingredients.

Bring to the boil then lower the heat to a gentle simmer.

Cook gently for at least 2–3 hours and ideally 6–8 hours.

Remove the chicken and place on a platter to cool. Once the chicken has cooled remove all meat from the carcass. (This can be used for a chicken salad.)

2 tbsp apple cider vinegar (optional)
2 tbsp coconut oil (optional)
Sea salt and black peppercorns

The stock can be strained at this stage or the vegetables can be put through a high-speed blender. For a richer stock, add the carcass and continue to cook for a further 4–5 hours. Alternatively, the carcass can be used to make an additional batch of lighter stock, following the recipe but using the carcass instead of the whole chicken.

This stock will keep in the fridge for 3–4 days or can be frozen for up to 1 month.

Butters and spreads

Utterly Buttery Creamy Spread

Simply combine a mixture of half organic virgin coconut oil and half ghee to produce a creamy spread. This is also perfect for cooking.

Nutritional information per tbsp

Calories 135kcal
Protein 0g
Carbohydrates 0g
Total fat 15g of which saturates 11.4g

Garlic Oil Spread

Blend coconut oil with a couple of cloves of garlic, crushed, and extra virgin olive oil to form a spreadable paste. Delicious on toasted bread.

Nutritional information per tbsp

Calories 110kcal
Protein 0.2g
Carbohydrates 0.4g of which sugars 0g
Total fat 12g of which saturates 7g

Gut Healing Creamy Butter

Blend together 400g/14oz ghee with 125ml/5fl oz olive oil, 2–3 tsp probiotic powder and 3 tsp colostrum powder (available from good health food shops and online). Unless you have a microbial imbalance in the gut (see Chapter 2), you could also include 3 tsp L-glutamine and 3 tsp raw honey or Manuka honey.

Nutritional information per tbsp

Calories 125kcal
Protein 0.4g
Carbohydrates 0.8g of which sugars 0.4g
Total fat 13.5g of which saturates 7.2g

Ghee

Ghee is clarified butter – that is, the oil of butter with the milk solids removed. Ghee tends to be less mucous-forming than butter and contains no lactose (milk sugar). It keeps longer than butter and does not require refrigeration. Organic ghee is now readily available but it is easy to make your own. Ghee contains a combination of saturated and unsaturated fats and includes short-chained fats, making it easily digestible. It is rich in butyric acid, a short-chain fatty acid that supports the health and healing of cells in the small and large intestines. Ghee also contains antioxidants, conjugated linoleic acid and fat-soluble vitamins A, D, E and K.

450g/1lb organic butter

Cut the butter into chunks and place in a pan. Melt the butter over a low heat.

When it begins to bubble, you will see white milk solids settling on the surface. After a couple of minutes these solids will clear from the surface.

Remove from the heat and let it cool. The solids will sink to the bottom of the pan.

Gently tip the pan without stirring and strain off the clear yellow liquid into a sterilised jar.

Nutritional information per tbsp

Calories 135kcal

Protein 0g

Carbohydrates 0g

Total fat 15g of which saturates 9.9g

Simple Nut Cheese

60g/2oz/½ cup pine nuts or cashew nuts
60g/2oz/½ cup macadamia nuts
2 tsp lemon juice
¼ tsp sea salt
2 tbsp nutritional yeast
3–4 tbsp water

Ideally, soak the nuts for 1–2 hours and then drain before using.

Place all the ingredients in a food processor or blender with just enough water to make a smooth cheese.

Nutritional information per 100g

Calories 34kcal

Protein 1g

Carbohydrates 0g

Total fat 3.3g of which saturates 0.5g

Sauces

Tomato Vegetable Sauce

- SERVES 4

1 tbsp olive oil or coconut oil
1 onion, chopped
1 garlic clove, crushed
1 stick celery, chopped
1 carrot, chopped
1 red pepper, chopped
400g/14oz canned plum tomatoes
1 tbsp tomato purée
1 tbsp balsamic vinegar

Heat the oil in a large saucepan. Sauté the onion and garlic for 2 minutes until softened.

Add the celery, carrot and pepper and stir for 1–2 minutes.

Add the rest of the ingredients. Cover and simmer for 15 minutes until the vegetables are tender.

Purée the sauce with a hand-held blender. Add a little water if needed to thin the sauce.

Nutritional information per serving

Calories 72kcal

Protein 2.2g

Carbohydrates 9.5g of which sugars 8.5g

Total fat 2.6g of which saturates 0.4g

Simple Watercress and Herb Sauce

This is delicious served with fish and shellfish or drizzled over steamed vegetables. Similar to a pesto, yet dairy free. Using walnuts and flaxseed oil is an easy way to increase the omega-3 content.

- SERVES 4

100g/3½oz watercress
30g/1oz fresh parsley
60g/2oz walnuts
4 tbsp flaxseed oil
100ml/3½fl oz olive oil
Zest of 1 lemon
1 tsp lemon juice
Pinch of xylitol to taste

Place the watercress, parsley and walnuts in a blender and pulse until finely chopped.

Gradually pour in the flaxseed oil and olive oil with the lemon zest, lemon juice and xylitol. Season to taste. Blend to form a smooth, thick sauce.

Chill in the fridge until needed, for up to 2 days.

Nutritional information per tbsp

Calories 94kcal

Protein 0.6g

Carbohydrates 0.3g of which sugars 0.2g

Total fat 9.9g of which saturates 1.2g

Supergreens Pesto

1 tsp supergreen powder (e.g. chlorella or spirulina)
30g/1oz/¼ cup walnuts
30g/1oz/¼ cup pine nuts
1 large handful of rocket (arugula) leaves
1 handful of fresh basil leaves
1–2 tbsp lemon juice
1–2 cloves garlic
1–2 tbsp nutritional yeast flakes
4–6 tbsp flaxseed or olive oil
Sea salt and freshly ground black pepper

In a food processor, place the supergreen powder and nuts and process until coarsely chopped. Add the rocket and basil leaves, lemon juice, garlic and nutritional yeast flakes and process to form a paste.

Gradually add enough oil to form a thick sauce. Season with sea salt and black pepper.

Nutritional information per tbsp
Calories 57kcal
Protein 1g
Carbohydrates 0.3g of which sugars 0.2g
Total fat 5.7g of which saturates 0.7g

Drinks and milks

Homemade Kefir

Kefir is a delicious probiotic drink, useful for improving gut microflora, if taken regularly (e.g. each morning). It is made with kefir 'grains', comprising a mother culture that digests sugar in a fermentation process. The easiest way to make it is to use a kefir starter kit. These are readily available online. Although cow's milk is traditionally used, kefir can be made with sheep's milk, soy, coconut, rice or nut milk or the liquid from young coconuts. Kefir has many benefits, including better digestion of fats, proteins and carbohydrates. It is an ancient cultured food rich in amino acids, enzymes, calcium, magnesium, phosphorus and B vitamins. Kefir contains several major strains of friendly bacteria (*Lactobacillus Caucasus, Leuconostoc, Acetobacter* species and *Streptococcus* species) and beneficial yeasts (such as *Saccharomyces Kefir* and *Torula Kefir*). Once you have made a batch, you can use some of this to make up to 6–7 more batches before you need to purchase more starter powder. Generally one starter kit will make about 1 litre/2 pints kefir but the exact amount will vary according to the size of the starter pack. It takes between 24–30 hours to ferment the cultures in milk at room temperature on colder days but less if it is warm. Once fermented, store it in the fridge and consume it within 4 days. You can then take 200ml/7fl oz of your freshly made kefir to make another 1 litre portion of kefir if desired.

1 starter kit
1 litre/2 pints milk or milk alternative or coconut water from young green coconuts
A clean, sterilised jar big enough to hold 1 litre/2 pints

Empty one starter culture sachet into a small glass, pour over a little of the milk and stir to make a smooth paste.

Gradually add more milk and keep stirring to ensure there are no lumps. Then pour all of the milk and culture into your prepared jar.

Cover the jar with cling film or put the lid on and leave the mixture to ferment at 23°C/72°F for at least 24 hours (up to 48 hours is needed for coconut water). The mixture should be pourable but still thick. Coconut water and rice milk will not thicken.

> **Nutritional information per cup (250ml) using low fat organic milk**
>
> **Calories 110kcal**
> **Protein 11g**
> **Carbohydrates 12g of which sugars 12g**
> **Total fat 2g of which saturates 1.5g**

Basic Nut Milk

While there are many alternative milk options now available, it is easy and delicious to make your own nut milks.

Almond or Cashew Milk

▪ SERVES 2

200g/7oz almonds or cashew nuts
   (soak overnight if desired)
600ml/21fl oz/2⅓ cup water
Pinch of stevia or 3–4 dates
¼ tsp natural vanilla extract
   (optional)

Put the ingredients in a blender. Process on high until smooth. If it looks a little grainy, strain the milk through muslin or a very fine sieve.

Best drunk straight away but can keep in the fridge covered for up to 1 day.

> **Nutritional information per cup (250ml)**
>
> **Calories 382kcal**
> **Protein 13.1g**
> **Carbohydrates 4.4g of which sugars 2.9g**
> **Total fat 34.7g of which saturates 2.8g**

Quick and Easy Sweet Milk

▪ SERVES 2

500ml/17fl oz/2 cups water
2 tbsp cashew nut butter or almond
   nut butter
Pinch of stevia or 3–4 dates

Place all the ingredients into a blender and process to form a creamy, smooth milk.

Serve immediately.

> **Nutritional information per cup (250ml)**
>
> **Calories 80kcal**
> **Protein 2g**
> **Carbohydrates 2.2g of which sugars 0.8g**
> **Total fat 7.7g of which saturates 0.7g**

Dressings

Simply whisk all the ingredients and chill until required. Most will keep in the fridge for 4–5 days.

Basic Vinaigrette

4 tbsp extra virgin olive oil
4 tbsp flaxseed oil
3 tbsp balsamic vinegar
4 tbsp water
1 tsp Dijon mustard
Black pepper
1 clove garlic, crushed

Nutritional information per tbsp

Calories 54kcal
Protein 0.1g
Carbohydrates 0.1g of which sugar 0.1g
Total fat 5.7g of which saturates 0.7g

Balsamic Vinaigrette

3 tbsp extra olive oil
6 tbsp flaxseed oil
2 tbsp balsamic vinegar
1 garlic clove, crushed
1 tsp Dijon mustard
Sea salt to taste

Nutritional information per tbsp

Calories 95kcal
Protein 0.1g
Carbohydrates 0.1g of which sugars 0.1g
Total fat 9.8g of which saturates 1.1g

Apple Cider Dressing

4 tbsp extra virgin olive oil
2 tbsp apple cider vinegar
¼ tsp Dijon mustard
Sea salt, pepper and herbs to taste

Nutritional information per tbsp

Calories 73kcal
Protein 0.1g
Carbohydrates 0.1g of which sugars 0.1g
Total fat 8g of which saturates 1.1g

Honey, Sesame and Ginger Dressing

Juice and zest of 2 limes
1 tsp freshly grated ginger
2 tbsp raw honey
2 tbsp soy sauce
2 tsp sesame oil
4 tbsp hemp oil, flaxseed oil or extra
    virgin olive oil

Nutritional information per tbsp

Calories 44kcal
Protein 0.1g
Carbohydrates 3.1g of which sugars 3.1g
Total fat 3.5g of which saturates 0.5g

Tofu Dressing

2 tsp xylitol or honey
1 tsp tabasco sauce or mustard to
    taste
5 tbsp silken tofu or soy yoghurt
2 tbsp cider vinegar
Freshly ground black pepper
A little water to thin if needed

Nutritional information per tbsp

Calories 42kcal
Protein 4.4g
Carbohydrates 3.4g of which sugars 1.3g
Total fat 1.6g of which saturates 0g

Tahini Soy Dressing

1 tbsp tahini (sesame seed paste)
Lemon juice to taste
1 tsp soy sauce
A little water to thin

Nutritional information per tbsp

Calories 49kcal
Protein 1.5g
Carbohydrates 0.2g of which sugars 0.1g
Total fat 4.7g of which saturates 0.7g

Lemon and Ginger Dressing

Grated rind and juice of ½ lemon
1 tsp raw or Manuka honey
1 tbsp extra virgin olive oil
1 tsp freshly grated root ginger
1 tbsp mint leaves, chopped

Nutritional information per tbsp

Calories 30kcal
Protein 0.1g
Carbohydrates 1.8g of which sugars 1.7g
Total fat 2.5g of which saturates 0.4g

Raspberry Walnut Vinaigrette

4 tbsp raspberry vinegar
1 tsp Dijon mustard
3 tbsp walnut oil
3 tbsp olive oil
Sea salt and freshly ground black
    pepper to taste

Nutritional information per tbsp

Calories 64kcal
Protein 0.1g
Carbohydrates 0.1g of which 0.1g
Total fat 6.9g of which saturates 0.8g

Almond Tomato Dressing

4 sundried tomatoes, drained
2 tomatoes
2 tbsp almond nut butter
1 tsp xylitol or honey (optional)
1 garlic clove
Pinch of sea salt
2 tsp lemon juice

Blend in a food processor adding a little water to thin as needed.

Nutritional information per tbsp
Calories 44kcal
Protein 1.2g
Carbohydrates 0.3g of which sugars 0.3g
Total fat 4.2g of which saturates 0.6g

Tofu Mayonnaise

150g/5oz silken tofu
1 tsp Dijon mustard
4 tbsp flaxseed oil
1 tsp honey to taste
2 tbsp lemon juice
4 tbsp water
1 small clove of garlic (optional)
Pinch of sea salt and freshly ground
    black pepper

Simply blend all the ingredients in a blender until smooth, adding enough water to create a thick sauce. Chill in the fridge for 2–3 days.

Nutritional information per tbsp
Calories 49kcal
Protein 3.5g
Carbohydrates 2g of which sugars 0.3g
Total fat 3g of which saturates 0.2g

Dill Ranch Nut Dressing/Dip

125g/4½oz/1 cup cashews, soaked
    for 1 hour or ideally overnight
    in the fridge, then rinsed and
    drained
1 tbsp nutritional yeast flakes
    (optional)
¼ tsp sea salt or garlic salt
1–2 garlic cloves, crushed
2 tbsp apple cider vinegar to taste
Pinch of xylitol to taste
2 tsp tomato purée
125ml/4fl oz/½ cup water
Large handful of fresh dill, chopped

Place all the ingredients except the dill in a blender with the water and process until smooth and creamy. Add a little more water if needed to reach the desired consistency. Keep it thicker if you are using it for a dip.

Stir in the chopped dill. Season to taste.

Nutritional information per tbsp
Calories 64kcal
Protein 2g
Carbohydrates 2g of which sugars 0.6g
Total fat 5.2g of which saturates 1g

Accompaniments

Homemade Sauerkraut

Pickled fermented vegetables make a delicious healthy addition to the diet. Unlike shop-bought versions, they are raw and therefore richer in beneficial enzymes. Not only does pasteurisation destroy these enzymes, but many commercial versions are also high in salt and other additives. Sauerkraut is based on shredded cabbage but there are many other variations of pickled fermented vegetables (e.g. kimchi). They can help populate the digestive tract with friendly bacteria and are traditionally thought to be alkalising. Aim to include these on a regular basis. To aid digestion we recommend having a few tablespoons 10–15 minutes before meals. The juice from the fermentation can also be used as a replacement for vinegar in salad dressings.

Use organic, fresh vegetables. Wash and dry them throughly. Vary the vegetables according to taste.

1 cabbage (e.g. savoy or napa or a mixture of white and red cabbage), shredded in a food processor
3 carrots, grated or chopped finely
2 shallots, finely chopped
2 tbsp sea salt
125ml/4fl oz/½ cup warm water
1 tbsp root ginger, peeled and grated
3 garlic cloves, peeled and chopped
2 tsp dill seed
2 tsp fennel seeds
Handful of washed, soaked sea vegetables, chopped (optional)

Place the vegetables in a large mixing bowl.

Place the sea salt and water in a separate small bowl and stir to dissolve. Pour over the vegetables and massage the mixture with your hands. Set aside at room temperature overnight to soften.

The following day, drain, reserving the salt water. Stir in the garlic, ginger, dill and fennel seeds to the cabbage mixture and the sea vegetables (if using). Mix well. Tightly pack the mixture into a large glass jar with a lid. Pour over the saved salt water and press it firmly so there is no trapped air and the cabbage is covered in its own juice. Tightly close the lid. Leave the jar in a warm, dark place for 3–4 days. It will take at least a week if left in a cool place.

Refrigerate after opening. This will keep for a couple of weeks in the fridge.

Nutritional information per tbsp
Calories 4kcal
Protein 0.3g
Carbohydrates 0.7g of which sugars 0.6g
Total fat 0.1g of which saturates 0g

Homemade Yoghurt and Soured Cream

When making your own yoghurt, we recommend organic milk only. Goat's yoghurt may be better tolerated by some people than cow's. Soy yoghurt can also be made in the same way. Goat's and soy yoghurt tend to contain more liquid than cow's yoghurt and may be better in drinks. To make your own yoghurt, you will need to introduce bacteria into the milk. You can buy commercially available yoghurt starter kits, but equally you can use 'live' yoghurt as a starter. After making the first batch you can use some of your yoghurt to make the next batch.

In a pan, bring 1 litre/2 pints milk (goat's, cow's or soy) to just below boiling point. Do not boil. Take off the heat and allow to cool down until the temperature is around 38–40°C/100–104°F. This should feel warm on the skin. Add the starter kit to the milk according to packet instructions or 3–4 tbsp live yoghurt. Stir well. You can place the mixture into a yoghurt maker or use a clean dry thermos flask. Ferment the yoghurt for 24 hours. After fermentation, place the yoghurt into a clean jug or bowl and refrigerate.

To thicken the yoghurt, you can strain off some of the liquid. Simply place a piece of muslin in a sieve set over a large bowl. Pour the yoghurt into the lined sieve and allow it to drip through for several hours. The longer you leave it to drip, the thicker the yoghurt will be, and you can also create a soft cottage-type cheese in this way.

To make soured cream, simply use organic cream instead of milk, and use either a starter kit or 200g/7oz live yoghurt and ferment as above for 24 hours.

Nutrient-Packed Salad

This is a simple and filling salad that can be varied according to taste. Romaine lettuce, collard greens, Swiss chard and kale are all robust enough for the dressing and are rich in carotenoids, vitamins C and K and the minerals magnesium, calcium, iron, manganese and potassium. If you prefer, you could use one of the other dressings in this chapter. For additional protein include more sprouted seeds or beans or accompany with some meat, fish or eggs.

▪ SERVES 4

Dressing
125g/4½oz/1 cup cashew nuts
100ml/3½fl oz water
2 tsp lemon juice or apple cider
    vinegar
Pinch of xylitol or stevia to taste
1 tbsp nutritional yeast flakes
    (optional)
1 garlic clove
1 tomato
½ tsp sea salt
Freshly ground black pepper

....

150g/5oz collard greens, kale or
    Swiss chard, shredded
1 romaine lettuce, chopped
1 ripe avocado, sliced
4 spring onions (scallions), chopped
Large handful of sprouted beans or
    seeds
12 cherry tomatoes, halved
1 nori sheet or 2 tsp seaweed
    sprinkles

For the dressing simply place all the ingredients in a blender and process until smooth and creamy – add a little more water if needed. This can be chilled in the fridge for 2–3 days.

Place the greens and lettuce in a large bowl. Spoon a small amount of the dressing over the leaves and toss to coat – this will help to soften the leaves.

Add the avocado, spring onions, sprouted beans and tomatoes and toss lightly. Crumble over the nori sheet or sprinkle over the seaweed flakes. Spoon over a little additional dressing if needed and serve.

Nutritional information per serving

Calories 253kcal
Protein 8.3g
Carbohydrates 7.7g of which sugars 3.4g
Total fat 20.8g of which saturates 4.1g

References

1. Bland, J. and Benum, S. (1999) 'Genetic Nutritioneering: How You Can Modify Inherited Traits and Live a Longer, Healthier Life.' Los Angeles, CA: Keats. Page 222.
2. Jones, D.S., Bland, J.S. and Quinn, S. (2005) 'What is Functional Medicine?' In D.S. Jones (ed.) *The Textbook of Functional Medicine*. Gig Harbor, WA: Institute for Functional Medicine. Page 5.
3. Ames, B. (2002) 'High dose vitamin therapy stimulates variant enzymes with decreased coenzyme binding affinity (increased Km): Relevance to genetic disease and polymorphisms.' *American Journal of Clinical Nutrition 75*, 616–58.
4. Heaney, R. (2003) 'Long-latency deficiency disease: Insights from calcium and vitamin D.' *American Journal of Clinical Nutrition 78*, 912–9.
5. McCann, J. and Ames, B. (2009) 'Vitamin K, an example of triage theory: Is micro-nutrient inadequacy linked to diseases of ageing?' *American Journal of Clinical Nutrition 90*, 889–907.
6. Ames, B. (2010) 'Prevention of mutation, cancer and other age-associated disease by optimising micronutrient intake.' *Journal of Nucleic Acids*, online. Available from www.ncbi.nlm.nih.gov/pubmed/20936173.
7. Institute for Functional Medicine (2012) 'What is functional medicine?' Available at www.functionalmedicine.org/about/whatisfm, accessed on 29 February 2012.
8. Buettner, D. (2008) *Blue Zones: Lessons for Living Longer from the People Who've Lived the Longest*. Washington, DS: National Geographic.
9. Pubmed: US National Library of Medicine, National Institutes of Health, www.ncbi.nlm.nih.gov/pubmed.
10. Nicolle, L. and Woodriff Beirne, A. (2010) *Biochemical Imbalances in Disease*. London: Singing Dragon.

2

Improving Gastro-Intestinal Health

In this chapter we discuss 'functional' gastro-intestinal (GI) problems. Despite being relatively common, with the propensity to cause extremely debilitating symptoms, the results of conventional medical tests typically appear normal in such cases, with no organic pathological condition being identified.

One or more underlying imbalance may be involved, some of the most prevalent being:

- hypo- or hyperchlorhydria (low or high gastric acid production)
- sub-optimal enzyme secretion, either from the pancreas and/or the villi in the small intestine (e.g. lactase required in the digestion of dairy foods)
- problems with the synthesis and/or flow of bile
- dysbiosis (an imbalance in the GI microflora), which can include yeast or bacterial overgrowth, parasitic infections and/or diminished levels of commensal ('friendly') microbes.
- intestinal hyperpermeability (commonly known as 'leaky gut').

Some typical signs and symptoms of GI dysfunction

- Abdominal bloating.
- Excessive burping or flatulence, often odorous.
- Gastric reflux, which may be accompanied by burning.
- Heartburn.
- Constipation, diarrhoea, or alternating between both.
- Gastritis and/or ulceration.
- Abdominal cramping.

- Nausea.

- Stools that are pale in colour and/or float (this may indicate fat malabsorption).

- A doctor's diagnosis of 'irritable bowel syndrome'.

- Increasingly restricting the variety of foods eaten, due to the fear of adverse reactions.

(Note that certain symptoms require the swift attention of a medic: severe pain in the stomach, abdomen and/or back/shoulder blade area; any persistent change in bowel habit; blood in the stool, sputum or vomit.)

These are just a sample of the most common presentations, but it is worth remembering that sometimes more unspecific, systemic symptoms may also be related to imbalances in the gut. Such symptoms include muscular and cognitive fatigue, low mood, painful joints, behavioural problems and/or headaches.

Laboratory tests that may be helpful in identifying functional GI imbalances include those that show abnormal:

- stool levels of bacteria, yeasts, parasites, short-chain fatty acids, inflammatory markers, such as calprotectin, white blood cells or mucous, occult blood, elastase, triglycerides, vegetable or meat fibres

- urinary levels of organic acids indicating a small intestinal bacterial overgrowth (such as indican, benzoate and hippurate) or yeast overgrowth (such as D-arabinitol)

- salivary levels of the mucous membrane antibody secretory IgA

- patterns of hydrogen or methane excretion in a breath test

- ratios of urinary or salivary lactulose and mannitol in a challenge test (indicating intestinal hyperpermeability).

What health conditions are GI imbalances linked to in the long term?

A great many systemic conditions of ill health have a GI-dysfunction component, as will be seen in this chapter and throughout this book. Thus, identifying and addressing GI imbalances is typically one of the first points of leverage used by healthcare advisers who practise personalised nutrition. Some specific long-term conditions include the following:

- Inflammatory bowel disease (IBD), such as Crohn's or ulcerative colitis. Irritable bowel syndrome (IBS) often has an inflammatory component[1, 2] and in recent years it has been suggested that IBS and IBD may be situated on one and the same continuum of GI pathology.[3]

- Systemic autoimmune disease, such as rheumatoid arthritis or lupus, due to dysbiosis and leaky gut (see Focus box 2.1).

- Conditions related to malabsorption, such as osteoporosis, muscle wasting and other symptoms of nutrient deficiency.

Key nutritional interventions to consider

The 5 'R' Approach

The recommendations below are designed to help bring back balance to the entire digestive system. In personalised nutrition, this is done by way of a five-stage programme, originally designed by the Institute for Functional Medicine (IFM).[4, 5] An adapted version, comprising solely dietary and lifestyle interventions, is suggested here:

1. *Removing* whatever is in excess, such as fat, alcohol, stress, allergens, sensitivities and problematic GI microbes.

2. *Replacing* dietary fibre, if necessary, to support gut transit time and motility, and replacing the factors necessary to optimise digestive secretions, if these are found to be low. For example, zinc is a crucial cofactor in hydrochloric acid (HCl) synthesis.

3. *Repopulating* the gut by using probiotic foods to bring the microflora back into balance and prebiotic foods to help the commensal bacteria to proliferate.

4. *Repairing* the lining of the gut to optimise absorption and immune tolerance (see Focus box 2.1). This requires eating foods rich in zinc, vitamins A, D and C and amino acids, particularly L-glutamine.

5. *Rebalancing* the mental, emotional and spiritual aspects of your life, in order to reduce the sympathetic, and increase the parasympathetic, drive in the autonomic nervous system.

Follow the basic healthy eating guidelines in Chapter 1, modifying them with the following recommendations.

What to eat and drink

- Eat an anti-inflammatory diet (see Chapter 8), including oily fish for the essential fats EPA and DHA (see Chapter 4). Inflammation contributes to leaky gut.[6]

- Include probiotic foods, such as *Homemade Yoghurt, Kefir* and *Sauerkraut* (Chapter 1), in your diet. By making these foods yourself, you can ensure that they contain live bacteria, whereas some commercial varieties are lacking. Probiotics have been found to reduce dysbiosis and certain types of diarrhoea and constipation. There are many studies indicating a role for probiotics in IBS symptoms.[7] For information on the many functions attributed to probiotics, see Trueman and Bold (2010).[8]

- Consume good levels of soluble fibre, including prebiotic foods, such as Jerusalem artichokes, asparagus, leeks, onions and garlic. Prebiotics help desirable bacteria to colonise the gut. If you are not used to eating these types of foods, increase them very gradually, as they may cause transient wind and bloating if dysbiosis is present.

- Soluble fibre is also found in oats, linseeds (flax), chia seeds and powder and most vegetables, including root vegetables, and it has a great many benefits for GI health. Soluble fibre stimulates GI motility, gives stools a looser consistency[7] and may help with reflux symptoms.[9] It also promotes the bacterial synthesis of a short-chain fatty acid called n-butyrate in the large intestine. N-butyrate is an important energy source for the intestinal epithelial cells, helping to inhibit colonic oxidative stress, inflammation and carcinogenesis.[10]

- Soaked linseeds or chia seeds can be particularly helpful for people with constipation. Try soaking 1–2 tsp of cracked linseeds in half a pint of room-temperature water overnight. Drink the mixture in the morning, followed by another half-pint of warm water. Leave at least 30 minutes before breakfast. Alternatively, try soaking 1 tbsp ground linseed in 125ml/4fl oz/½ cup 100 per cent prune juice overnight, then eating it in the morning with a spoon, followed by a glass of water. (Note that fruit juices, including prune juice, may not suit you if you have a GI microbial imbalance.) To use chia seeds, place 2 tbsp in 250ml/8fl oz/1 cup water and leave to soak for 15–30 minutes, stirring with a whisk to prevent clumping. This can then be added to smoothies or raw soups.

- Instead of linseeds or chia seeds, you could try psyllium husks, another source of soluble fibre. Mix 2 tsp into a glass of warm water first thing in the morning. Follow with another glass of warm water.

- Eating stewed apples with raisins (or sultanas) and cinnamon is a tasty way to increase soluble fibre and immune-enhancing polyphenols. Used regularly, anecdotal evidence suggests that this type of dish may aid GI function, including mucosal immune system tolerance (see Focus box 2.1).[11]

(Be mindful that if you have a microbial imbalance, the sugar content of too much dried fruit could exacerbate wind and bloating in some people.)

- Anecdotally, some people find that drinking aloe vera juice and/or mixing slippery elm into a warm drink can help to soothe an irritated gut. Discuss this with your nutrition adviser.

- Eat antimicrobial-rich foods, such as garlic (allium), clove, oregano, liquorice, curcumin, olive oil and coconut oil.

- Bitter leaves, such as chicory (endive), watercress, dandelion and rocket (arugula), may help to stimulate digestive secretions.

- Lemon juice and apple cider vinegar help to acidify the digestive tract and may therefore help with protein digestion.

- Eat enzyme-rich foods, such as sprouted seeds, pineapple and papaya.

- Consume zinc-rich foods, such as oysters, beef, crab, pork and chicken. Vegan sources include seeds, sea vegetables and wholegrains. Zinc is an important cofactor for gastric acid synthesis and also for the health of the taste buds. It is also required for tissue healing. Zinc deficiency predisposes to leaky gut.[12]

- Fennel has long been used as a digestive aid. It also contains the anti-inflammatory phytonutrient anethole, which may help reduce the risk of colon cancer.[13] If you suffer from excess wind, try chewing some fennel seeds after eating.[14]

- Foods containing micronutrients that may help to heal the gut lining include:

  ○ Fish, poultry and/or eggs. Eat at least seven eggs or a serving of organic liver every week. These high-protein foods contain zinc and the amino acid L-glutamine. L-glutamine is food for the intestinal epithelial cells and increasing its intake has been shown to help improve leaky gut.[15]

    Eggs and liver also contain vitamin A, needed for the health of all mucous membranes in the body. It's important to get vitamin A in the diet because deficiency predisposes to gut mucosal damage[12] and up to 45 per cent of healthy individuals may be poor converters of beta-carotene (its precursor) to the active vitamin.[16]

  ○ Meat broths, such as *Chicken Stock* (Chapter 1), which make tasty bases for soups, casseroles, sauces and gravies. Meat broths are excellent sources of collagen, which is a key protein within the gut lining.

  ○ Salad greens, broccoli, peppers and berries. These foods are rich in vitamin C, which is vital for collagen synthesis.

Deeply coloured berries (blueberries, strawberries, raspberries, cranberries, blackcurrants) also contain phytochemicals called anthocyanins, which may inhibit collagen-damaging enzymes called matrix metalloproteinases (MMPs).[17]

What not *to eat and drink*

- If you feel you may be sensitive to certain types of food, you could undertake a three- to four-week elimination diet. This is an experiment to see which foods may be affecting you, either through an immune response or for other reasons. This type of intervention has been found to help in many gut and systemic conditions.[18, 19, 20] Such diets are best designed and supervised by a nutrition expert and are not suitable for everyone – for example, in pregnancy or in individuals who have suffered from an eating disorder or who are underweight.

  Examples of elimination diets include the following:

  ○ Avoidance of foods that more commonly cause sensitivity reactions: gluten grains (especially wheat bran), dairy, soy, corn, beef, pork, shellfish, oranges, peanuts, refined sugars and eggs.[21] Some individuals may also want to experiment with temporarily avoiding beans and pulses, raw onions, leeks and cruciferous vegetables and raw fermentative fruits (apples, pears, plums).

  ○ Acid reflux cases may want to experiment with avoiding chocolate, coffee, tea and mint, as these reduce the muscular tone of the sphincter that connects the stomach to the oesophagus.[22] Reduce caffeine gradually – for example, by replacing half the coffee with alternatives, such as dandelion and/or chicory coffee, or with (organic) decaffeinated coffee. The latter option enables caffeine-sensitive individuals to continue benefitting from the healthful polyphenols in coffee (as described in Chapter 3).

  ○ Avoidance of a single food type only, such as dairy, if you suspect a lactase insufficiency, or gluten grains, if you suspect a gluten sensitivity. It is now recognised that gluten sensitivity can exist separately from coeliac disease.[23, 24]

  ○ Avoidance of foods that you may have been consuming in excess, and to which you may have become addicted.

- Avoid regular high fat intake (such as often occurs with low-carb, or ketogenic, diets), as this is associated with acid reflux[9] and, anecdotally, with both constipation and diarrhoea.

- Moderate your alcohol consumption to at least within government guidelines and include two alcohol-free days a week. GI bacterial overgrowths have been found to be far more common in heavy drinkers.[25]

- Don't overeat, as this can overwhelm the supply of hydrochloric acid (HCl), bile and digestive enzymes.

- Limit your intake of sugars and refined carbohydrates, as these can cause excessive fermentation in the gut if the microflora is imbalanced. If you suffer from excess wind and bloating, and you suspect a GI dysbiosis (see above), you may find it helpful to reduce your fruit intake (to a maximum of two pieces a day) and, where fruit is eaten, to have it before, rather than after, other food. This is because fruit is quick to pass through the digestive tract. If it gets stuck behind other, more slowly digestible foods, it is prone to fermentation, worsening the symptoms of a microflora imbalance. However, we recommend stewed apple and cinnamon (see above) on an empty stomach, for its therapeutic effect. If appropriate, replace the fruit recipes in the meal plan below with the stewed apple option (also in the meal plan).

- Some individuals with GI problems find it helpful to avoid the sugar substitutes sorbitol and xylitol, as they are poorly absorbed.[26] If you think xylitol may be affecting you, you can use stevia (see Focus box 5.2) as an alternative in the recipes in this chapter. Stevia is many times sweeter than xylitol, so you only need a very small amount.

- Although soluble fibre is generally helpful (see above), you may want to experiment with limiting your intake of *in*soluble fibre – for example, from wheat bran.

- Don't drink too much (of anything) while eating, as this may dilute the digestive juices. A few sips throughout the meal is generally well tolerated.

Lifestyle

- Manage the stress in your life. The GI tract is connected to the central nervous system (CNS) via serotonergic and cholinergic nerves. These pathways comprise the enteric nervous system (ENS), or the gut–brain axis.[7] Hence the gut is sometimes referred to as a neurological organ.[27]

    Many studies show that bloating and other GI symptoms correlate with depression, anxiety and stress.[7] Such psychological factors not only affect GI motility via the ENS, but also contribute to intestinal permeability[28] and act as mediators in GI inflammation.[2]

Ways to reduce stress and anxiety include the following:

- ◦ 'Mindful eating' – slowing down the eating experience is psychologically calming and it enhances digestion. See 'How to eat' below.

- ◦ Ensuring that you get enough (high-quality) sleep. If you have trouble sleeping, make sure your bedroom is completely dark and well-ventilated, switch off all the electrics at the plug sockets and keep the two hours prior to bedtime free of computers, television, intense exercise, caffeine and bright lighting. Relax in a warm bath with chamomile or lavender essential oils added.

- ◦ Reflecting on your mental, emotional and spiritual balance. Do you think you could benefit from some therapeutic support? Cognitive behavioural therapy, hypnotherapy and acupuncture have all been found helpful in IBS symptoms.[7]

- Take regular, moderate (not excessive) exercise, as this may improve acid reflux,[9] constipation[29] and other functional GI symptoms, such as bloating.[7]

- Lose weight if you are carrying too much. Abdominal obesity plays a role in gastroesophageal reflux[9] and it also predisposes to inflammation (see Chapter 8).

- With the help of your doctor, review the intake of certain drugs:

  - ◦ antibiotics, as they disrupt the gut microflora

  - ◦ non-steroidal anti-inflammatory drugs, as they contribute to intestinal permeability

  - ◦ proton pump inhibitors, as their inhibition of gastric acid can contribute to a bacterial overgrowth in the small intestine.[30]

- Prepare your kitchen. Make sure you have it well stocked with foods you can eat, and that you have thrown out or given away any foods you are excluding.

- Get sunshine daily, to help improve your vitamin D levels. Vitamin D is required for the immune system in the gut (see Focus box 2.1).

How to eat

Good digestion is just as much about *how* you eat as *what* you eat. Follow the general dietary guidelines in Chapter 1. In addition:

- Take time to anticipate and enjoy meals, as this triggers hormonal responses that prepare the GI system to better digest and absorb the nutrients.[31] This includes chewing your food well. Aim to chew each mouthful 30 times. This will seem like an impossibly dull task at first, and will considerably extend the time taken to eat a meal, but it will soon become habit and you will feel better for it. Incompletely chewed food is harder to digest. It can also lead to the food bolus moving too slowly through the GI tract because it has not had a chance to mix with sufficient volumes of saliva to keep it lubricated. Saliva also contains amylase enzymes, which start the digestive process.

- Some people find it helpful to adopt 'food combining', so that animal proteins are not eaten at the same meal as starchy foods. If you want to experiment with this, it is best to work with a nutrition adviser, in order to minimise the risk of compromising blood glucose control (see Chapter 5).

- If you have a tendency towards acid reflux, eat with an upright posture (rather than slouching, slumping or lounging) and leave at least two hours before retiring to bed.

Focus box 2.1   Gut-immune – what's the link?

It is often said that 75 per cent of the immune system resides in the gut. The gut is an important site for the development and maintenance of immune tolerance (see Chapter 8). Here are two examples of gut-related immune functions:

- It is in the gut (as well as the thymus gland) that we see significant production and activation of a particular type of T helper cell called T regulatory cells. (These are also known as Treg or Th cells.) Treg cells balance the T helper cell subsets Th1, Th2 and Th17. An unbalanced ratio of these Th cell subsets leads to an inappropriate immune response to allergens, gut contents or to one's own body, which can then contribute to inflammatory disorders. For example, autoimmune conditions such as rheumatoid arthritis (RA), inflammatory bowel disease (IBD), psoriasis and coeliac disease are associated with an inappropriate Th1 response, while allergies, including asthma and eczema, are classed as Th2 diseases.[32] (Note that the situation is complex and that both Th1- and Th2-mediated diseases can exist within the same individual.)

- The gut mucosa also produces and maintains optimal levels of the antibody secretory IgA (sIgA). This keeps the mucosa tolerant to harmless molecules (such as the commensal bacteria), while also neutralising toxins and pathogenic microbes and helping to prevent the development of leaky gut.[33]

Optimising immune tolerance via the gut
Thus, many experts believe that the starting point in improving systemic immune health and inflammation should be by manipulating the mucosal immunology, specifically through optimising the microflora balance and the integrity of the mucous membranes.

MICROFLORA BALANCE
The gut microflora and the administration of certain strains of probiotics (i.e. preparations of 'friendly' microorganisms that confer health benefits) have been found to improve immune tolerance by, for example, increasing Treg,[34] increasing sIgA[35] and inducing the anti-inflammatory cytokine IL-10, which inhibits inflammatory IL-17.[32]

Research has shown links between dysbiosis (gut and urinary) and various autoimmune inflammatory diseases. For example, there is an association between *Helicobacter pylori* infection and cardiovascular disease.[36, 37] There is also a likely involvement of *Klebsiella pneumoniae* infection in the aetiology of the autoimmune condition ankylosing spondylitis,[38] and of an upper urinary tract *Proteus* infection in the development of rheumatoid arthritis in genetically susceptible individuals.[39] Early-life dysbiosis may also be a factor in the development of asthma and other allergies.[40]

Thus, it is becoming increasingly recognised that disturbances in the GI microbiota may underlie systemic immune system problems. Not only does our immune system control microorganisms, it is itself controlled by microorganisms.[41]

THE INTEGRITY OF THE GI MUCOUS MEMBRANE
The presence of a leaky gut (LG) is associated with various autoimmune diseases, both GI-related and systemic.[42]

Common causes of leaky gut are nutrient deficiencies (such as L-glutamine, zinc and vitamin A), stress and the use of certain medications, especially non-steroidal anti-inflammatory drugs (NSAIDs).

Leading on from this, it is thought that potential exists for arresting autoimmune inflammatory processes by re-establishing intestinal barrier function, as this would prevent inflammatory triggers (see Chapter 8) from gaining access to the body's adaptive immune system.[43]

Recent research also indicates that a microbial imbalance (dysbiosis) and/or food-derived environmental triggers (especially gluten) can cause dysfunction of the tight junctions, by activating the zonulin pathway. This leads to LG and consequent inflammation, autoimmunity and/or cancer.[44] (Zonulin is a human protein that helps to regulate the intercellular tight junctions in the GI epithelia, controlling the entry of proteins and other potential allergens.) Food-derived lectins can also contribute, particularly those found in wheatgerm and soy (see 'What *not* to eat and drink' in Chapter 8).

We have seen that dysbiosis may be a trigger for LG, and indeed many experts believe that we should see ourselves as 'human-microbe hybrids' rather than simply as human bodies in isolation.[31] This makes sense when we consider that the microorganisms resident in the human body outnumber our cells by 10 to 1 and that the human microbiome is estimated to encode 100 times more unique genes than our own genome.[45] The crucial importance of this was recognised with the launch in 2008 of the five-year Human Microbiome Project, which is mapping patterns of human microbial populations in health and disease and includes the metagenomic sequencing of gut flora.[46, 47] Our resident bacteria have powerful roles to play in our health, and we should be mindful that diet and lifestyle influence the expression not only of our human genes but also of our bacterial genes.

Refer to Ash (2010)[32] for a more detailed discussion of the gut's influence on immune function, and to Trueman and Bold (2010)[8] for a fuller discussion of the roles of the human microflora in health and disease.

Focus box 2.2   Going gluten-free – what can I eat?

Gluten grains are wheat, spelt, kamut, rye and barley. If your nutrition consultant has suggested an experimental period of gluten-free eating, there are plenty of healthy alternatives to choose from.

According to the Codex Standard for food for special dietary use for persons intolerant to gluten (CODEX STAN11-1979), oats can be tolerated by most, but not all, gluten-sensitive individuals. However, a major concern is the potential contamination of oats with wheat, rye or barley during grain harvesting, transport, storage and processing. For this reason, it is best to select certified gluten-free oats.

Recent research suggests that the suitability of oats depends not only on the individual susceptibility (some people tolerate higher amounts of gluten than others) and on the purity of the product, but also on the variety of the oats consumed.[48] Other research suggests that cross-reactivity of other non-gluten grains, such as maize, may be a problem for some people who are sensitive to gluten, including those with coeliac disease.[49] Cross-reactivity happens when the body mistakes another food for gluten and reacts accordingly. A range of different foods may cause cross-reactivity. Cross-reactivity testing is now available; please seek advice from your nutrition practitioner.

The only way you are really going to find out which grains are affecting you is by avoiding the suspects for a few weeks and then reintroducing them one at a time, monitoring your symptoms. Bear in mind, however, that many people who are sensitive to gluten are asymptomatic.

We recommend that if you intend to test for coeliac disease and/or gluten sensitivity, you do so prior to starting a gluten-free diet. This is because blood levels of gliadin immunoglobulins gradually diminish during gluten avoidance; and this can lead to false negative test results.

Here are some suggestions for gluten-free alternatives – it is important to check labels carefully and be mindful that cross-reactivity may occur with some of these alternatives:

- gluten-free oats (porridge, oatmeal, oat cakes)
- corn (cornflour/cornstarch, corncakes, corn pasta)
- buckwheat (blinis, udon noodles)
- amaranth (grain, flakes and flour, bread)
- rice (brown basmati, brown short grain, carmague red, wild rice, rice pasta/noodles, rice cakes and crackers, rice flour and bread)
- millet (flakes, grain, flour, bread and pasta)
- quinoa (grain, flakes, flour and bread)
- sweet potatoes
- potatoes (vegetable and flour)
- yam and cassava

- kelp or shirataki noodles as pasta alternatives

- sago and tapioca

- pumpkins and squashes

- spiralised courgette (zucchini)

- pulses (e.g. gram flour and pasta, pea and/or soy flour and breads)

- nuts (e.g. coconut, almond, chestnut flours).

See our recipes for gluten-free *Pecan Banana Bread, Breakfast Muesli Muffins, Crunchy Berry Granola* and *Buckwheat and Almond Bread* (Chapter 11).

Three ways to choose your gluten-free food

On 1 January 2012 new UK legislation on gluten-free foods came into effect and this has led to changes in the way food is labelled.

The new law gives consumers different ways to help make choices about selecting gluten-free foods:

- Foods labelled 'gluten-free' must contain no more than 20 parts per million (ppm) gluten.

- Foods labelled 'very low gluten' have between 21 and 100 ppm gluten.

- 'No gluten-containing ingredients' denotes foods that are made with ingredients that do not contain gluten and where cross-contamination controls are in place. This term is not covered by the law. These foods will have very low levels of gluten but have not been tested to the same extent as those labelled gluten-free or very low gluten.

Where will I see these labels?

The new law applies to both pre-packed and loose foods labelled gluten-free. It will therefore apply to all food that is labelled gluten-free and sold in supermarkets, restaurants, cafés, shops and any other food outlet.

Three-day meal plan

Dishes and snacks in italics are supported by recipes in this chapter or other chapters as indicated.

Day 1

Breakfast: *Pecan Banana Bread* spread with *Gut Healing Creamy Butter* (Chapter 1)

Snack: Handful of blueberries

Lunch: *Asian Chicken Soup*

Snack: *Homemade Kefir* (Chapter 1)

Dinner: *Coconut and Coriander Dahl with Chickpea Pancakes*

Day 2

Breakfast: *Breakfast Muesli Muffins*, spread with *Gut Healing Creamy Butter* (Chapter 1)

Snack: Vegetable sticks with *Dill Ranch Nut Dip* (Chapter 1) or *Simple Nut Cheese* (Chapter 1)

Lunch: *Curried Baked Fish* with green salad or steamed fish with *Simple Watercress and Herb Sauce* (Chapter 1)

Snack: *Stewed Apple with Cinnamon*: cut apples of choice into chunks and stew in water with cinnamon and a few sultanas or raisins for 15 minutes. Eat hot or cold. To enhance the therapeutic effect, this can be eaten twice a day as a snack. If eaten cold, pro- and prebiotic powders and gut healing support supplements can be added (discuss with your healthcare practitioner)

Dinner: Two-egg omelette, with chopped fresh herbs, served with *Beetroot Carpaccio with Sweet Sherry Vinegar Dressing* and green salad

Day 3

Breakfast: *Papaya Fruit Salad with Lemongrass Dressing* and a handful of mixed seeds

Snack: *Homemade Yoghurt* (Chapter 1). Add 1 tbsp finely chopped crystallised ginger unless your symptoms include wind and bloating from a GI microbial imbalance

Lunch: *Chicory, Fennel and Sprouted Bean Salad with Lemon Sesame Dressing* (add a few prawns for additional protein if needed)

Snack: Vegetable sticks with *Homemade Sauerkraut* (Chapter 1)

Dinner: *Baked Sea Bass with Red Onion Chutney* and bitter leaf salad

Drinks

- Increase the standard 1.5 litres/3 pints of water (and/or non-caffeinated herbal teas) to 2 litres/4 pints if you are constipated or have diarrhoea. Drink water warm, as cold drinks can cause muscle contraction in the gut.

- Reduce or avoid carbonated drinks (including fizzy water).

- If you have constipation, drink the cracked linseeds every morning, on rising, or the prune juice mix (see page 36) or use chia seeds in a smoothie.

- Herbal teas: peppermint (concentrated peppermint oil is used as a GI antispasmodic), ginger, fennel, liquorice, cinnamon, valerian and chamomile.

- With the agreement of your nutrition adviser, add aloe vera juice to water and drink it throughout the day, or add it to green juices.

- Slippery elm in various preparations acts as a demulcent, emollient, expectorant and diuretic. The mucilaginous substance in the inner bark is soothing to irritated mucous membranes in the GI tract. It can be made into warm malted drinks (with hot water or milk, including non-dairy milks, and spices) or a porridge/oatmeal. It is also available as lozenges and teas.

Recipes

Breakfast

Pecan Banana Bread

This high-protein, grain-free bread makes a delicious breakfast option or snack and is suitable for those following the Specific Carbohydrate Diet (SCD). (The SCD aims to rebalance the gut flora, reduce inflammation and help heal the gut lining, through the avoidance of 'specific carbohydrates' that are more difficult to digest. For information, see Gotschall 1994.)[50] You'll need a food processor or blender to grind the pecan nuts to form a flour-like consistency. The bread is best served warm or toasted, spread with a little coconut oil or nut butter (or see the spreads in Chapter 1).

- MAKES 1LB LOAF, ABOUT 10–12 SLICES

300g/10½oz/scant 3 cups pecan nuts
½ tsp cream of tartar
½ tsp baking soda
1 tsp cinnamon
4 free-range eggs
1 large ripe banana
2 tbsp light olive oil
1 tbsp honey

Place the pecan nuts in a grinder or blender and process to form a fine meal. Place in a bowl with the other dry ingredients.

Place the eggs, banana, oil and honey in a blender and process until smooth.

Pour into the dry ingredients and mix thoroughly.

Spoon into a lined loaf pan. Bake at 180°C/350°F, gas mark 4, for 40–45 minutes until firm to touch. Allow to cool for 5 minutes before turning out.

Slice and serve warm with coconut oil or nut butter.

Nutritional information per slice (10 slices)
Calories 278kcal
Protein 5.4g
Carbohydrates 4.8g of which sugars 4.3g
Total fat 26.3g of which saturates 2.8g

Breakfast Muesli Muffins

Forget café muffins and cakes which are often loaded with sugars and saturated fats. This tasty, healthy version is gluten-free and low in sugar. It is also packed with soluble fibre, from the oats, flaxseed and dried fruit, to support bowel health and aid elimination. Baking the milled flaxseed does not harm the vulnerable fatty acids as would be the case if the isolated oil were used (see Chapter 4 for more information). If you do not have rice and potato flour, substitute with a commercial (wholegrain) gluten-free flour mix instead.

▪ MAKES 8 MUFFINS

100g/3½oz/½ cup brown rice flour
50g/1¾oz/¼ cup potato flour
100g/3½oz/1 cup gluten-free (sugar-free) muesli mix
1 tbsp ground flaxseed
½ tsp xanthum gum
2 tsp baking powder
1 tsp ground cinnamon
4 eggs
4 tbsp/60ml light olive oil or melted coconut oil
1 large ripe banana
50g/1¾oz xylitol/scant ⅓ cup (or, alternatively, a little stevia) to taste
1 tsp vanilla extract
60g/2oz dried unsweetened berries

Topping
4 tbsp chopped pecan nuts
1 tsp ground cinnamon
1 tbsp xylitol (or a little stevia) to taste

Preheat the oven to 190°C/375°F, gas mark 5. Grease 8 large muffin moulds.

Place the flours and muesli in a bowl with the flaxseed, xanthum gum, baking powder and ground cinnamon.

Place the eggs, oil, banana, xylitol (or stevia) and vanilla into a blender and process until smooth. Stir into the flour with the berries and stir thoroughly to mix.

Spoon the mixture into 8 large muffin moulds.

For the topping, mix together the nuts, cinnamon and xylitol (or stevia). Sprinkle over each muffin.

Place in the oven and bake for 20–25 minutes until risen and golden brown.

Allow to cool in the tin before removing.

Nutritional information per muffin
Calories 280kcal
Protein 7.2g
Carbohydrates 40.2g of which sugars 16.6g
Total fat 10.8g of which saturates 2g

Papaya Fruit Salad with Lemongrass Dressing

Papaya is rich in papain, an enzyme that helps digest proteins. This enzyme is especially concentrated in the fruit when it is unripe. This light Asian-flavoured dish also includes fresh pineapple, the core of which contains bromelain, a similar enzyme to aid protein digestion. Using apple juice as the main sweetener means that the syrup is relatively low in sugar. Lemongrass adds a refreshing citrus taste and fragrance.

▪ SERVES 4

Dressing
250ml/8fl oz apple juice
2 stems lemongrass, halved and
    bashed with a rolling pin
2 star anise
Strips of fresh ginger root (optional)

....

2 papaya, peeled, seeds removed,
    flesh sliced
¼ fresh pineapple, including the
    core, cut into chunks
8 fresh lychees, halved, stones
    removed
1 ripe avocado, diced

Place the apple juice, lemongrass, star anise and ginger in a pan. Bring to the boil and simmer for 5 minutes until syrupy.

Turn off the heat and set aside for 5–10 minutes – the lemongrass will add flavour as it cools.

Place the fruit in a large bowl. Strain the syrup over the fruit. Chill before serving.

Nutritional information per serving
Calories 125kcal
Protein 1.6g
Carbohydrates 17.8g of which sugars 13.9g
Total fat 5.1g of which saturates 1.1g

Lunch

Asian Chicken Soup

This is a soothing soup, combining chicken and coconut milk with Asian spices and herbs. Ginger and turmeric may reduce inflammation in the gut and ease spasms, while garlic is well known for its antimicrobial properties. Use fresh organic chicken stock to make this recipe. For a lighter option, replace the coconut milk with additional chicken stock. Some people find corn difficult to digest, in which case replace the baby sweetcorn with a handful of sprouted seeds.

▪ SERVES 4

Spice paste
1 large red chilli, seeded
1 tbsp fresh ginger, grated
1 tsp ground turmeric
3 garlic cloves, crushed
½ onion, roughly chopped

Soup
1 tbsp coconut oil
400g/14oz can coconut milk
400ml/14fl oz/scant 1⅔ cups
    Chicken Stock (Chapter 1)
1 tbsp fish sauce
2 tsp xylitol (or, alternatively, a little
    stevia, to taste)
2 organic chicken breasts, skinless,
    cubed

Make the spice paste. Put all of the ingredients into a food processor. Add 4 tbsp of the coconut milk and process to form a paste.

Heat the coconut oil in a large pan, add the spice paste and cook for 1–2 minutes. Add the remaining coconut milk, stock, fish sauce and xylitol (or stevia). Bring to the boil, then gently simmer for 7–10 minutes.

Add the chicken and sweetcorn to the soup and cook for 2–3 minutes. Add the spinach leaves and sugar snap peas and cook for a further minute.

Ladle the soup into bowls and sprinkle over the coriander and spring onions to serve.

8 baby sweetcorn, sliced
Large handful baby spinach leaves
Handful sugar snap peas, halved
Handful of coriander leaves
 (cilantro), chopped
4 spring onions (scallions), sliced

Nutritional information per serving
Calories 158kcal
Protein 21.8g
Carbohydrates 9g of which sugars 8.5g
Total fat 4.4g of which saturates 2.6g

Curried Baked Fish

An easy baked fish dish lightly spiced with turmeric, ginger, garlic and curry paste and baked in coconut milk to create a delicious creamy sauce. Use white fish, such as snapper, sea bream, haddock, cod and grey mullet. The sauce can also be used to bake chunks of vegetables and tofu for a vegetarian option.

▪ SERVES 4

400g/14oz can coconut milk
1 tbsp cornflour (cornstarch)
100ml/3½fl oz/scant ½ cup
 vegetable stock
2 tsp curry paste
½ tsp ground turmeric
1 garlic clove, crushed
4 white fish fillets, boned
1 red pepper, cut into chunks
Handful of cherry tomatoes, halved
Sea salt and freshly ground pepper
Handful of chopped coriander leaves
 (cilantro)

Preheat oven to 180°C/350°F, gas mark 4.

Mix a little of the coconut milk with the cornflour to make a paste. Mix into the rest of the coconut milk, vegetable stock, curry paste and spices and pour into a shallow ovenproof dish.

Add the fish and red pepper and bake for 20 minutes.

Add the tomatoes and cook for a further 10 minutes.

Season to taste. Sprinkle over the coriander leaves to serve.

Nutritional information per serving
Calories 154kcal
Protein 19.6g
Carbohydrates 14.2g of which sugars 7.7g
Total fat 2.1g of which saturates 0.4g

Chicory, Fennel and Sprouted Bean Salad with Lemon Sesame Dressing

Bitter greens like chicory (endive) are a great addition to any salad as they help stimulate digestive secretions. Fennel may reduce gut inflammation (see above). Sprouted beans and seeds provide protein and additional enzymes to promote healthy digestion, while the dressing contains lemon juice to stimulate digestion. (Note that grapefruit may be best avoided if you are taking certain medications – see Chapter 3.) Serve this salad as a light lunch or as an accompaniment to fish dishes.

▪ SERVES 4

Dressing
2 tsp white wine vinegar
2 tbsp lemon juice
5 tbsp walnut oil
1 tbsp tahini
Sea salt and freshly ground black
    pepper to taste

....

1 medium fennel bulb
1 grapefruit
1 red apple (or carrot, courgette/
    zucchini or green papaya, if you
    are prone to wind and bloating
    and want to reduce the sugar
    content)
100g/3½oz sprouted mixed beans
2 heads chicory (endive), leaves
    separated

To make the dressing, whisk all the ingredients together to form a creamy thick dressing. Add a little water if needed to thin as necessary. Season to taste. This can be kept in the fridge for 3–4 days.

Remove the outer layer from the fennel and shred it finely – a mandolin is perfect, or use an attachment in a food processor.

Top and tail the grapefruit and cut between the membrane to release the segments.

Quarter the apple and remove the core. Cut into thin slices. Place in a bowl with the grapefruit, fennel and sprouted beans and toss lightly.

Place the chicory leaves on a platter. Scatter over the fennel mixture. Drizzle with the dressing just before serving.

Nutritional information per serving
Calories 235kcal
Protein 2.7g
Carbohydrates 6.6g of which sugars 6.2g
Total fat 22.1g of which saturates 2.2g

Dinner

Coconut and Coriander Dahl with Chickpea Pancakes

Coriander (cilantro) has antimicrobial properties and is ideal in Asian-inspired dishes and curries like this creamy dahl recipe. We have included plenty of turmeric, which is an anti-inflammatory spice and has been shown to possess anti-cancer properties. The chickpea pancakes are a high-protein, gluten-free alternative to naan bread. Instead of large pancakes, you could reduce the amount of water and make little blinis to serve alongside the dahl.

▪ MAKES 6 PANCAKES

Dahl
150g/5oz red split lentils
Pinch of sea salt
250ml/8fl oz/1 cup *Chicken Stock* or
    Vegetable Stock (Chapter 1)
1–2 tsp ground turmeric
1 tbsp coconut oil
1 red onion, diced
2 tsp cumin seeds
150ml/5fl oz/scant ⅔ cup coconut
    milk

To make the dahl, rinse the lentils. Heat the stock and turmeric in a pan until boiling. Add the lentils, season with sea salt and bring to the boil. Reduce the heat and simmer on a very low heat, covered, for 15–20 minutes or until the lentils are tender. Add a little water if it gets too dry.

Melt the coconut oil in a pan and sauté the onion and cumin seeds for 3–4 minutes. Add the cooked lentils, coconut milk, coriander and tomato and cook for a further 2 minutes. Stir in the spinach and allow to wilt. Keep warm.

Handful of coriander leaves
    (cilantro)
1 tomato, diced
100g/3½oz baby spinach leaves

Chickpea pancakes
150g/5oz/scant 1¼ cups gram/
    chickpea flour
1 egg
200ml/7fl oz/generous ¾ cup water
Coconut oil for frying

Meanwhile make the pancakes. Sieve the flour in a bowl. Add the egg and then stir in enough water to make a smooth batter. You may find using an electric whisk is helpful to remove the lumps. Use less water if making little thick blinis.

Heat a little coconut oil in a frying pan. Add a spoonful of the batter and cook until the edges are turning golden. If you are making little blinis, place dessertspoonfuls into the pan. Flip over and cook for another minute. Remove from the pan and keep warm while you repeat to make another 5 pancakes.

To serve, either present the dahl alongside the blinis or pancakes or spoon a little of the dahl into the centre of each pancake and roll up.

Nutritional information per pancake with dahl
Calories 200kcal
Protein 12.4g
Carbohydrates 26.6g of which sugars 2.9g
Total fat 5g of which saturates 2.2g

Beetroot Carpaccio with Sweet Sherry Vinegar Dressing

Beetroot is well known for its ability to support bile secretions. Its fibre content may also benefit overall digestive health. If you are not a fan of raw beetroot, try this dish, which uses precooked beetroots (without vinegar), sliced very thinly and dressed with an omega-rich sweet dressing. This is a delicious accompaniment to a lunch dish or main meal, or can be eaten on its own as a snack.

▪ SERVES 4

Dressing
3 tbsp sherry vinegar (can substitute
    lemon juice if you suffer from
    excessive wind and bloating
    and have been diagnosed with
    dysbiosis)
4 tbsp walnut oil
½–1 tsp Dijon mustard to taste
2 tsp raw honey
Seasoning to taste

....

4 medium/large cooked and peeled
    beetroots
Handful of rocket (arugula) leaves

Mix all the dressing ingredients together.

Thinly slice the beetroots either by hand or using a mandolin and arrange overlapping each other on a platter. Season.

Drizzle the dressing over the beetroot and garnish with a handful of rocket leaves.

Nutritional information per serving
Calories 170kcal
Protein 1.2g
Carbohydrates 6.6g of which sugars 6.4g
Total fat 15.2g of which saturates 1.4g

Baked Sea Bass with Red Onion Chutney

Most white fish have negligible levels of omega-3 fatty acids, but sea bass and halibut contain a small amount, as well as vitamin A, which is important for gut health and healing. This simple recipe is easy to prepare and looks absolutely stunning. Ask your fishmonger to butterfly the fish for you to make it easier to stuff with the chutney. If you do not have time to make your own chutney, you can use a good-quality shop-bought version, but be aware that this is likely to be higher in sugar. The bitter leaf salad may help stimulate digestion.

▪ SERVES 4

Chutney
2 tsp coconut oil
½ red onion, chopped
2 garlic cloves, crushed
1 tsp finely grated root ginger
400g/14oz can chopped plum tomatoes
2 tbsp xylitol (or, alternatively, a little stevia) to taste
½ tsp ground cumin
Pinch of cinnamon
3 tbsp cider vinegar
Pinch of smoked paprika

....

2 x 500g/1lb 2oz sea bass
1 tbsp olive oil
Bitter leaf salad to serve (e.g. rocket/arugula, chicory/ endive, watercress)
1 carrot (optional)

Heat the coconut oil in a pan and sauté the onion, garlic and ginger for 2 minutes until softened. Add the remaining chutney ingredients and bring to a simmer. Cook uncovered over a low heat for 40 minutes until thick and chunky. Stir occasionally to prevent it sticking to the pan.

Allow to cool. The chutney can be stored in the fridge for up to 1 week.

Mix 2–3 tbsp chutney mixture with the olive oil. Brush the chutney mixture all over the sea bass and set aside to marinate for 20–30 minutes.

Preheat the oven to 180°C/350°F, gas mark 4.

Spoon 3–4 tbsp chutney into the cavities of the sea bass. Place the stuffed sea bass on to a baking tray and bake them in the oven for 15–20 minutes, or until the flesh of each sea bass is opaque.

Serve the sea bass with a bitter leaf salad. Add carrot strips for sweetness if desired. Alternatively, serve with the *Nutrient-Packed Salad* (Chapter 1).

Nutritional information per serving
Calories 323kcal
Protein 49.4g
Carbohydrates 10.8g of which sugars 10.1g
Total fat 10.2g of which saturates 2.6g

References

1. Pimentel, M. and Chang, C. (2011) 'Inflammation and microflora.' *Gastroenterology Clinics of North America 40*, 1, 69–85.
2. Spiller, R. and Garsed, K. (2009) 'Infection, inflammation and the irritable bowel syndrome.' *Digestive and Liver Disease 41*, 12, 844–9.
3. Bercik, P., Verdu, E.F. and Collins, S.M. (2005) 'Is IBS a low-grade inflammatory bowel disease?' *Gastroenterology Clinics of North America 34*, 2, 235–45.

4. Hanaway, P. (2011) *Impaired Intestinal Permeability and Other Gut Dysfunctions*. Presentation given at the Advance Functional Medicine in Clinical Practice (AFMCP) symposium, October 2011. London: IFM.

5. Lukaczer, D. (2005) 'The 4R Programme.' In D. Jones (ed.) *The Textbook of Functional Medicine*. Gig Harbor, WA: Institute for Functional Medicine.

6. Swidsinski, A., Loening-Baucke, V., Theissig, F., Engelhardt, H. *et al.* (2006) 'Comparative study of intestinal mucous barrier in normal and inflamed colon.' *Gut 56*, 3, 343–50.

7. Yoon, S., Grundmann, O. and Koepp, L. (2011) 'Management of IBS in adults: Conventional and complementary/alternative approaches.' *Alternative Medicine Review 16*, 2, 134–51.

8. Trueman, L. and Bold, J. (2010) 'Gastro-Intestinal Imbalances.' In L. Nicolle and A. Woodriff Beirne (eds) *Biochemical Imbalances in Disease*. London: Singing Dragon.

9. Festi, D., Scaioli, E., Baldi, F., Vestito, A. *et al.* (2009) 'Body weight, lifestyle, dietary habits and gastroesophageal reflux disease.' *World Journal of Gastroenterology 15*, 14, 1690–701.

10. Hamer, H.M., Jonkers, D., Venema, K., Vanhouvin, S., Troost, F.J. and Brummer, R.J. (2008) 'Review article: The role of butyrate on colonic function.' *Alimentary Pharmacology and Therapeutics 27*, 2, 104–19.

11. Ash, M. (2011) 'Is this a perfect functional meal for mucosal tolerance?' Nutri-link Clinical Education. Available at www.nutri-linkltd.co.uk/documents/apple_tolergenic_food.pdf, accessed on 3 March 2012.

12. Davidson, G., Kritas, S. and Butler, R. (2007) 'Stressed mucosa.' *Nestle Nutrition Workshop Series, Paediatric Programme 59*, 133–42.

13. Chainy, G.B., Manna, S.K., Chaturvedi, M.M. and Aggarwal, B.B. (2000) 'Anethole blocks both early and late cellular responses transduced by tumor necrosis factor: Effect on NF-kappaB, AP-1, JNK, MAPKK and apoptosis.' *Oncogene 8*, 19, 25, 2943–50.

14. Willcox, D.C., Willcox, B.J., Todoriki, H. and Suzuki, M. (2009) 'The Okinawan diet: Health implications of a low-calorie, nutrient-dense, antioxidant-rich dietary pattern low in glycemic load.' *Journal of the American College of Nutrition 28*, Suppl., 500–516S.

15. Rapin, J.R. and Wiernsperger, N. (2010) 'Possible links between intestinal permeability and food processing: A potential therapeutic role of glutamine.' *Clinics (Sao Paulo) 65*, 6, 635–43.

16. Leung, W.C., Hessel, S., Méplan, C., Flint, J. *et al.* (2009) 'Two common SNPs in the gene encoding beta-carotene 15,15'-monooxygenase alter beta-carotene metabolism in female volunteers.' *Journal of the Federation of American Societies for Experimental Biology 23*, 4, 1041–53.

17. Shin, D.Y., Lu, J.N. and Kim, G.Y. (2011) 'Anti-invasive activities of anthocyanins through modulation of tight junctions and suppression of matrix metalloproteinase activities in HCT-116 human colon carcinoma cells.' *Oncology Reports 25*, 2, 567–72.

18. Stefanini, G.F., Saggioro, A., Alvisi, V., Angelini, G. *et al.* (1995) 'Oral cromolyn sodium in comparison with elimination diet in the irritable bowel syndrome, diarrheic type: Multicenter study of 428 patients.' *Scandinavian Journal of Gastroenterology 30*, 6, 535–41.

19. Van den Bogaerde, J., Kamm, M.A. and Knight, S.C. (2001) 'Immune sensitization to food, yeast and bacteria in Crohn's disease.' *Alimentary Pharmacology and Therapeutics 15*, 10, 1647–53.

20. Millichap, J.G. and Yee, M.M. (2003) 'The diet factor in pediatric and adolescent migraine.' *Pediatric Neurology 28*, 1, 9–15.

21. Lukaczer, D. (2011) *Prescribing an Elimination Diet*. Presentation given at the Advance Functional Medicine in Clinical Practice (AFMCP) symposium, October 2011. London: IFM.

22. Castell, D.O. (1975) 'Diet and the lower esophageal sphincter.' *American Journal of Clinical Nutrition 28*, 11, 1296–8.

23. Brown, A.C. (2012) 'Gluten sensitivity: Problems of an emerging condition separate from celiac disease.' *Expert Review of Gastroenterology and Hepatology 6*, 1, 43–55.

24. Sapone, A., Bai, J.C., Ciacci, C., Dolinsek, J. *et al.* (2012) 'Spectrum of gluten-related disorders: Consensus on new nomenclature and classification.' *BMC Medicine 10*, 1, 13.

25. Hauge ,T., Persson, J. and Danielsson, D. (1997) 'Mucosal bacterial growth in the upper gastrointestinal tracts in alcoholics (heavy drinkers).' *Digestion 58*, 6, 591–5.

26. Heizer, W.D., Southern, S. and McGovern, S. (2009) 'The role of diet in symptoms of irritable bowel syndrome in adults: A narrative review.' *Journal of the American Dietetic Association 109*, 7, 1204–14.

27. Holzer, P., Schicho, R., Holzer-Petsche, U. and Lippe, I.T. (2001) 'The gut as a neurological organ.' *Wiener Klinische Wochenschrift 113*, 17–18, 647–60.

28. Spiller, R.C. (2009) 'Overlap between irritable bowel syndrome and inflammatory bowel disease.' *Digestive Diseases 27*, Suppl. 1, 48–54.

29. De Schryver, A.M., Keulemans, Y.C., Peters, H.P., Akkermans, L.M. *et al.* (2005) 'Effects of regular physical activity on defecation patterns in middle-aged patients complaining of chronic constipation.' *Scandinavian Journal of Gastroenterology 40*, 4, 422–9.

30. Lombardo, L., Foti, M., Ruggia, O. and Chiecchio, A. (2010) 'Increased incidence of small intestinal bacterial overgrowth during proton pump inhibitor therapy.' *Clinical Gastroenterology and Hepatology 8*, 6, 504–8.

31. Power, M.L. and Schulkin, J. (2008) 'Anticipatory physiological regulation in feeding biology: Cephalic phase responses.' *Appetite 50*, 2–3, 194–206.

32. Ash, M. (2010) 'Dysregulation of the Immune System: A Gastro-Centric Perspective.' In L. Nicolle and A. Woodriff Beirne (eds) *Biochemical Imbalances in Disease.* London: Singing Dragon.

33. Johansen, F.E., Pekna, M., Norderhaug, I.N., Haneberg, B. *et al.* (1999) 'Absence of epithelial immunoglobulin A transport, with increased mucosal leakiness, in polymeric immunoglobulin receptor/secretory component-deficient mice.' *Journal of Experimental Medicine 190*, 7, 915–22.

34. Issazadeh-Navikas, S., Teimer, R. and Bockermann, R. (2012) 'Influence of dietary components on regulatory T cells.' *Molecular Medicine 18*, 1, 95–110.

35. Kabeerdoss, J., Shobana Devi, R., Mary, R.R., Prabhavathi, D. *et al.* (2011) 'Effect of yoghurt containing Bifidobacterium lactis Bb12® on faecal excretion of secretory immunoglobulin A and human beta-defensin-2 in healthy adult volunteers.' *Nutrition Journal 10*, 1, 138.

36. Figura, N., Franceschi, F., Santucci, A., Bernardini, G., Gasbarrini, G. and Gasbarrini, A.. (2010) 'Extragastric manifestations of Helicobacter pylori infection.' *Helicobacter 15*, Suppl. 1, 60–8.

37. Khodaii, Z., Vakili, H., Ghaderian, S.M., Najar, R.A. and Panah, A.S. (2011) 'Association of Helicobacter pylori infection with acute myocardial infarction.' *Coronary Artery Disease 22*, 1, 6–11.

38. Nicola, P. (2011) 'Is ankylosing spondylitis linked to Klebsiella?' *Advancing Nutrition 6*, 24–5.

39. Ebringer, A., Rashid, T. and Wilson, C. (2010) 'Rheumatoid arthritis, Proteus, anti-CCP antibodies and Karl Popper.' *Autoimmunity Reviews 9*, 4, 216–23.

40. Kozyrskyi, A.L., Bahreinian, S. and Azad, M.B. (2011) 'Early life exposures: Impact on asthma and allergic disease.' *Current Opinion in Allergy and Clinical Immunology 11*, 5, 400–6.

41. Round, J.L. and Mazmanian, S.K. (2009) 'The gut microbiota shapes intestinal immune responses during health and disease.' *Nature Reviews Immunology 9*, 5, 313–23.

42. Fasano, A. (2012) 'Leaky gut and autoimmune diseases.' *Clinical Reviews in Allergy and Immunology 42*, 1, 71–8

43. Fasano, A. and Shea-Donohue, T. (2005) 'Mechanisms of disease: The role of intestinal barrier function in the pathogenesis of gastrointestinal autoimmune diseases.' *Nature Clinical Practice Gastroenterology and Hepatology 2*, 9, 416–22.

44. Fasano, A. (2011) 'Zonulin and its regulation of intestinal barrier function: The biological door to inflammation, autoimmunity and cancer.' *Physiological Reviews 91*, 1, 151–75.

45. Qin, J., Li, R., Raes, J., Arumugam, M. *et al.* (2010) 'A human gut microbial gene catalogue established by metagenomic sequencing.' *Nature 464*, 7285, 59–65.

46. NIH/National Human Genome Research Institute (2010) 'Human Microbiome Project: Diversity of human microbes greater than previously predicted.' *Science Daily.* Available at www.sciencedaily. com/releases/2010/05/100520141214.htm, accessed on 6 January 2012.

47. Smeets, P.A., Erkner, A. and de Graaf, C. (2010) 'Cephalic phase responses and appetite.' *Nutrition Reviews 68*, 11, 643–55.

48. Comino, I., Real, A., de Lorenzo, L., Cornell, H. *et al.* (2011) 'Diversity in oat potential immunogenicity: Basis for the selection of oat varieties with no toxicity in coeliac disease.' *Gut 60*, 7, 915–22.

49. Cabrera-Chávez, F. Iametti, S., Miriani, M., de la Barca, A.M., Mamone, G. and Bonomi, F. (2012) 'Maize prolamins resistant to peptic-tryptic digestion maintain immune-recognition by IgA from some celiac disease patients.' *Plant Foods for Human Nutrition* 67, 1, 24–3

50. Gotschall, E. (1994) *Breaking the Vicious Cycle: The Specific Carbohydrated Diet.* Baltimore, ON: Kirkton Press.

3

Supporting Detoxification

We are what we eat, drink, breathe, touch and can't eliminate.[1]

While there are many different definitions of detoxification, this chapter focuses on the process of 'biotransforming' potentially harmful molecules into metabolites that can be safely excreted.

Normal body processes produce myriad compounds (such as hormones, neurotransmitters and cytokines), all of which need to be safely deactivated and disposed of, once they have done their job. In addition, the food, drink and medications that we consume need to be detoxified, as do all the other molecules to which we are exposed on a daily basis. These include toxic metals, traffic pollution, bacteria, alcohol, cleaning chemicals and cigarette smoke, to name but a few (see Focus box 10.2 in Chapter 10). We are, each and every one of us, gradually accumulating hundreds of chemicals, as we go through life.[1]

The extent to which such toxicants (now commonly referred to as 'toxins') affect our health depends not only on our level of exposure but on how well our detoxification systems are functioning. Many organs are involved, the main ones being the liver, the gastro-intestinal mucosa, the skin, the lungs and the kidneys. These organs make use of various enzymes, transporters and elimination pathways to recognise and disable toxins. It is the liver that undertakes by far the greatest share of the work, through a process technically known as hepatic biotransformation (see Focus box 3.2).

For a fuller discussion of the sources of different types of toxins and the ways in which detoxification processes work, see Muller and Yeoh (2010).[2]

Some typical signs and symptoms of excessive toxic load

Symptoms are usually rather unspecific, so look for a cluster from the following:

- Headaches.

- Night sweats.

- Fatigue and sluggishness.

- Skin eruptions.

- Low mood and irritability.

- Poor cognition.

- Chemical, odour or pollution sensitivities, such as sneezing, wheezing, nasal drip and/or dermatitis.

- Adverse reactions to foods and/or food additives, such as sulphites (found in wine, salad bar food, dried fruit and many processed foods).

- Excessive recovery time required after anaesthesia.

- Bloating, excess wind and constipation.

- Chronic itching.

Various laboratory evaluations can be used to help identify a need for detoxification support:

- Tests to assess the level of toxic load. These include hair, urine and/or blood levels of toxic metals, porphyrins and xenobiotics.

- Tests assessing detoxification potential. These include challenges with drugs, such as aspirin and paracetamol; and measurements of urine and/or blood levels of essential detoxification nutrients, such as amino acids, B vitamins and glutathione. (Note that the challenge test can only be prescribed by a medic because it uses drugs.)

- Tests indicating liver function. These include levels of liver enzymes (alkaline phosphatase (ALP) and aspartate transaminase (AST)).

Abnormal levels of certain urinary organic acids (namely 2-methylhippurate, benzoate, hippurate, orotate, glucarate, alpha-hydroxybutyrate and/or pyroglutamate) can also indicate the functional effects of certain toxins, as well as the status of particular nutrients required for detoxification.[3]

What health conditions is a high toxic load linked to in the long term?

Toxicity leads to a range of physiological problems, such as oxidation (see Chapter 9) and inflammation (see Chapter 8), and is thought to contribute to many of today's degenerative diseases, such as:

- Cancer. Endocrine disrupting pollutants, for example (see Chapter 7), may increase the risk of oestrogen-driven breast cancers.[4] What's more, toxicants have been found to become more carcinogenic in cases where the detoxification enzymes are sub-optimal.[5] Studies indicate that phase 2 enzyme induction (see Focus box 3.2) reduces susceptibility to carcinogens.[6]

- Fibromyalgia, chronic fatigue syndrome, Parkinson's disease[7] and other neurodegenerative diseases.[8]

- Autoimmune diseases. Environmental toxins may be possible triggers for these conditions.[9] Mercury – for example, from dental amalgam – may be a risk factor for autoimmune thyroiditis in some individuals.[10] Poor oestrogen detoxification may increase disease activity in systemic lupus erythematosus (SLE).[11]

- Cardiovascular disease. Long-term exposure to inorganic arsenic, for example, has been found to contribute.[12]

Biomarkers of reduced detoxification capacity have also been found in autism.[13] It has even been hypothesised that exposure to toxins may disrupt human weight control systems[14] and that this may explain why some individuals appear not to respond to normally successful obesity interventions.[15]

Key nutritional interventions to consider

Overall aims

- Minimise toxins from foods and drinks.

- Ensure a good supply of antioxidants to help disable the free radicals produced from phase 1 biotransformation (see Focus box 3.2).

- Consume plant bioactives that support phase 2 conjugation (see Focus box 3.2).

- Get regular amino acids for the phase 2 conjugates, especially the sulphur amino acids methionine, cysteine and taurine.

- Get a good supply of B vitamins and other cofactor nutrients for the detoxification process.

- Optimise gastro-intestinal (GI) function. This may help to minimise the production of toxic gasses (from dysbiosis), prevent toxic molecules from translocating across the gut membrane into the bloodstream (from leaky gut) and promote regular elimination (constipation can lead to the reabsorption of toxins). See Chapter 2 for more information on these and for GI dietary and lifestyle support.

What to eat and drink

- Eat organic or wild foods, where possible, to minimise exposure to pesticides, antibiotics, growth promoters and other drugs.

- Consume a wide range of brightly coloured fruits, vegetables, herbs and spices, for their important phytochemicals (see Chapter 9). Many of these reduce the activity of certain phase 1 enzymes and/or up-regulate the function of certain phase 2 enzymes, enabling toxicants to be more efficiently disabled. This ability to alter detoxification function is thought to be a key mechanism by which certain phytochemicals may reduce the risk of cancer.[16]

  Key foods in this respect are cruciferous vegetables (see Focus box 3.3),[17] pomegranate juice,[18] berries,[19] green tea,[20] coffee,[21] turmeric,[22] ginger,[23] onions and garlic,[23] a range of common culinary herbs, such as coriander (cilantro), dill, parsley, rosemary and mint,[23] citrus zest[24, 25, 26] and beetroot.[27, 28]

  The phytochemicals in these plants also act as antioxidants, which help to disable the 'free radicals' produced from phase 1 detoxification reactions (see Focus box 3.2). Chapter 9 has more information on antioxidant-rich foods.

Focus box 3.1   Should we be drinking coffee?

The detrimental effects of excessive caffeine intake are well known and can include dependency, gastric upset and disrupted sleep. But a substantial body of recent research indicates that in some cases the benefits of regular coffee consumption may outway the risks.

Caffeine enhances exercise endurance,[29, 30] mood and cognition[31, 32] and preliminary data indicates it may even reduce the risk of Alzheimer's disease[31, 32, 33] and Parkinson's disease.[31, 34]

Moreover, coffee is rich in polyphenols, the most well-researched being chlorogenic acid. Through their antioxidant activity, and their ability to modulate insulin sensitivity, intracellular signalling and other biochemical pathways, coffee polyphenols appear to reduce the risk of type 2 diabetes,[35, 36, 37] liver diseases,[38, 39] certain cancers and other age-related diseases[31] in a dose-dependent manner.

We believe that it is time to reassess our negative assumptions about coffee; and that the level and type of coffee consumption should be set according to your unique set of needs, including your individual caffeine threshold. Decaffeinated (organic) varieties would be a better option for those who are caffeine sensitive.

- Eat high-quality protein, as this contains sulphur amino acids required for the phase 2 pathways and for glutathione synthesis (see Focus box 3.2).[40] Good choices are lean organic or wild meat, game, poultry, fish and eggs. Vegetarian sources of sulphur amino acids are eggs, nuts, seeds, beans and pulses.

- These protein foods provide the range of B vitamins required as detoxification cofactors. Wholegrains are also good sources of some B vitamins. Gluten-free grains are preferable, due to gluten's negative effect on the gastro-intestinal mucous membrane (see Chapter 2).

- Olive oil or other monounsaturated fats (MUFAs) should be your main source of fat. Also add polyunsaturated fats (PUFAs) from oily fish, nuts, seeds and cold-pressed seed oils. MUFAs and PUFAs have been found to increase bile production,[41] which is helpful for excreting the toxic conjugates produced from the phase 2 enzyme system.

- For gut health, eat probiotic and prebiotic foods (see Chapter 2).

- It is also worth noting that an iron deficiency may affect the functioning of phase 1, as iron is a vital component of the cytochrome P450 enzymes.[42] The most bioavailable iron is haem iron from lean red meat, especially liver and the darker meat from game, poultry and oily fish, as well as eggs. Vegetarian iron, which is less bioavailable, is found in beans, pulses, dark green leafy vegetables and dried fruit. It is better absorbed when eaten with foods rich in vitamin C, such as fruit and raw or lightly cooked vegetables. (Note that some raw green leaves, such as spinach, beet greens, Swiss chard, okra and parsley, contain oxalic acid, which can impair mineral absorption in humans. Boiling and steaming reduces the oxalate load to some extent.[43])

What not to eat and drink

- Avoid alcohol, as it rapidly depletes glutathione stores in the liver. Alcohol's phase 1 metabolite acetaldehyde (which causes hangover symptoms) is far more toxic than alcohol itself and is linked to increased cancer risk.[44, 45] The World Cancer Research Fund recommends avoiding alcohol for cancer prevention.[46]

- Minimise your intake of well-done meat, which contains potentially carcinogenic heterocyclic amines and, if barbecued, polycyclic aromatic hyrdrocarbons (PAHs) (see Chapter 9). Keeping cooking temperatures to below 200°C/400°F, pre-microwaving meat prior to conventional cooking and eating high-fibre foods at the same meal, may help to prevent the activation of these toxic compounds.[4]

- Avoid damaged fats: *trans-*, oxidised or hydrogenated (see Chapter 4).

- Reduce the intake of saturated fat (full-fat dairy and fatty meat products). Excessive saturated fat may reduce bile acid production, leading to increased cholesterol[41] and less efficient excretion of toxins. See Chapter 4 for more on fats.

- Don't eat processed foods, as these can contain chemical additives, such as colourings, preservatives, sweeteners and other flavour enhancers, in addition to high levels of salt.

- Note that grapefruit interacts with many commonly used medications, including calcium channel blockers, statins and antihistamines.[47] Grapefruit bioflavonoids affect the activity of certain drug metabolising enzymes and transporters, thus altering the bioavailability of these and other drugs.[48] If you are taking medication you should ask your doctor about such potential interactions and in cases of doubt, grapefruit should be avoided.

How to eat

- Follow the general dietary guidelines in Chapter 1.

- Treat commercially marketed 'detoxification programmes' with caution. In particular, it can be counterproductive to fast for periods of more than 48 hours. During a lengthy fast, as the body's storage of fat is broken down to release energy, toxins are released from the adipocytes into the bloodstream. This puts an additional burden on the detoxification pathways, which, in turn, require more amino acids from protein and a whole array of micronutrients (as seen) to function well. Thus, a nutrient-rich diet is crucial for optimal detoxification. Lack of these detoxification nutrients is a key cause of the headaches, nausea, skin eruptions, severe fatigue, low mood, slow cognition and irritability that are often experienced during a fast. (In addition, fasting can be extremely problematic for anyone with less than optimal blood glucose control.)

Lifestyle

- Reduce your exposure to environmental pollutants in the home, at work and when out of doors. For more information see Focus box 10.2 and the free access article from Crinnion (2010).[49]

- If you need to lose weight, do it gradually, so as to temper the rate at which any stored toxins are released from adipocytes into the bloodstream.

- Reduce or avoid smoking and recreational drugs. As nicotine is so strongly addictive, many people find hypnotherapy and/or psychotherapy helpful.

- Discuss with your doctor the extent to which it may be possible to reduce your intake of medical drugs.

- Pay attention to oral hygiene, brushing and flossing correctly twice a day. Have regular dental check-ups and professional cleans – agree the frequency with your dentist.

- Make sure you are physically active on a daily basis. For example, aim to walk five miles a day. Sweating, from exercise, saunas and infrared saunas and/or steam baths, can promote toxin elimination through the skin.

- Try not to use cling film or tin foil – switch to baking parchment. Use glass storage, rather than plastic. Switch to glass, iron or ceramic cookware, rather than non-stick, aluminium or stainless steel. Use glass or china in the microwave, rather than plastic.

Focus box 3.2   Hepatic biotransformation – what's actually going on?

Your liver detoxification capacity depends on your genetic inheritance, as well as your age, gender, diet and lifestyle.

Genetic inheritance is important because the liver is highly 'polymorphic'. In other words, there are wide genetic variations in liver enzyme function, meaning that individuals metabolise molecules at very different rates. Hence, for example, some people are more affected by caffeine than others. Similarly, certain compounds in well-cooked meat are more carcinogenic in people with particular genetic polymorphisms in their phase 2 'glucuronic acid' pathway (see below).[4]

There are two phases of hepatic biotransformation. In simple terms, their role is to transform a fat-soluble compound into a water-soluble compound, attaching it to another molecule (a 'conjugate'), so that it can be safely excreted. Without this process, fat-soluble toxins remain in the body and are generally stored in fatty tissue. (But note that not all toxins are fat-soluble – thus, not all require both phases in order to be eliminated.)

The enzymes in phase 1 start the process. The most common phase 1 enzymes are known as the cytochrome P450 family, or CYP enzymes. They use either oxidation, reduction or hydrolysis to form a reactive site on the toxic molecule. This can make the toxin more potentially dangerous than it was prior to entering phase 1 and it therefore needs to be swiftly taken up by the phase 2 system. Enzymes in phase 2 add a water-soluble conjugate to the reactive site, enabling the toxin to be excreted in the bile or urine. The main conjugates are sulphate, glutathione, glycine, glucuronide and acetyl and methyl groups; they require dietary amino acids in order to remain in good supply.

Note that there are also support systems to phases 1 and 2, such as the 'anti-porter' system and the metallothioneins. In the anti-porter system, sometimes referred to as 'phase 3 detoxification', special transporters pump toxins out of the cell. The metallothioneins bind toxic metals to transfer them out of the cell.

Phase 1 is generally up-regulated by exposure to toxins (although there are exceptions). However, if phase 1 starts working faster than phase 2, phase 2 may become unable to ring-fence all the activated metabolites from phase 1, and this could result in an increased toxic load. Reactive oxygen species produced during phase 1 can cause tissue damage, leading to degenerative diseases (see Chapter 9). Thus, the aim should be to optimise both phases 1 and 2.[1, 50, 51]

A useful graphic illustrating the process can be found in Liska, Lyon and Jones (2005, p.278).[50]

Focus box 3.3   Cruciferous vegetables

Cruciferous vegetables are particularly important components of a detoxification diet. Key vegetables to include are broccoli (especially broccoli sprouts), cauliflower, kale, watercress, rocket (arugula), cabbage, turnips, Brussels sprouts, turnips, radish, pak choi, spring greens, collard greens, Chinese cabbage, daikon and kohlrabi.

Large population studies suggest that eating cruciferous vegetables may be more effective than other fruits and vegetables at reducing cancer risk.[5, 52] These vegetables contain glucosinolates, which are converted to isothiocyanates, including sulforaphane, through the processes of chopping, chewing and being acted upon by gut flora.[5, 52]

The isothiocyanates are able to down-regulate phase 1 enzymes (preventing excessive production of toxic intermediates), and induce certain phase 2 enzymes.[52] In turn, these phytochemicals have been found to reduce susceptibility to carcinogens[5] and reduce cellular levels of toxic metals, such as arsenic[53] and mercury.[54]

Sulforaphane has also been shown to influence other processes involved in cancer growth, namely inducing cancer cell apoptosis, suppressing cell cycle progression and inhibiting angiogenesis and inflammation.[55] In addition, another active component of broccoli, indole-3-carbinol, may offer protection from cardiovascular and neurodegenerative disease.[56]

November 2011 saw the launch of a new 'superbroccoli', marketed as Beneforte.[57] Eating the superbroccoli has been found to result in 2–4 times the level of sulforaphane in the blood than when eating standard broccoli. This, in turn, enhances the glutathione S-transferase (GST) phase 2 liver detoxification enzyme, especially in individuals with a particular GST genetic variation (polymorphism).[52]

See the three-day meal plan for some ideas of how to incorporate more cruciferous vegetables into your daily diet, even as tasty between-meal snacks.

Three-day meal plan

Dishes and snacks in italics are supported by recipes in this chapter or other chapters as indicated.

Day 1

Breakfast: 2 eggs scrambled with a little coconut oil and mixed with wilted (very lightly steamed) chopped baby pak choi drizzled with a little *Supergreens Pesto* (Chapter 1)

Snack: *Green Herb Cleanser*

Lunch: *Apple and Borscht Soup* with an optional piece of lightly toasted *Buckwheat and Almond Bread* (Chapter 11). Optional dessert: *Green Tea Poached Pears*

Snack: 1 tbsp *Roasted Garlic and Bean Dip with Crudités*

Dinner: *Grilled Sardines with Salsa Verde*. Serve with a *Cauliflower Tahini Mash*: steam a head of cauliflower until tender. Place in a food processor with a little tahini and process to form a mash, seasoning it to taste

Day 2

Breakfast: *Supergreens Berry Smoothie*

Snack: Handful of raw, mixed nuts

Lunch: *Watercress and Celeriac Soup with Sprouted Seeds*, optional rice cake or gluten-free oat cake

Snack: *Baked Cauliflower with Curry Spices and Turmeric*: toss cauliflower florets in a little coconut oil, curry powder and turmeric; bake in the oven for 20–30 minutes at 180°C/350°F, gas mark 4, turning half way through (may be prepared in advance and eaten hot or cold)

Dinner: *Salmon Kedgeree* with a side of steamed broccoli and salad

Day 3

Breakfast: Porridge made with gluten-free oats, sugar-free almond or hemp milk and 1 tsp of ground sprouted flaxseed for extra fibre and essential fatty acids. Top with a handful of berries or pomegranate seeds. Or *Soaked Muesli*: place 3 tbsp porridge oats (oatmeal), and a handful each of nuts, seeds and dried fruit in a bowl and cover with a little apple juice and almond or hemp milk. Soak overnight in the fridge. Add chopped fruit and a spoonful of natural yoghurt to serve

Snack: *Alkaline Detox Broth* or fresh beetroot juice

Lunch: *Warm Artichoke and Feta Salad with Lemon Dressing*

Snack: *Tangy Kale Crisps* (Chapter 7)

Dinner: *Balsamic and Soy Marinated Veggies* served with mixed beans or shredded cooked chicken. Optional dessert: *Citrus Salad* with *Flaxseed and Almond Biscuits*

Drinks

- It is important to keep up fluid intake. Drinking water is best filtered if possible. Plumbed-in filters are preferable to jug filters, to minimise the likelihood of bacterial growth during storage.

- The *Alkaline Detox Broth* can be sipped throughout the day. Herbal teas include dandelion, milk thistle, lemon and ginger, nettle, chamomile, fennel, liquorice. Use aloe vera in water, coconut water, green vegetable juices and occasionally beetroot juice.

Recipes

Breakfast

Supergreens Berry Smoothie

A simple breakfast option or snack, this cleansing smoothie contains supergreen powder and probiotics to provide additional nutrients to support detoxification and gut health. (Note that this smoothie may not be suitable for individuals with GI dysbiosis – see Chapter 2.) A scoop of protein powder has been included to make it more substantial but this can be omitted if desired.

- SERVES 1

250ml/8fl oz/1 cup water or coconut water
Handful of raspberries or frozen berries
1 apple, cored and chopped
2 large handfuls of baby spinach or kale
1 scoop protein powder, vanilla or plain
1 tsp supergreen powder (optional)
1 tsp probiotic powder (optional)
1 tsp glutamine powder (optional)

Blend all the ingredients in a blender until smooth and creamy.

Best drunk immediately.

Nutritional information per serving
Calories 187kcal
Protein 12.8g
Carbohydrates 22.8g of which sugars 16.5g
Total fat 4.6g of which saturates 1g

Lunch

Apple and Borscht Soup

A lovely vibrant soup. Beetroots contain phytonutrients called betalains, including betanin and vulgaxanthin, which may provide antioxidant, anti-inflammatory and detoxification support. This wonderful combination of earthy beetroots and sweet apple is delicious served hot or cold.

▪ SERVES 4

1 tbsp coconut oil
1 tsp cumin seeds
1 onion, chopped
¼ red cabbage, chopped
2 eating apples, peeled, cored and chopped
4 medium-sized beetroots, washed and grated
660ml/23¼fl oz vegetable stock
1 star anise
Sea salt and pepper
Lemon juice or apple cider vinegar

Melt the coconut oil in a large pan over medium heat. Add the cumin seeds and onion and sauté for 1–2 minutes.

Add the cabbage, apple and beetroot and sauté for 5 minutes until the vegetables start to soften.

Pour in the stock, add the star anise and bring to the boil. Cover and simmer for 10 minutes.

Remove the star anise and purée the soup with a hand-held blender until smooth. Add a little water to thin if needed.

Season to taste; add a little lemon juice or apple cider vinegar to taste.

Nutritional information per serving
Calories 61kcal
Protein 1.6g
Carbohydrates 8g of which sugars 7.4g
Total fat 2.8g of which saturates 2g

Watercress and Celeriac Soup with Sprouted Seeds

Watercress, like other cruciferous vegetables, contains sulphur compounds to assist liver function and the production of glutathione. This delicious soup is rich and creamy, with the addition of celeriac, and contains soluble fibre, useful for supporting elimination. Adding the watercress at the end of the cooking time helps preserve its nutrients and creates a wonderful vibrant green soup. Top with broccoli sprouts for an additional supply of glucosinolates. Accompany with oat cakes or gluten-free bread if desired.

▪ SERVES 4

1 tbsp coconut oil
1 onion, roughly chopped
1 garlic clove, crushed
275g/9¾oz celeriac, peeled and chopped
550ml/1 pint vegetable or chicken stock
200g/7oz watercress, roughly chopped
Sea salt and freshly ground black pepper
Handful of broccoli sprouts

Heat a frying pan and melt the coconut oil. Sauté the onion and garlic until softened, about 2–3 minutes.

Add the celeriac to the pan and stir to coat in the oil. Pour over the stock and bring to the boil.

Reduce the heat and simmer for 15 minutes, until the celeriac is just tender.

Add the watercress and simmer for a further minute.

Purée the soup with a hand blender or in a jug blender until smooth and creamy.

Return the soup to the pan and season with sea salt and freshly ground black pepper, to taste.

Top with broccoli sprouts to serve.

Nutritional information per serving
Calories 83kcal
Protein 3.1g
Carbohydrates 4.8g of which sugars 3.5g
Total fat 5.6g of which saturates 4g

Warm Artichoke and Feta Salad with Lemon Dressing

Globe artichokes have traditionally been used to support liver function. They increase bile flow from the liver to the gallbladder, aiding the digestion of fats, and are also a good source of soluble fibre. Anecdotally, artichoke is thought to help protect the liver from the occasional overindulgence in alcohol. Baby artichokes are widely available and are the easiest to use, as their undeveloped chokes require minimal preparation. If you are short of time, you could substitute fresh artichokes with those marinated in olive oil. This delicious Mediterranean-style salad includes bitter greens, such as rocket (arugula) (a cruciferous salad leaf), which can help stimulate digestive juices. Include plenty of zest in the lemon dressing to provide limonene, which may support phase 2 detoxification pathways.

■ SERVES 4

Lemon oil dressing
Juice and zest of 1 lemon
1 tbsp honey
3 tbsp flaxseed oil or an omega-blended oil
2 tbsp extra virgin olive oil
Freshly ground black pepper

If using raw artichokes, fill a large bowl with water and add the lemon juice.

Trim the stems of the artichokes and peel them to remove the outer tough parts. Trim the tops off the outer coarse leaves.

Scoop out the choke (if present) inside with a teaspoon or melon baller.

Slice the artichokes in half and place them in the acidulated water.

Juice of 2 lemons
12 baby artichokes or artichoke
    hearts marinated in olive oil
400ml/14fl oz/scant 1⅔ cup chicken
    or vegetable stock
250g/9oz rocket leaves or mixed
    bitter greens (e.g. watercress,
    rocket/argula, baby spinach)
Handful of chopped fresh basil
    leaves
200g/7oz cherry tomatoes, halved
12 black olives, halved
200g/7oz feta cheese, cut into
    chunks
Handful of broccoli sprouts or other
    sprouted seeds (e.g alfalfa)

Place the chicken stock or vegetable stock in a pan and bring to the boil. Add the artichokes and simmer, covered, for 15 minutes, or until the artichokes are tender. Leave in the pan to keep warm.

Whisk all the dressing ingredients together.

Place the rocket leaves and basil on a platter and scatter over the cherry tomatoes, olives, feta cheese and sprouts. Spoon out the artichokes from the pan, or use the artichokes in oil, drained, and add to the salad. Drizzle over the lemon oil dressing to serve.

Nutritional information per serving (with 1 tbsp dressing)

Calories 179kcal
Protein 10.7g
Carbohydrates 3.7g of which sugars 3.5g
Total fat 13.6g of which saturates 7.4g

Dinner

Grilled Sardines with Salsa Verde

Salsa verde is packed with flavour and nutrients. Parsley is a rich source of antioxidants, particularly flavonoids, vitamin C and beta-carotene. It also contains folic acid, important for methylation. This delicious sauce is perfect as a dressing over baked fish, seafood and poultry. Accompany with a simple mixed salad for a healthy lunch or light dinner dish, or with a cauliflower mash for something more substantial. Instead of sardines you could also use 4 mackerel fillets.

▪ SERVES 4

8 fresh sardines, gutted and cleaned
Sea salt and freshly ground black
    pepper

Salsa verde
1 large bunch of flat leaf parsley
Handful of basil leaves
2 garlic cloves, crushed
1 tbsp fresh mint leaves, chopped
2 anchovies, rinsed
2 tbsp capers, rinsed

Preheat the grill to high.

Remove the heads from the sardines, then cut open along the belly from the head end to the tail and open out, flesh side down. Press down along the body with the heel of your hand, then turn the fish over and lift out the bones. Some fishmongers will do this for you.

Place the sardines on to a grill tray skin side down and season with sea salt and freshly ground black pepper. Place under the grill for 3–4 minutes, or until completely cooked through.

2 tbsp red wine vinegar
1 tsp Dijon mustard
3 tbsp flaxseed oil
4 tbsp extra virgin olive oil
½ red onion, finely chopped

For the salsa verde, simply place in a food processor all the ingredients except the oils and onion. Process the mixture until chunky, then slowly add the oils and mix thoroughly. Stir in the red onion. Spoon the salsa verde over the sardines to serve.

Nutritional information per serving
Calories 417kcal
Protein 26.6g
Carbohydrates 0.9g of which sugars 0.4g
Total fat 34g of which saturates 6g

Salmon Kedgeree

This is perfect for a weekend brunch but also makes a tasty, light dinner dish. Although smoked haddock is traditionally used, we have included salmon to provide omega-3 fats. Mackerel or trout could also be used.

▪ SERVES 4

450ml/16fl oz/generous 1¾ cups
    fish stock (homemade – Chapter
    1 – or chilled ready-prepared fish
    stock)
250g/9oz salmon fillets, skin on
200g/7oz hot smoked salmon,
    flaked
2 tbsp fresh dill, chopped
1 tbsp coconut oil
1 medium onion, finely chopped
1 tsp curry powder
½ tsp turmeric
175g/6oz brown basmati rice
3 spring onions (scallions), finely
    sliced
1 tbsp lemon juice
Handful of watercress, trimmed
Sea salt and freshly ground black
    pepper
3 hard-boiled eggs, halved

Bring the fish stock to the boil in a medium saucepan. Reduce the heat to a simmer and add the fresh salmon. Poach for 6–8 minutes, then carefully remove with a slotted spoon, reserving the fish stock.

Remove the skin from the poached salmon. Flake into a bowl with the hot smoked salmon. Add the dill.

For the rice, melt the coconut oil in a large saucepan and fry the onion for 4–5 minutes, or until softened. Stir in the spices and rice and fry for a further minute. Add the reserved fish stock and bring to the boil. Cover with a lid, reduce the heat and simmer for 10–12 minutes. Remove the pan from the heat and set aside to steam for 10 minutes.

Gently stir in the spring onions, lemon juice, salmon and watercress, and season to taste. Spoon on to plates and garnish with the hard-boiled eggs.

Nutritional information per serving
Calories 317kcal
Protein 22.7g
Carbohydrates 28.6g of which sugars 0.7g
Total fat 12.4g of which saturates 4.2g

Balsamic and Soy Marinated Veggies

This is a great way to serve vegetables. Pouring the marinade over the warm vegetables allows them to soak up the lovely tangy flavours. This is best prepared the day before you wish to eat it to really let the flavours develop.

▪ SERVES 4

Marinade
6 tbsp extra virgin olive oil
3 tbsp balsamic vinegar
2 tbsp tamari soy sauce
2 cloves garlic, crushed
Freshly ground black pepper

1 head of broccoli, broken into
   florets
1 head of cauliflower, broken into
   florets
150g/5oz green beans, trimmed
225g/8oz button mushrooms, halved

Mix all the marinade ingredients together.

Steam the broccoli, cauliflower and green beans for 2–3 minutes until only just tender but still crunchy.

Place in a large bowl with the mushrooms and pour over the marinade. Toss to coat thoroughly.

Marinate overnight. Serve at room temperature.

Nutritional information per serving
Calories 209kcal
Protein 6.5g
Carbohydrates 4.6g of which sugars 3.7g
Total fat 18g of which saturates 2.7g

Snacks and desserts

Green Herb Cleanser

Juices are simple and quick to prepare and an easy way to boost your intake of nutrients in an easily absorbable form. Although best drunk immediately, you can store them in the fridge covered for 24 hours. When juicing leafy vegetables, it is better to use a masticating juicer, as this will extract more of the juice and nutrients. Parsley and coriander (cilantro) are useful herbs to support detoxification. They contain beta-carotene, vitamins C and K, and a range of volatile oil components and flavonoids, including myristicin, limonene, eugenol and linalool. Coriander also contains caffeic and chlorogenic acids. These herbs have diruretic properties, useful for easing fluid retention. The apples provide a little sweetness to the juice.

▪ MAKES 1 LARGE GLASS

Large handful each of parsley and
   coriander (cilantro)
2 green apples
1 lemon
2 sticks celery
½ cucumber

Simply place all the ingredients through a juicer alternating between soft and hard ingredients.

Best drunk immediately.

Nutritional information per serving
Calories 89kcal
Protein 2.5g
Carbohydrates 19.5g of which sugars 19.3g
Total fat 0.6g of which saturates 0g

Green Tea Poached Pears

A refreshing, lightly spiced dish, rich in antioxidants from the green tea, the berries and the citrus rind. Use a peeler or zester to remove the rind from the lemon and lime. This is best served warm as a dessert or a breakfast dish, with a little natural yoghurt or nut cream.

▪ SERVES 4

400ml/14fl oz/scant 1⅔ cups apple juice
2 green tea bags
2 star anise
2 cinnamon sticks
Rind of 1 lemon and 1 lime
4 firm pears, peeled, halved and core scooped out with a spoon
Handful fresh or frozen berries
Natural yoghurt or nut cream to serve (optional)

Place the apple juice, tea bags, spices, lemon and lime rind into a big saucepan and bring to the boil. Stir well, then add the pear halves. Cover and simmer for 12–15 mins until the pears are just tender.

Lift out the pears, then turn up the heat and add the berries. Boil for a few minutes until syrupy. Discard the tea bags. Serve the pears with the warm syrup poured over.

Add a spoonful of yoghurt or nut cream if desired.

Nutritional information per serving

Calories 100kcal
Protein 0.6g
Carbohydrates 25.4g of which sugars 25.4g
Total fat 0.3g of which saturates 0g

Roasted Garlic and Bean Dip with Crudités

This creamy homemade dip makes a delicious alternative to hummus and is an ideal snack or lunch option with salad. Roasting the garlic mellows and sweetens its flavour.

▪ SERVES 8

1 garlic bulb
Olive oil for drizzling
400g/14oz can cannellini beans or butter beans, drained
Zest and juice of ½ lemon
½ tsp smoked paprika
2–3 tbsp extra virgin olive oil
Sea salt and freshly ground black pepper
Selection of vegetable crudités to serve (e.g. carrots, peppers, cucumber, celery, mange tout/ snow peas, cauliflower and broccoli florets)

Preheat the oven to 180°C/350°F, gas mark 4. Place the garlic bulb on a large piece of foil, drizzle on a little olive oil and tightly seal the foil. Roast for 45 minutes. Remove from the oven, open the foil and allow to cool slightly.

Squeeze out the garlic pulp and place in a food processor. Add the remaining ingredients and process until smooth and creamy. Season to taste.

Serve with a selection of vegetables.

The dip can be stored in the fridge for 2–3 days or frozen for up to 1 month.

Nutritional information per serving (2 tbsp)

Calories 63kcal
Protein 2g
Carbohydrates 4g of which sugars 0.4g
Total fat 4.3g of which saturates 0.6g

Alkaline Detox Broth

This is a great electrolyte-rich broth to drink throughout the day. The concept of diet-induced acidosis is gaining interest as a possible contributing factor to chronic disease, although more studies are needed. Increasing your levels of electrolytes, such as potassium and magnesium, may help to improve the acid–alkaline balance of body fluids.[58] For something more substantial, you can blend the vegetables and serve it as a soup.

▪ SERVES 4

3 stalks celery
2 carrots
1 onion
2 cloves garlic, crushed
3 small potatoes, unpeeled
Handful of fresh spinach leaves
Bunch of fresh parsley, finely
   chopped
1 litre/2 pints filtered water
2 bay leaves

Coarsely chop all the vegetables. Cover with water and place in a pan. Add the bay leaves.

Bring to the boil, reduce heat and allow to simmer, covered, until the broth has a rich flavour, about 20 minutes.

Strain and drink hot or cold throughout the day as a snack, or, alternatively, blend the soup with all the ingredients and eat for lunch.

Nutritional information per serving
Calories 57kcal
Protein 2.2g
Carbohydrates 10.9g of which sugars 3.4g
Total fat 0.5g of which saturates 0.1g

Citrus Salad

A simple cleansing fruit salad rich in vitamin C and lycopene. It also contains limonoids, phytonutrients that promote the formation of the detoxification enzyme glutathione S-transferase. (Note that grapefruit may be best avoided if you are taking certain medications – see page 61.) This salad is delicious served with yoghurt or nut cream and makes an ideal breakfast or snack option.

▪ SERVES 4

1 red grapefruit, peeled
2 clementines or tangerines, peeled
4 oranges, peeled
½ tsp ground cinnamon
2 tbsp crystallised ginger, chopped

Cut the grapefruit, clementines and 3 of the oranges into thin slices. Place into a bowl.

Juice the remaining orange and pour the juice into the bowl with the cinnamon and ginger.

Allow to marinate to enhance the flavours.

Flaxseed and Almond Biscuits

A wonderful light biscuit, delicious as a snack to help satisfy sweet cravings. These biscuits are gluten-free and grain-free and provide a good source of protein and fibre.

▪ MAKES 12 BISCUITS

125g/4½oz/1 cup almonds
Pinch of sea salt
3 tbsp ground flaxseed
½ tsp bicarbonate of soda
3 tbsp sesame seeds
65g/2½oz/⅓ cup tahini
1 tbsp olive oil
2 tbsp yacon syrup, maple syrup or
     honey
1 tbsp xylitol
Zest of 1 orange
1 free-range egg
2 tsp vanilla extract

Preheat the oven to 180°C/350°F, gas mark 4.

Place the almonds in a food processor and process to form a fine flour.

Place in a bowl with a pinch of sea salt, the flaxseed, bicarbonate of soda and sesame seeds.

In a separate bowl, mix together the remaining ingredients.

Add the wet ingredients to the almonds and mix well.

Using a dessertspoon, place spoonfuls of the dough on to a lined baking sheet, spacing apart as they will expand a little on cooking.

Bake in the oven for 10–15 minutes until golden. Cool on a wire rack to firm up.

The dip can be stored in the fridge for 2–3 days or frozen for up to 1 month.

Nutritional information per biscuit
Calories 161kcal
Protein 5.3g
Carbohydrates 4.2g of which sugars 3.2g
Total fat 13.8g of which saturates 1.7g

References

1. Roundtree, R. (2011) *Genetic and Environmental Determinants: Toxins, Toxicity and Biotransformation.* Presentation given at the Advance Functional Medicine in Clinical Practice (AFMCP) symposium, October 2011. London: IFM.

2. Muller, A. and Yeoh, C. (2010) 'Compromised Detoxification.' In L. Nicolle and A. Woodriff Beirne (eds) *Biochemical Imbalances in Disease.* London: Singing Dragon.

3. Lord, S. and Bralley, J. (2008) 'Clinical applications of urinary organic acids. Part 1: Detoxification markers.' *Alternative Medicine Review 13*, 3, 205–15.

4. Kortenkamp, A. (2006) 'Breast cancer, oestrogens and environmental pollutants: A re-evaluation from a mixture perspective.' *International Journal of Andrology 29*, 1, 193–8.

5. Felton, J.S. and Malfatti, M.A. (2006) 'What do diet-induced changes in phase I and phase II enzymes tell us about prevention from exposure to heterocyclic amines?' *Journal of Nutrition 136*, 10, Suppl., 2683–4S.

6. Talalay, P. and Fahey, J.W. (2001) 'Phytochemicals from cruciferous plants protect against cancer by modulating carcinogen metabolism.' *Journal of Nutrition 131*, 11, Suppl., 3027–33S.

7. Liska, D.J. (1998) 'The detoxificaiton enzyme systems.' *Alternative Medicine Review 3*, 3, 187–98.

8. Williams, A.C., Steventon, G.B., Sturman, S. and Waring, R.H. (1991) 'Hereditary variation of liver enzymes involved with detoxification and neurodegenerative disease.' *Journal of Inherited Metabolic Disease 14*, 4, 431–5.

9. Hess, E.V. (2002) 'Environmental chemicals and autoimmune disease: Cause and effect.' *Toxicology 181–2*, 65–70.

10. Bártová, J., Procházková, J., Krátká, Z., Benetková, K., Venclíková, Z. and Sterzl, I. (2003). 'Dental amalgam as one of the risk factors in autoimmune diseases.' *Neuroendcrinology Letters 24*, 1–2, 65–7.

11. McAlindon, T.E., Gulin, J., Chen, T., Klug, T., Lahita, R. and Nuite, M. (2001) 'Indole-3-carbinol in women with SLE: Effect on estrogen metabolism and disease activity.' *Lupus 10*, 11, 779–83.

12. Wang, C.H., Jeng, J.S., Yip, P.K., Chen, C.L. *et al.* (2002) 'Biological gradient between long-term arsenic exposure and carotid atherosclerosis.' *Circulation 105*, 15, 1804–9.

13. Adams, J.B., Audhya, T., McDonough-Means, S., Rubin, R.A. *et al.* (2011) 'Nutritional and metabolic status of children with autism vs. neurotypical children, and the association with autism severity.' *Nutrition and Metabolism 8*, 1, 34.

14. Baillie-Hamilton, P. (2002) 'Chemical Toxins: a hypothesis to explain the global obesity epidemic.' *Journal of Alternative and Complementary Medicine 8*, 2, 185–92.

15. Hyman, M. (2007) 'Systems biology, toxins, obesity and functional medicine.' *13th International Symposium of the Institute for Functional Medicine*, 134-139. Available at http://drhyman.com/downloads/Toxins-and-Obesity.pdf, accessed on 25 July 2012.

16. Moon, Y.J., Wang, X. and Morris, M.E. (2006) 'Dietary flavonoids: Effects on xenobiotic and carcinogen metabolism.' *Toxicology in Vitro 20*, 2, 187–210.

17. Talalay, P. and Fahey, J.W. (2001) 'Phytochemicals from cruciferous plants protect against cancer by modulating carcinogen metabolism.' *Journal of Nutrition 131*, 11, Suppl., 3027–33S.

18. Faria, A., Monteriro, R., Azevedo, I. and Calhau, C. (2007) 'Pomegranate juice effects on cytochrome P450s expression: In vivo studies.' *Journal of Medicinal Food 10*, 4, 643–9.

19. Duthhie, S.J. (2007) 'Berry phytochemicals, genomic stability and cancer: Evidence for chemoprotection at several stages in the carcinogenic process.' *Molecular Nutrition and Food Research 51*, 6, 665–74.

20. Yuan, J.M. (2011) 'Green tea and prevention of esophageal and lung cancers.' *Molecular Nutrition and Food Research 55*, 6, 886–904.

21. Huber, W.W. and Parzefall, W. (2005) 'Modification of N-acetyltransferases and glutathione S-transferases by coffee components: Possible relevance for cancer risk.' *Methods in Enzymology 401*, 307–41.

22. Osawa, T. (2007) 'Nephroprotective and hepatoprotective effects of curcuminoids.' *Advances in Experimental Medicine and Biology 595*, 407–23.

23. Craig, W.J. (1999) 'Health-promoting properties of common herbs.' *American Journal of Clinical Nutrition 70*, 3, Suppl., 491–9S.

24. Crowell, P.L. and Gould, M.N. (1994) 'Chemoprevention and therapy of cancer by d-limonene.' *Critical Reviews in Oncology 5*, 1, 1–22.

25. Van Leishout, E.M., Posner, G.H., Woodard, B.T. and Peters, W.H. (1998) 'Effects of the sulforaphane analog compound 30, indole-3-carbinol, D-limonene or relafen on glutathione S-transferases and flutathione peroxidase of the rat digestive tract.' *Biochimica et Biosphysica Acta 1370*, 3, 325–36.

26. Van der Logt, E.M., Roelofs, H.M., van Lieshout, E.M., Nagengast, F.M. and Peters, W.H. (2004) 'Effects of dietary anticarcinogens and nonsteroidal anti-inflammatory drugs on rat gastrointestinal UDP-glucuronosyltransferases.' *Anticancer Research 24*, 2B, 843–9.

27. Lee, C.H., Wettasinghe, M. and Bolling, B.W. (2005) 'Betalains, phase II enzyme-inducing components from red beetroot (beta vulgaris L.) extracts.' *Nutrition and Cancer 53*, 1, 91–103.
28. Georgiev, V.G., Weber, J., Kneschke, E.M., Denev, P.N., Bley, P.T. and Pavlov, A.I. (2010) 'Antioxidant activity and phenolic content of betalain extracts from intact plants and hairy root cultures of the red beetroot Beta vulgaris cv. Detroit dark red.' *Plant Foods for Human Nutrition 65*, 2, 105–11.
29. Ryu, S., Choi, S.K., Joung, S.S. *et al.* (2001) 'Caffeine as a lipolytic food component increases endurance performance in rats and athletes.' *Journal of Nutritional Science and Vitaminology (Tokyo) 47*, 2, 139–46.
30. Conger, S.A., Warren, G.L., Hardy, M.A. *et al.* (2011) 'Does caffeine added to carbohydrate provide additional ergogenic benefit from endurance?' *International Journal of Sports Nutrition and Exercise Metabolism 21*, 1, 71–84.
31. Downey, M. (2012) 'Discovering coffee's unique health benefits.' *Life Extension Magazine, January.* Available at www.lef.org/magazine/mag2012/jan2012_Discovering-Coffees-Unique-Health-Benefits_01.htm, accessed on 25 July 2012.
32. Eskelinen, M.H. and Kivipelto, M. (2010) 'Caffeine as a protective factor in dementia and Alzheimer's disease.' *Journal of Alzheimer's Disease 20*, Suppl 1, S167–74.
33. Rosso, A., Mossey, J. and Lippa, C.F. (2008) 'Caffeine: neuroprotective functions in cognition and Alzheimer's disease.' *American Journal of Alzheimer's Disease and Other Dementias 23*, 5, 417–22.
34. Prediger, R.D. (2010) 'Effects of caffeine in Parkinson's disease: from neuroprotection to the management of motor and non-motor symptoms.' *Journal of Alzheimer's Disease 20*, Suppl 1, S205–20.
35. Zhang, Y., Lee, E.T. and Cowan, L.D. (2011) 'Coffee consumption and the incidence of type 2 diabetes in men and women with normal glucose tolerance: the Strong Heart Study.' *Nutrition, Metabolism and Cardiovascular Diseases 21*, 6, 418–23.
36. Muley, A., Muley, P. and Shah, M. (2012) 'Coffee to reduce risk of type 2 diabetes? A systematic review.' *Current Diabetes Reviews.*
37. Natella, F. and Scaccini, C. (2012) 'Role of coffee in modulation of diabetes risk.' *Nutrition Reviews 70*, 4, 207–17.
38. Masterton, G.S. and Hayes, P.C. (2010) 'Coffee and the liver: a potential treatment for liver disease?' *European Journal of Gastroenterology and Hepatology 22*, 11, 1277–83.
39. Muriel, P. and Arauz, J. (2010) 'Coffee and liver diseases.' *Fitoterapia. 81*, 5, 297–305.
40. Hunter, E.A. and Grimble, R.F. (1997) 'Dietary sulphur amino acid adequacy influences glutathione synthesis and glutathione-dependent enzymes during the inflammatory response to endotoxin and tumour necrosis factor-alpha in rats.' *Clinical Science 92*, 3, 297–305.
41. Li, Y., Hou, M.J., Ma, J., Tang, Z.H., Zhu, H.L. and Ling, W.H. (2005) 'Dietary fatty acids regulate cholesterol induction of liver CYP7alpha1 expression and bile acid production.' *Journal of Lipids 40*, 5, 455–62.
42. Enns, C.A. and Zhang, A.S. (2009) 'Iron homeostasis: Recently identified proteins provide insight into novel control mechanisms.' *Journal of Biological Chemistry 284*, 2, 711–5.
43. Chai, W. and Liebman, M. (2005) 'Effect of different cooking methods on vegetable oxalate content.' *Journal of Agricultural and Food Cheimistry 53*, 8, 3027–30.
44. Coronado, G.D., Beasley, J. and Livaudais, J. (2011) 'Alcohol consumption and the risk of breast cancer.' *Salud Pública de México 53*, 5, 440–7.
45. Testino, G., Ancarani, O. and Scafato, E. (2011) 'Alcohol consumption and cancer risk.' *Recenti Progressi in Medicina 102*, 10, 399–406.
46. World Cancer Research Fund (2011) 'Alcohol and cancer prevention.' Available at www.wcrf-uk.org/cancer_prevention/recommendations/alcohol_and_cancer.php, accessed on 18 January 2012.
47. Hare, J.T. and Elliott, D.P. (2003) 'Grapefruit juice and potential drug interactions.' *The Consultant Pharmacist 18*, 5, 466–72.

48. Hanley, M.J., Cancalon, P., Widmer, W.W. and Greenblatt, D.J. (2011) 'The effect of grapefruit juice on drug disposition.' *Expert Opinion on Drug Metabolism and Toxicology 7*, 3, 267–86.

49. Crinnion, W.J. (2010) 'The CDC fourth national report on human exposure to environmental chemicals: What it tells us about our toxic burden and how it assist environmental medicine physicians.' *Alternative Medicine Review 15*, 2, 101–9.

50. Liksa, D., Lyon, M. and Jones, D. (2005) 'Detoxification and Biotransformation Imbalances.' In D.S. Jones (ed.) *The Textbook of Functional Medicine.* Gig Harbor, WA: Institute for Functional Medicine. Page 278.

51. Liska, D. (1998) 'The detoxification enzyme systems.' *Alternative Medicine Review 3*, 3, 187–98.

52. Gasper, A., Al-Janobi, A., Smith, J., Bacon, J.R. *et al.* (2005) 'Glutathione-S-transferase M1 polymorphism and metabolism of sulforaphane from standard and high-glucosinolate broccoli.' *American Journal of Clinical Nutrition 82*, 6, 1283–91.

53. Shinkai, Y., Sumi, D., Fukami, I., Ishii, T. and Kumaqai, Y. (2006) 'Sulforaphane, an activator of Nrf2, suppresses cellular accumulation of arsenic and its cytotoxicity in prmary mouse hepatocytes.' *FEBS Letters 580*, 7, 1771–4.

54. Toyama, T., Shinkai, Y., Yasutake, A., Uchida, K., Yamamoto, M. and Kumaqai, Y. (2011) 'Isothiocyanates reduce mercury accumulation via an Nrf2-dependent mechanism during exposure of mice to methylmercury.' *Environmental Health Perspectives 119*, 8, 1117–22.

55. Juge, N., Mithen, R.F. and Traka, M. (2007) 'Molecular basis for chemoprevention by sulforaphane: A comprehensive review.' *Cellular and Molecular Life Sciences 64*, 9, 1105–27.

56. Jeffery, E. and Araya, M. (2009) 'Physiological effects of broccoli consumption.' *Phytochemistry Reviews 8*, 1, 283–98.

57. John Innes Centre (2011) 'British research leads to UK launch of Beneforte broccoli.' Available at http://news.jic.ac.uk/2011/10/british-research-leads-to-uk-launch-of-beneforte-broccoli, accessed on 17 January 2012.

58. Pizzorno, J., Frassetto, L. and Katzinger, J. (2009) 'Diet-induced acidosis: Is it real and clinically relevant?' *British Journal of Nutrition 103*, 8, 1185–94.

4

Supporting Essential Fatty Acid
and Eicosonoid Balance

While the title of this chapter suggests a nutrient imbalance, essential fatty acid (EFA) ratios are key determinants of a biochemical process that has powerful and wide-ranging effects on health and disease: that of eicosonoid metabolism. This chapter will discuss the eicosonoids and other important roles of EFAs, giving guidance on the intake of EFAs and other dietary fats.

What is a fatty acid imbalance?

Technically speaking, fatty acids are long hydrocarbon chains with a carboxyl group at one end. Once absorbed from the digestive tract, fatty acids are used as building blocks for more complex fat structures, such as triglycerides (in which fatty acids are stored for energy), phospholipids (anchoring fatty acids within cell membranes), cholesterol and steroids (for hormones and bile). Fatty acids also have important roles in cell membrane structure and function, gene expression and, as seen, eicosonoid synthesis.

Natural dietary fatty acids are either saturated (SFAs), monounsaturated (MUFAs) or polyunsaturated (PUFAs). The latter comprise the omega-3 and omega-6 PUFAs, the food sources and metabolism of which can be seen in Figure 4.1.

All natural fatty acids can be synthesised in the human body except for the omega-3 PUFA alpha-linolenic acid (ALA) and the omega-6 PUFA linoleic acid (LA). These have to be obtained from the diet and are therefore classed as 'essential'. Today's diet also contains manmade fats, such as hydrogenated, *trans-* and oxidised fats, which are considered detrimental to health.

Because all these fatty acids have powerful effects on biochemical processes, we need to ensure that their relative levels within the body are appropriately balanced. This is highly determined by diet and lifestyle. UK and international guidelines on fat intake exist for the purposes of public health (see 'What to eat and drink' below). However, a *personalised* nutrition plan will take account of your long-term dietary and lifestyle patterns and the existing ratios of fatty acids in your membrane phospholipids. (In the future, it is likely to take account of your genetic polymorphisms that influence how you metabolise fats.)

For a more detailed discussion of PUFA metabolism and the role of PUFAs in health and disease, see Nicolle and Hallam (2010).[1]

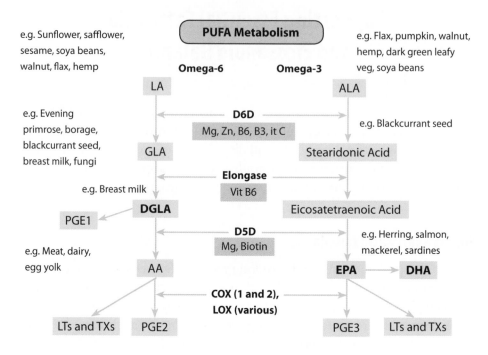

Figure 4.1   *Food sources and metabolism of essential fatty acids to highly unsaturated fatty acids (HUFAs) and eicosonoids*

Key: AA = arachidonic acid; ALA = alpha-linolenic acid; COX = cyclooxygenase; D5D = delta-5-desaturase; DGLA = dihomo-gamma-linolenic acid; D6D = delta-6-desaturase; DHA = docosahexaenoic acid; EPA = eicosapentaenoic acid; GLA = gamma-linolenic acid; LA = linolenic acid; LOX = lysyl oxidase; LTs = leukotrienes; PGE = prostaglandin E; TXs = thromboxanes

Signs and symptoms

Some possible signs of PUFA deficiency and/or imbalances between omega-6 and omega-3 include itchy, dry skin and scalp, brittle nails, atopic symptoms, including asthma and eczema, excessive thirst and urination, behavioural problems, including aggression and violence, low mood, anxiety, having a tendency towards inflammatory conditions and hormonal imbalances (including cortisol, thyroid hormones and insulin). PUFA balance is important for every physiological process and it therefore features in every chapter of this book (refer to individual chapters for more detail).

The most relevant laboratory evaluation is an erythrocyte membrane test showing the ratios between the fatty acids present in the phospholipids. Abnormal ratios both between fatty acid classes and between individual fatty acids within the same family can indicate a range of situations, such as overall deficiencies and excesses, and problems of EFA metabolism to the longer-chain eicosapentaenoic acid (EPA), docosahexaenoic acid (DHA) and gamma-linolenic acid (GLA) (see Figure 4.1).

Functional B vitamin and mineral testing can also be undertaken to identify deficiencies in cofactor nutrients required for fatty acid metabolism.

Serum triglycerides, cholesterol (both low-density lipoprotein cholesterol (LDL-c) and high-density lipoprotein cholesterol (HDL-c) and, where possible, the relative proportions of their sub-units) provide useful information in assessing the general efficiency of fat metabolism.

What health conditions are fatty acid imbalances linked to in the long term?

Historically, SFAs have been labelled as the 'baddie' but, although they can raise triglycerides and LDL-c when eaten in excess, they are the most stable (and therefore healthy) fats to cook with. Most people should be able to consume them safely in moderation. Of more concern to health are:

- the intake of trans-fats (TFAs), as these can contribute to cardio-metabolic problems that are precursors to diabetes and cardiovascular disease (CVD) (see Focus box 4.3)

- an excessively high intake of omega-6 PUFAs compared to omega-3 PUFAs, as this has been associated with chronic inflammation and a range of degenerative diseases (see Focus box 4.2)

- poor conversion of essential fats to the longer-chain EPA, DHA and GLA (see Figure 4.1). In such cases, lack of omega-6 GLA can be just as problematic as lack of the omega-3 derivatives (see Focus box 4.2).

Key nutritional interventions to consider

Overall aims

- To eat a healthy balance of SFA, MUFAs and PUFAs and minimise the intake of processed and damaged fats.

- To optimise the ratio of omega-6 and omega-3 PUFAs (see Focus box 4.2). Many studies recommend a ratio of 4:1, lower if you need to redress a long-term imbalance.

- To ensure sufficient intake of the nutrient cofactors required for EFA metabolism.

- To minimise dietary and lifestyle factors that can hinder EFA metabolism.

What to eat and drink

- Eat a maximum of 30–35 per cent of your daily calories as fat.

- The majority of this fat should be in the form of MUFAs (see Focus box 4.3). These are found in olive oil, rapeseed oil, rice bran oil, avocados, most nuts (including macadamias, hazelnuts, pecans, almonds, cashews, pistachios), sesame and organic, free-range poultry.

   When choosing olive oil, opt for one that is organic, virgin, cold-pressed and unfiltered, as these are higher in the health-promoting polyphenols. To prevent oxidation, keep the bottle in a cool, dark cupboard – not the fridge because the low temperature will cause it to set – and use it in dressings and for cooking at lower temperatures. You can add it to simmering liquids, such as casseroles, curries and tagines, but ideally don't use it for frying or for sealing meat.

   Rapeseed oil has recently become popular and we recommend it for dressings and dips. It may not be the best choice for cooking because, although it contains MUFAs, it is also high in omega-3 PUFAs, which may be damaged if heated to high temperatures. As above, choose organic, cold-pressed oils.

- Saturated fat can be included in a healthy diet, but preferably well under the government-set ceiling of 10 per cent of total calories, or about 20g per day for women and 30g per day for men.

   Saturated fat is useful for cooking because it is the most stable fat and thus the least likely to become damaged. If you are going to roast or stir-fry vegetables, for example, it would be healthier to use coconut fat, butter or lard in small quantities than to use a vegetable oil, a seed oil or olive oil.

   You'll see that coconut fat is our cooking fat of choice in our recipes, as there is evidence that this is a healthier saturated fat (see Focus box 4.3). If cost is an issue, butter, lard, ghee, goose fat or olive oil would be alternatives, depending on the temperature of the cooking and on your particular health issues. (Discuss with your healthcare practitioner.)

- Eat foods containing natural omega-6 PUFAs (linoleic acid). The best sources are raw seeds, especially sunflower, pumpkin, chia, sesame and hemp seeds, and their organic, cold-pressed oils. Keep the oils in the fridge. It is best not to heat them, as this can damage the delicate PUFAs. Nowadays, you can also buy 'butters' made from pumpkin and other seeds. Raw nuts also contain some linoleic acid. Aim to eat a tablespoon of raw seeds or their oils every day. See Table 4.1 for more on the EFA content of nuts and seeds.

Table 4.1 Average fat content of nuts and seeds

Nuts and seeds	LA (g/100g)	ALA (g/100g)	SFA (g/100g)
Almonds	12.20	0.00	3.90
Brazil nuts	20.50	0.05	15.10
Cashews	7.70	0.15	9.20
Hazelnuts	7.80	0.09	4.50
Macadamia nuts	1.30	0.21	12.10
Peanuts	15.60	0.00	6.80
Pecans	20.60	1.00	6.20
Pine nuts	33.20	0.16	4.90
Pistachios	13.20	0.25	5.40
Walnuts	38.10	9.08	6.10
Flaxseeds (linseed)	4.32	18.12	3.20
Pumpkin seeds	20.70	0.18	8.67
Seasame seeds (hulled)	23.58	0.42	7.67
Sunflower seeds	32.78	0.07	5.22

Source: Nicolle and Hallam 2010[1]

- Eat foods containing natural omega-3 PUFAs. Rapeseed oil, linseeds (flax), chia, hemp seeds, pumpkin seeds and walnuts contain the EFA alpha-linolenic acid (ALA). As for the omega-6 EFAs, these should be eaten daily but preferably not heated.

You can see from Figure 4.1 that these fatty acids are converted in the body to highly unsaturated fatty acids (HUFAs), which are precursors to the eicosonoids. Most of the evidence for the health benefits of omega-3 fatty acids is based on studies of EPA and DHA (see Focus box 4.2), which are HUFAs synthesised from ALA. However, this conversion process is highly inefficient (see Focus box 4.1 below). Thus it is important for optimal health to consume EPA and DHA in the diet – the best source being oily fish.

Focus box 4.1   Why do we need to eat EPA and DHA?

The HUFAs EPA and DHA are synthesised from the essential fat ALA. But there are problems with this:[2, 3, 4]

- The conversion process is highly inefficient, with only 0.3–8 per cent EPA being produced from ALA in men and the conversion to DHA in males often negligible.

- The conversion rate is better in women, in some cases being as high as 21 per cent conversion to EPA and 9 per cent to DHA, but there is significant variability between individuals, even when background diets are similar.

- Vegans tend to have lower levels of EPA and DHA than omnivores.

- Eating the omega-6 LA (which is a valuable part of a healthy diet) can further inhibit the conversion process.

- Researchers have concluded that the only *reliable* way to increase EPA and particularly DHA is to get them in the diet.

- Most of the studies of PUFAs in chronic diseases have looked at EPA, DHA and GLA, rather than their precursors.

Aim to eat 2–4 portions of oily fish a week. If you are pregnant or breastfeeding, this should be reduced to 1–2 portions a week, due to the concern about the possible contamination with methylmercury, dioxins and polychlorinated biphenyls.[5] The most polluted fish are the larger varieties, such as shark, swordfish, marlin and tuna, and these should be avoided, especially during pregnancy. According to Sustain (the not-for-profit alliance for better food and farming), smaller fish, such as sprats, sardines, pilchards and trout, carry minimal pollution risk as they do not live long enough to accumulate the toxicants.[6] These fish are also in the most plentiful supply.

See Table 4.2 for the Ω3 PUFA content of some oily fish.

Table 4.2 Oily fish and their Ω3 PUFA content

Type of fish	EPA (g/100g)	DHA (g/100g)	Total Ω3 FA (g/100g)
Fresh salmon	0.50–1.20	0.40–1.30	2.70
Fresh mackerel	0.71	0.12–1.10	1.93
Canned sardines	0.55–0.89	0.10–0.86	1.57
Canned and smoked salmon	0.55	0.85	1.54
Fresh tuna	0.30	1.10	1.50
Herring	0.51	0.11–0.69	1.31
Fresh trout	0.23	0.09–0.8.3	1.15

Source: *Adapted from Jackson et al. 2004[5] and Massaro et al. 2008[7]*

- Many countries, including the UK, recommend at least 500mg EPA and DHA a day, although Norway recommends 1–2g.[3] UK guidelines are that total natural PUFA intake should comprise 6–10 per cent of total daily calories, in a ratio of approximately 5:1 omega-6:omega-3.[8] A ratio of 1:1 to 3:1 is estimated in hunter-gatherer diets and some authors propose this as a more ideal ratio for today.[3, 9, 10] In an individualised approach to nutritional health, the optimal ratio will vary. However, many people may benefit initially from a reduction in omega-6 PUFAs and an increase in omega-3 PUFAs, as the typical modern diet is heavily skewed towards omega-6, at the expense of omega-3.[3]

- When eating meat and dairy products, opt for organic, grass-fed varieties, as a greater proportion of their fat content is PUFAs, with a lower omega-6:omega-3 ratio.[11, 12]

- Eat foods containing the nutrient cofactors for the enzymes used in the conversion of the EFAs ALA and LA to the HUFAs EPA, DHA and GLA and eventually to the eicosonoids (see Figure 4.1). These are the desaturase enzymes (delta-6-desaturase and delta-5-desaturase) and the elongases. As you can see from Figure 4.1, key cofactors are:[1]

  - Magnesium. Good food sources are lightly cooked Swiss chard and spinach, kelp, squash, pumpkin seeds, steamed broccoli, halibut and, to a lesser extent, other green vegetables, nuts and seeds.

  - Zinc and B vitamins. Eat lean cuts of beef, pork, venison and lamb, crab, poultry, calf's liver, seeds, sea vegetables and wholegrains.

  - Biotin. Eggs are a good source.

  - Vitamin C. Eat salad greens, broccoli, bell peppers and fresh fruits, especially strawberries and citrus fruits.

- Eat a wide range of brightly and deeply coloured fruits and vegetables for their antioxidant content (see Chapter 9 for more on antioxidants). PUFAs are vulnerable to oxidation – hence when increasing their intake, it is also wise to ensure a good intake of antioxidants to help preserve the delicate double bonds in their chemical structure. Antioxidants that help prevent lipid peroxidation are alpha lipoic acid (made in the body but some is found in beef, liver and dark green leafy vegetables), vitamin E (wheatgerm, seeds and avocado) and CoQ10 (made by the liver but an increased intake may be required if you are taking statin medication).

What not *to eat and drink*

- Avoid hydrogenated and TFAs. These fats are manmade – the double bonds in the hydrocarbon chains of MUFAs and PUFAs are saturated with hydrogen, as this extends the shelf life of the fats and hardens them for ease of use in food manufacturing. Thus, these fats are found in most processed foods, especially margarines, baked goods, sauces and salad dressings. These fats are extremely harmful to health (see Focus box 4.3).

  Because of the lack of TFA information on food labels in many countries (see Focus box 4.3), it may be best to avoid all processed foods that contain vegetable fats or other oils from plant sources (except coconut or palm oils), unless they are clearly stated to be 'unhydrogenated'.

- Avoid oxidised PUFAs and MUFAs. These are produced when vegetable, nut and seed oils are:

  - used for frying, grilling or baking at high temperatures

  - left out in light and/or heat

  - consumed in processed foods, even organic, that are grilled or fried (such as falafel, pies and vegetarian sausages).

Using the whole seed does not appear to cause so much oxidation. When the omega-3 fat ALA is baked within the seed, for example, it seems that it can withstand the temperatures of baking. One study found that heating both whole and milled flax (linseeds) at either 100°C or 350°C (212°F or 660°F) for one hour had little effect on fatty acid composition or oxidation. Nor was there any evidence of new *trans-* forms of ALA.[13] Other studies have also found the ALA in milled flaxseed to be stable when baked in muffin mixes (at 180°C/350°F) and when boiled within flax-enriched spaghetti.[14]

We therefore support the use of whole or milled flaxseed in baking, especially as it also increases the content of protein, fibre, lignans, potassium and magnesium of the recipes, making them more nourishing. We find that flax binds together other ingredients particularly well and helps to keep baked goods moist.

- Reduce your intake of sugar, by swapping all white starches to wholegrain alternatives and avoiding foods with added sugar. Check labels for added sugars under other names (see Focus box 5.3). As much as 15–20g of fat can be synthesised in the body every day, simply by eating more carbohydrates than are required for energy production.[15]

What's more, diets high in starches or sugars lead to poor conversion of EFAs to HUFAs.[16, 17] Excessive insulin affects the conversion enzymes so that more GLA is converted to inflammatory arachidonic (AA), rather than to anti-inflammatory prostaglandin E1 (PGE1).[18]

- Take steps to minimise your consumption of fructose. Excessive fructose is converted to fat in the liver and is implicated in elevated serum triglyceride levels, non-alcoholic and fatty liver disease and insulin resistance.[19, 20, 21] Although most of the detrimental fructose effects come from its consumption as 'high fructose corn syrup' in processed foods (see Focus box 5.2), it is wise to limit your fruit intake to 2–3 pieces a day and to use fruit juices only sparingly. Juices are concentrated sources of sugar because the fruit's fibre content has been removed and also because it can take 3–5 portions of fruit to make one large glassful of juice.

- Moderate your alcohol intake. Alcohol leeches B vitamins, which are important cofactors in EFA metabolism.

Lifestyle

- Stop smoking – not only is it inflammatory, but it may inhibit the D6D enzyme in EFA metabolism.[16, 17] As nicotine is so strongly addictive, many people find hypnotherapy and/or psychotherapy helpful.

- Take steps to lose weight if you are carrying too much. Being overweight leads to high levels of triglycerides and LDL-c in the bloodstream, increasing the risk of CVD. What's more, excess fat around the abdomen produces inflammatory adipocytokines (see Focus box 8.1). This leaves you with a greater requirement for anti-inflammatory eicosonoids.

- Improve your response to stress (see Chapter 6), as stress has been hypothesised to inhibit EFA metabolism.

- Try to avoid taking non-steroidal anti-inflammatory drugs (NSAIDs), as these inhibit eicosonoid synthesis. If you are on prescription NSAIDs, do not alter your intake until you have discussed with your doctor the risks and benefits of reducing them.

- Ensure you are physically active every day. Exercise helps with weight management and reduces stress levels. What's more, the PUFA conversion enzymes may be suppressed by lack of exercise.[16, 17]

Focus box 4.2   What do EFAs do?

Cell membrane structure and function

The long-chain EFA derivatives EPA, DHA, AA and GLA (see Figure 4.1) are incorporated into the phospholipid bilayer of every cell membrane in the body. Here, they work together to keep the membrane appropriately fluid, so that its receptors and enzymes can work well. In general, omega-3 HUFAs increase fluidity, while omega-6 PUFA, SFAs and *trans*-fats reduce fluidity.[22]

Eicosonoid synthesis

The HUFAs are also metabolised into eicosonoids. These are short-lived, hormone-like chemicals, such as prostaglandins, thromboxanes and leukotrienes, and the more recently discovered resolvins, docosatrienes, neuroprotectins and endocannabinoids. Good health requires an optimal balance between all the different eicosonoids, as this regulates arterial constriction, platelet aggregation, tumour growth, appetite, weight gain and inflammation.[3, 23, 24]

Gene expression (cellular signalling and transcription)

Some of PUFAs' effects occur through their ability to alter gene expression. For example, AA up-regulates a nuclear transcription factor called nuclear factor kappa B (NF-κB), which triggers the production of inflammatory cytokines. Conversely, EPA inhibits NF-κB.[25]

Studies on PUFAs in health and disease

Studies have found that poor EFA conversion to EPA, DHA and GLA (see Figure 4.1) is detrimental to health. It is thought to be a factor in the aetiology of atopic eczema and multiple sclerosis;[26] and may be a key reason for South Asians being at higher risk of insulin resistance, metabolic syndrome and CVD.[16] Such inefficient EFA conversion may also contribute to non-alcoholic fatty liver disease.[17]

By far the most studied PUFAs in human health are EPA and DHA. In general, a high AA:EPA ratio has been associated with diseases such as CVD, cancer,[27] Alzheimer's disease (and milder forms of cognitive impairment)[28] and other chronic inflammatory conditions.[3, 29, 30]

Conversely, a higher EPA and DHA intake has been shown to improve various markers of cardiovascular health (including levels of inflammation, triglycerides and LDL-c particle size)[31] and reduce the risk of death from cardiac events;[32, 33] improve insulin sensitivity[34, 35] and reduce the risk of metabolic syndrome progressing to type 2 diabetes;[36] reduce the risk of certain cancers, such as breast and colon;[27] improve the effects of chemotherapy and surgery[27] and help to maintain weight and muscle mass in cancer patients;[27, 37] improve signs and symptoms of multiple sclerosis[38, 39] and rheumatoid arthritis;[40, 41] help reduce bone loss in low-oestrogen conditions;[42] improve learning and behaviour in under-achieving children;[43] be helpful in depression;[44] and enhance the recall, attention and processing speed in individuals diagnosed with CIND (cognitive impairment no dementia).[45]

Most of the evidence is for fatty acid supplementation, rather than using diet as the sole source, but it shows the wide-ranging effects of these PUFAs on physiological processes and the importance of not becoming deficient.

There is also evidence for the omega-6 fat GLA reducing inflammation and improving signs and symptoms of multiple sclerosis, rheumatoid arthritis, osteoporosis[1] and learning and behavioural disorders.[43] GLA can be metabolised to anti-inflammatory prostaglandin E1 (PGE1) (see Figure 4.1). Thus, omega-6 is just as important in the diet as omega-3, as long as it is not eaten in excess. GLA itself is not readily available in the diet but can be obtained from specially formulated 'omega-blended' oils, which you can use in dips, dressings or smoothies.

Focus box 4.3   More on the non-essential fats

Monounsaturated fatty acids (MUFAs)

MUFAs are a healthy addition to the diet and are less prone to oxidation than are PUFAs because they only have one double bond in their chemical structure.

MUFAs are most commonly consumed as oleic acid in olive oil. (Other MUFA sources include rapeseed oil, rice bran oil, avocados, most nuts (including macadamias, hazelnuts, pecans, almonds, cashews, pistachios), sesame and organic, free-range poultry.) Olive oil is the basis of the Mediterranean diet, which has long been associated with lower risks of obesity, cardiovascular disease, metabolic syndrome, type 2 diabetes and cancer and with healthier ageing[46] (see Chapter 5). Olive oil's polyphenol content gives it antioxidant properties that help protect against age-related cognitive decline, as well as improve endothelial function and inhibit lipid peroxidation.[46] (LDL-c becomes atherogenic if it is oxidised.) Some of its health benefits may be due to its ability to down-regulate pro-atherogenic genes.[47]

Saturated fatty acids (SFAs)

Although SFAs are unhelpful when consumed in excess, they have a place in the diet because they are more stable (and thus healthier) than MUFAs and PUFAs when they are heated (see above). Moreover, the long-held belief that SFAs cause chronic diseases is now being challenged: the incidence of such diseases has been rising, despite the replacement of much dietary animal fat with higher levels of starches and vegetable fats (including TFAs).[48]

Coconut oil appears to be a healthier SFA than animal fat (as found in lard and full-fat dairy, for example) because, although (in excess) it can raise LDL-c, it is associated with higher levels of protective HDL-c.[49, 50] Coconut fat contains medium-chain triglycerides (MCTs), which are less likely than animal fats to be stored in adipose tissue. Indeed, MCTs may increase the use of fats for energy expenditure, as well as reduce food intake and beneficially alter body composition.[51] Thus, using MCTs as the main type of saturated fat in the diet may help to promote weight loss.[52]

One of coconut oil's beneficial fatty acids is lauric acid, which is also found in human breast milk. Lauric acid converts in the body to a compound called monolaurin, which may help support the immune system. Other fatty acids include capric and capyrilic acids, which have antimicrobial properties. Coconut oil and its components have been shown to have antimicrobial action against a number of different pathogens, including *Candida albicans*, MRSA, *Helicobacter pylori* and *Staphylococcus aureus*.[53, 54, 55]

Trans-fatty acids (TFAs)

Industrially produced TFAs are harmful to health, leading to unwanted weight gain, insulin resistance, inflammation, endothelial dysfunction and thus an increased risk of CVD and other chronic diseases.[56, 57, 58, 59] Replacing TFAs with SFAs, MUFAs and PUFAs has been shown to reduce various blood markers indicative of CVD risk and inflammation.[60]

Observational studies have also linked higher TFAs with increased risks of certain cancers, such as breast[56] and ovarian.[61]

Recognising the potential dangers of TFAs, US legislation now stipulates that TFA content in foods must be clearly labelled. Denmark has gone a step further by imposing a maximum level of 2g TFAs per 100g total fat. This has resulted in processed foods in Denmark containing negligible amounts of TFAs,[62] without any noticeable effect on availability, price and perceived 'quality' of the affected foods.[63]

Three-day meal plan

Dishes and snacks in italics are supported by recipes in this chapter or other chapters as indicated.

Day 1

Breakfast: *Berry Chia Breakfast Pudding*

Snack: A few cherry tomatoes

Lunch: *Honey-Glazed Spiced Mackerel* with leafy green salad

Snack: *Walnut Cacao Fudge*

Dinner: *Asian Omelette with Chilli Cucumber Salad*

Day 2

Breakfast: Porridge oats (oatmeal) cooked with sugar-free almond milk, a grated apple, 1 tbsp each of ground flaxseeds and ground chia seeds and some ground cinnamon to taste

Snack: Celery with low-fat cottage cheese or *Dill Ranch Dip* (Chapter 1) or *Simple Nut Cheese* (Chapter 1)

Lunch: *Mixed Bean Salad with Pumpkin Seed Pesto Dressing*

Snack: Handful of mixed seeds and goji berries or *Hemp Milkshake*

Dinner: *Seared Salmon with Puy Lentils and Warm Mustard Dressing* and mixed salad

Day 3

Breakfast: *Crunchy Berry Granola* with coconut, almond or oat milk

Snack: A few olives

Lunch: *Thai Beef Salad*

Snack: *Homemade Yoghurt* (Chapter 1) with a handful of seeds

Dinner: *Roasted Mustardy Vegetables with Chicken or Tofu*

Drinks

- Water and/or a range of herbal teas, including green and white teas for their antioxidant content.

Recipes

Breakfast

Berry Chia Breakfast Pudding

Chia seeds are a rich source of omega-3 (ALA) fatty acids and antioxidants. They are perfect for adding to desserts, smoothies and bars, as well as for this grain-free breakfast pudding. Rich in soluble fibre, they form a gel when added to water or juice that helps slow down the rate of digestion, keeping you feeling satisfied through the morning. In addition, the sesame seeds in the tahini contain omega-6 (LA) fatty acids.

- SERVES 4

50g/1¾oz/½ cup chia seeds
250ml/8fl oz/1 cup 100 per cent unsweetened pomegranate juice
2 tbsp tahini
12 pitted dates, chopped
Pinch of sea salt
Pinch of cinnamon
225g/8oz raspberries

Place the chia seeds in the pomegranate juice and leave to soak for 20 minutes. The seeds should swell up and thicken the liquid.

Place all the ingredients but only half of the raspberries into a blender. Process until smooth and creamy. Add a little water if too thick. Stir in the remaining raspberries.

Spoon into bowls and serve.

Nutritional information per serving
Calories 197kcal
Protein 5.2g
Carbohydrates 22.6g of which sugars 17.5g
Total fat 10g of which saturates 1.3g

Crunchy Berry Granola

Most commercial cereals are packed with fats and sugars, yet granola is simple to make yourself. This version includes nuts and seeds for healthy monounsaturated and omega-3 and omega-6 essential fatty acids (ALA and LA). It is cooked at a lower temperature than commercial granolas, in order to preserve the essential fats. Instead of added sugar, apple juice is combined with a little coconut oil to form a healthy crunchy cereal.

• SERVES 8–10

125g/4½oz/1¼ cups gluten-free porridge oats (oatmeal)
125g/4½oz/1¼ cups buckwheat flakes
60g/2oz/½ cup flaked almonds
60g/2oz/½ cup pecans, roughly chopped
60g/2oz/½ cup walnuts, chopped
60g/2oz/½ cup sunflower seeds
60g/2oz/½ cup pumpkin seeds
2 tbsp flaxseeds
1 tsp ground cinnamon
4 tbsp melted coconut oil
125ml/4fl oz/½ cup apple juice
115g/4oz dried unsweetened mixed berries or dried cherries

Preheat the oven to 150°C/300°F, gas mark 2.

Place the oats, buckwheat flakes, nuts, seeds and cinnamon in a large mixing bowl.

Mix together the melted coconut oil and apple juice. Stir into the dry ingredients. Mix thoroughly to combine, adding a little water to form a moist mixture.

Spread the mixture on to a large baking tray and bake for 40–50 minutes until golden, stirring halfway through.

Leave to cool, then stir in the dried fruit. Store in an airtight container for up to 2 weeks.

Nutritional information per serving (10 servings)
Calories 366kcal
Protein 9.3g
Carbohydrates 27.3g of which sugars 10.3g
Total fat 24.5g of which saturates 6.1g

Lunch

Honey-Glazed Spiced Mackerel

This dish includes a simple, quick marinade, which is delicious on oily fish, such as mackerel and sardines. The mackerel can be served hot or cold and makes an easy evening meal. Leftovers can be used cold in a salad the following day.

• SERVES 4

2 tbsp runny honey or maple syrup
1 tbsp umeboshi paste/plum paste (available from specialist Japanese grocers)
1 tbsp mirin
Pinch of ground ginger

Preheat the grill.

Place the honey into a bowl with the umeboshi paste and mirin. Season with sea salt and pepper.

Make several diagonal scores in the skin of the mackerel, going across the length of each fillet to stop them from curling up during cooking.

Sea salt and freshly ground black
pepper
4 x 100g/3½oz mackerel fillets, skin
on

Spoon the honey marinade over the mackerel fillets, coating thoroughly. Leave to marinate for 20 minutes.

Place the mackerel fillets on a lined baking sheet and grill for 5 minutes or until cooked through.

Nutritional information per serving
Calories 244kcal
Protein 18.9g
Carbohdyrates 5.8g of which sugars 5.8g
Total fat 16.1g of which saturates 3.3g

Mixed Bean Salad with Pumpkin Seed Pesto Dressing

Packed with vitamins and fibre, beans provide a great alternative to traditional leafy green salads. They are robust enough to soak up the tangy flavours of this delicious creamy pesto dressing which combines omega-rich pumpkin seeds, flaxseed oil and peppery watercress. For a vegan dressing, use nutritional yeast flakes instead of parmesan. By using tinned beans, you can create this salad in under 15 minutes. The pesto dressing can be prepared ahead and stored in the fridge for 2–3 days. It is delicious drizzled over steamed or roasted vegetables and potatoes too.

▪ SERVES 4

225g/8oz green beans, sliced in half
400g/14oz can cannellini beans,
    drained and rinsed
400g/14oz can borlotti beans,
    drained and rinsed
400g/14oz can chickpeas, drained
    and rinsed
1 red pepper, diced
1 red onion, finely diced
8 cherry tomatoes, halved
Sea salt and freshly ground black pepper

Pesto dressing
1 garlic clove, chopped
Pinch of sea salt
15g/½oz basil leaves
15g/½oz watercress
1 tbsp lemon juice
30g/1oz pumpkin seeds
2 tbsp extra virgin olive oil
3–4 tbsp flaxseed/hemp oil or
    omega-3–6–9 balance oil
15g/½oz freshly grated parmesan
    cheese or 1 tbsp nutritional yeast
    flakes

Bring a pan of water to the boil and blanch the green beans for 2 minutes until al dente. Drain and rinse under cold water.

Place all the beans and chickpeas in a large bowl with the pepper, onion and tomatoes. Toss lightly.

To make the pesto dressing, place the garlic, sea salt, basil, watercress, lemon juice and pumpkin seeds in a food processor or blender and process until coarsely ground. Slowly add enough of the oils to create a thick dressing. Stir in the parmesan cheese or nutritional yeast flakes.

Pour the dressing over the beans and mix well. Season to taste.

Nutritional information per serving
Calories 410kcal
Protein 16.3g
Carbohydrates 27.7g of which sugars 5.6g
Total fat 25.9g of which saturates 3.7g

Thai Beef Salad

This zesty, spicy salad is perfect for a lunch or evening meal, served with some wholemeal noodles. Use organic, grass-fed beef, as this can be 2–4 times richer in healthy omega-3 fats than grain-fed meat. It also contains more beta-carotene and vitamin E.[64] We have included plenty of colourful vegetables to increase the range of antioxidants in this salad but you can vary the selection according to taste. Using flaxseed oil or an omega-3–6–9 oil blend in the dressing is an easy way to sneak in some additional healthy fats. The dressing will keep in the fridge for 2–3 days and can be drizzled over prawns or fish too. In this recipe, the beef is seared on the outside, leaving it pink and tender on the inside. However, if you prefer your beef more thoroughly cooked, you can use a beef fillet (500g/1lb 2oz) instead and slow-roast it in the oven. To do this, preheat the oven to 60°C/140°F, gas mark ¼. Sear the fillet in the pan until browned all over. Remove the beef from the pan and set aside to cool. Wrap the fillet in non-PVC, heat-safe cling film and roast in the oven for 40 minutes. Test the meat with a digital meat thermometer – it should be at least 57–59°C (135–138°F). For extra tender beef, try marinating it in the fish sauce and oil for 1–2 hours.

- SERVES 4

1 tbsp Thai fish sauce
1 tbsp melted coconut oil or olive oil
500g/1lb 2oz sirloin steaks, trimmed of fat (or beef fillet if slow-roasting)
Freshly ground black pepper
Handful of chopped roasted cashew nuts to serve (roasted at 150°C/300°F, gas mark 2, for 15 minutes)

Dressing
4 tbsp tamari soy sauce
2 tbsp honey
3 tbsp flaxseed oil or an omega-blended oil
1 red chilli, deseeded and diced
1 garlic clove, crushed
1 tsp freshly grated ginger
Juice and zest of 2 limes
1 tbsp rice vinegar

....

150g/5oz sprouting broccoli, cut into small pieces
1 carrot, cut into julienne
1 red onion, thinly sliced

Mix together the fish sauce and coconut oil. Rub the steaks with the mixture and season on both sides. Allow the steaks to stand at room temperature for 5 minutes before cooking.

Heat a frying pan. Sear both sides of the steak for 3 minutes on each side. Take off the heat and leave to stand for 5–10 minutes. (Alternatively, slow-roast a beef fillet – see Introduction for instructions.) Slice thinly and set aside.

To make up the dressing, simply whisk all the ingredients together and set aside.

Blanch the broccoli for a couple of minutes in boiling water until al dente. Drain and rinse under cold water.

Put all the vegetables and herbs in a large bowl and toss lightly with a little of the dressing. Add the strips of beef and drizzle over a little more dressing, then sprinkle over the toasted nuts to serve.

Nutritional information per serving
Calories 427kcal
Protein 34.6g
Carbohydrates 18.7g of which sugars 16.8g
Total fat 23.5g of which saturates 4.7g

200g/7oz cherry tomatoes, halved
Handful of mange tout (snow peas)
   sliced lengthways
1 red pepper, cut into long strips
Handful of coriander leaves
   (cilantro), chopped
Handful of mint leaves, chopped

Dinner

Asian Omelette with Chilli Cucumber Salad

This layered omelette dish could be eaten at any meal, including as a high-protein breakfast option. Use either organic or omega-3-rich eggs (available from good supermarkets). We have added in a few shitake or enoki mushrooms and a dash of tamari for additional flavour. The salad is simple to assemble and the dressing can be prepared in advance and kept in the fridge for 2–3 days.

▪ SERVES 4

Dressing
Juice and zest of 4 limes
1 tbsp xylitol
1 garlic clove, crushed
1 small red chilli, deseeded and
   diced
1 tbsp fish sauce to taste
1 tsp tamari soy sauce
Handful of chopped coriander leaves
   (cilantro)

. . . .

½ red onion, finely chopped
1 cucumber, peeled, deseeded and
   cut into long strips
2 plum tomatoes, deseeded and
   diced
2 tbsp coconut oil
4 shitake or handful of enoki
   mushrooms, stalks removed and
   chopped
6 organic or free-range omega-rich
   eggs
1 tbsp tamari soy sauce

Make up the dressing by whisking all the ingredients together.

Place the onion, cucumber and tomatoes in a bowl and drizzle over some of the dressing. Toss to coat.

Heat 1 tbsp coconut oil in a pan and fry the mushrooms until soft. Remove from the pan.

Beat the eggs with the tamari.

Heat the remaining coconut oil in the frying pan. Pour ¼ of the egg mixture into the pan and swirl around the pan to coat. Sprinkle over a few of the mushrooms. Once the mixture is just setting roll up the omelette to one side of the pan. Pour in the next ¼ of the mixture and swirl to coat the pan – it should attach to the rolled-up omelette. Sprinkle over a few more mushrooms. Once set, start from the existing rolled omelette and roll it towards the other side of the pan like a Swiss roll. Repeat two more times with the remaining mixture rolling it backwards to form a large roll.

Once cooked, remove from the pan. Cut into slices. Serve with the salad and drizzle over a little more of the dressing.

Nutritional information per serving

Calories 189kcal
Protein 10.7g
Carbohydrates 8g of which sugars 6.9g
Total fat 13.2g of which saturates 6.3g

Seared Salmon with Puy Lentils and Warm Mustard Dressing

Fresh Alaskan salmon is one of the best food sources of the longer-chain omega-3 fats EPA and DHA. Here salmon fillets are lightly seared in coconut oil, but you could also bake the fillets in parchment paper with a little lemon juice. The fish is accompanied with earthy puy lentils and a tangy warm mustard dressing. Puy lentils hold their shape well and soak up the delicious flavours from the pan. For speed, you could substitute dried puy lentils for a can of cooked puy lentils and skip the first step in the recipe method. This makes an easy after-work meal but is equally tasty served cold the next day for lunch.

▪ SERVES 4

150g/5oz dried puy lentils
1 garlic clove, crushed
2 tbsp red wine vinegar
1 tbsp Dijon mustard
5 tbsp olive oil
1 tsp coconut oil
4 salmon fillets, boneless
Juice of 1 lemon (optional)
½ red onion, finely chopped
200g/7oz cherry tomatoes, halved
Sea salt and freshly ground black pepper
1 tbsp fresh dill, finely chopped
1 tbsp fresh flat leaf parsley, chopped

Place the lentils in a pan. Add water to cover. Bring to the boil and simmer for 8–10 minutes until al dente. Drain well.

Mix together the garlic, red wine vinegar, mustard and oil.

Heat the coconut oil in a frying pan and place the salmon fillet skin side down in the pan. Cook gently on both sides for 3–4 minutes until the skin is golden and the fish is just cooked through. Remove from the pan and keep warm. Alternatively, for lower-temperature cooking, place the salmon fillets in baking parchment with a little seasoning and lemon juice and bake in the oven at 180°C/350°F, gas mark 4 for 15–20 minutes until tender and cooked through.

Add the red onion and puy lentils to the pan and stir to coat in the pan juices. Add the tomatoes and oil and mustard dressing and allow the mixture to simmer for 1–2 minutes. Place the salmon on top of the lentils in the pan to warm through.

Season to taste and sprinkle over the herbs to serve.

Nutritional information per serving

Calories 399kcal

Protein 30.2g

Carbohydrates 19.5g of which sugars 2.6g

Total fat 22g of which saturates 4g

Roasted Mustardy Vegetables with Chicken or Tofu

This is an easy one-pan dinner. The tangy mustardy marinade imparts a wonderful flavour to the array of antioxidant-rich Mediterranean vegetables. If using chicken try and choose organic as it contains higher levels of polyunsaturated (PUFA) fatty acids compared to conventionally fed chicken. For a vegetarian/vegan option use firm tofu, which is not only rich in protein but also provides a good source of omega-3 essential fats. Serve with a mixed salad.

- SERVES 4

60g/2oz organic virgin coconut oil
1 garlic clove, crushed
1 tsp honey or xylitol
1 tbsp Dijon mustard
2 tbsp tamari soy sauce
Juice of 1 lemon
1 sweet potato, peeled and cut into chunks
2 red onions, cut into wedges
2 red peppers, cut into large chunks
2 yellow peppers, cut into large chunks
2 courgettes, cut into thick slices on the diagonal
4 chicken breasts, boneless and skinless or 400g/14oz firm tofu cut into chunks
2 tbsp chopped mint and coriander to serve
Sea salt and freshly ground black pepper

Melt the coconut oil and add the garlic, honey, mustard, tamari and lemon juice.

Place the vegetables in a roasting dish with the chicken breasts or tofu and drizzle over spiced oil. Season with sea salt and black pepper. Ensure the vegetables and chicken or tofu are thoroughly coated. If possible leave to marinate for 30 minutes.

Heat the oven to 180°C/350°F, gas mark 4.

Bake in the oven for 30–40 minutes until tender and cooked through. Stir half way through cooking.

Nutritional information per serving (chicken)
Calories 409kcal
Protein 34.7g
Carbohydrates 26.7g of which sugars 15.9g
Fat 18.1g of which saturates 13.7g

Nutritional information per serving (tofu)
Calories 356kcal
Protein 12.9g
Carbohydrates 29.8g of which sugars 18.6g
Total fat 20.5g of which saturates 13.7g

Snacks

Walnut Cacao Fudge

This protein-packed fudge uses walnut butter and ground walnuts to provide omega-3 and omega-6 (ALA and LA) fats. Flaxseeds also contain good levels of the omega-3 ALA. The recipe uses raw cacao powder, which has a mild chocolate flavour and is rich in antioxidants.

- MAKES 24 SQUARES

125g/4¼oz/1 cup walnut halves
125g/4¼oz/1 cup pecan nuts
2 tbsp ground flaxseeds
10 large Medjool dates or 20 pitted
  dates
80g/3oz walnut butter
60g/2oz coconut oil, melted
60g/2oz raw cacao powder

Place the walnuts and pecan nuts in a food processor and process until fine. Add the rest of the ingredients and process until the mixture starts to form a dough.

Line a square 20cm/8in shallow tray bake tin with non-stick baking parchment paper. Tip the dough into the tin and use your hands to press the mixture down into the tin firmly. Place in the freezer for 1–2 hours to firm up.

Cut the fudge into small squares to serve.

Store the fudge in the fridge for up to 4–5 days.

Nutritional information per square
Calories 147kcal
Protein 2.6g
Carbohydrates 6.1g of which sugars 3.8g
Total fat 12.6g of which saturates 3.2g

Hemp Milkshake

A creamy milkshake rich in omega-3 and omega-6 essential fats from the hemp seeds. If possible, soak the seeds for 1–2 hours, then strain before using. Hemp seeds are also rich in protein, dietary fibre and calcium and make a wonderful snack and can also be added to cereals, smoothies and baked dishes. The green tea powder is optional but provides a useful source of antioxidants. A teaspoon of a supergreen powder could also be added (available from good health food stores). For a chilled milkshake, chop and freeze the banana, then add it to the blender and process.

▪ SERVES 1

30g/1oz/¼ cup shelled hemp seeds
250ml/8fl oz/1 cup water
½ tsp green tea powder (optional)
½–1 tsp supergreen powder
  (optional)
Pinch of cinnamon
1 banana

Place all the ingredients in a blender and process until smooth and creamy.

Nutritional information per serving
Calories 269kcal
Protein 12.4g
Carbohydrates 23.7g of which sugars 19.9g
Total fat 13.9g of which saturates 1g

References

1. Nicolle, L. and Hallam, A. (2010) 'PUFA Imbalances.' In L. Nicolle L and A. Woodriff Beirne (eds) *Biochemical Imbalances in Disease*. London: Singing Dragon.
2. Arterburn, L.M., Hall, E.B. and Oken, H. (2006) 'Distribution, interconversion and dose response of Ω3 fatty acids in humans.' *American Journal of Clinical Nutrition 83*, 6, Suppl., 1467–76S.

3. Gomez Candela, C., Bermejo Lopez, L.M. and Loria Kohen, V. (2011) 'Importance of a balanced omega 6/omega 3 ratio for the maintenance of health: Nutritional recommendations.' *Nutricion Hospitalaria 26*, 2, 323–9.

4. Anderson, B.M. and Ma, D.W. (2009) 'Are all Ω3 polyunsaturated fatty acids created equal?' *Lipids in Health and Disease 10*, 8, 33.

5. Jackson, A., Key, T., Williams, C., Hughes, I. *et al.* (2004) *Scientific Advisory Committee on Nutrition. Advice on Fish Consumption: Benefits and Risks.* Committee on Toxicity. London: The Stationery Office.

6. Sustain (2005) 'Like shooting fish in a barrel.' Available at www.sustainweb.org/foodfacts/like_shooting_fish_in_a_barrel/, accessed on 25 April 2012.

7. Massaro, M., Scoditti, E., Carluccio, M.A., *et al.* (2008) 'Omega-3 fatty acids, inflammation and angiogenesis: Nutrigenomic effects as an explanation for anti-athergoenic and anti-inflammatory effects of fish and fish oils.' *Journal of Nutriegenetics and Nutrigenomics 1*, 4–23.

8. Committee on the Medical Aspects of Food Policy (1991) *Dietary Reference Values for Food Energy and Nutrients for the UK. Report of the Panel on DRVs of the COMA.* London: Department of Health.

9. Cordain, L., Boyd Eaton, S., Sebastian, A., Mann, N. *et al.* (2005) 'Origins and evolution of the Western diet: Health implications for the 21st century.' *American Journal of Clinical Nutrition 81*, 341–54.

10. Simopoulos, A.P. (2008) 'The importance of the omega-6/omega-3 fatty acid ratio in cardiovascular disease and other chronic diseases.' *Experimental Biology and Medicine 233*, 6, 674–88.

11. Ellis, K.A., Innocent, G., Grove-White, D., Cripps, P. *et al.* (2006) 'Comparing the fatty acid composition of organic and conventional milk.' *Journal of Dairy Science 89*, 6, 1938–50.

12. Daley, C.A., Abbott, A., Doyle, P.S., Nader, G.A. and Larson, S. (2010) 'A review of fatty acid profiles and antioxidant content in grass-fed and grain-fed beef.' *Nutrition Journal 10*, 9–10.

13. Ratnayake, W.M.N., Behrens, W.A., Fischer, P.W.F., L'Abbé, M., Mongeau, R. and Beare-Rogers, J. (1992) 'Chemical and nutritional studies of flaxseed (variety Linott) in rats.' *Journal of Nutritional Biochemistry 3*, 232–40.

14. Manthey, F.A., Lee, R.E. and Hall III, C.A. (2002) 'Processing and cooking effects on lipid content and stability of α-linolenic acid in spaghetti containing ground flaxseed.' *Journal of Agricultural and Food Chemistry 50*, 1668–71.

15. Quistorff, B. and Grunnett, N. (2003) 'Transformation of sugar and other carbohydrates into fat in humans.' *Ugeskrift for Laeger 165*, 15, 1551–2.

16. Das, U.N. (2010) 'A defect in delta 6 and delta 5 desaturases may be a factor in the initiation and progression of insulin resistance, the metabolic syndrome and ischemic heart disease in South Asians.' *Lipids in Health and Disease 9*, 130.

17. Das, U.N. (2011) 'A defect in the activities of delta 5 and delta 6 desaturases and pro-resolution bioactive lipids in the pathobiology of non-alcoholic fatty liver disease.' *World Journal of Diabetes 2*, 11, 176–88.

18. Culp, M. (2010) 'The Metabolic Syndrome.' In L. Nicolle and A. Woodriff Beirne (eds) *Biochemical Imbalances in Disease.* London: Singing Dragon.

19. Samual, V.T. (2011) 'Fructose induced lipogenesis: From sugar to fat to insulin resistance.' *Trends in Endonocrinology and Metabolism 22*, 2, 60–5.

20. Dekker, M.J., Su, Q., Baker, C., Rutledge, A.C. and Adeli, K. (2010) 'Fructose: A highly lipogenic nutrient implicated in insulin resistance, hepatic steatosis, and the metabolic syndrome.' *American Journal of Physiology: Endocrinology and Metabolism 299*, 5, E685–94.

21. Seneff, S., Wainwright, G. and Mascitelli, L. (2011) 'Is the metabolic syndrome caused by a high fructose, and relatively low fat, low cholesterol diet?' *Archives of Medical Science 7*, 1, 8–20.

22. Lord, R. and Bralley, J. (2008) 'Fatty Acids.' In R. Lord and J. Bralley (eds) *Laboratory Evaluations for Integrative and Functional Medicine*, Second Edition. Duluth, GA: Metametrix Institute.

23. Roynette, C.E., Calder, P.C., Dupertuis, Y.M. and Pichard, C. (2004) 'Ω3 Polyunsaturated fatty acids and colon cancer prevention.' *Clinical Nutrition 23*, 139–51.

24. Calder, P.C. (2009) 'PUFAs and inflammatory processes: New twists in an old tale.' *Biochimie 91*, 6, 791–5.

25. Wahle, K.W.J., Rotondo, D. and Heys, S.D. (2003) 'Polyunsaturated fatty acids and gene expression in mammalian systems.' *Proceedings of the Nutrition Society 62*, 349–60.

26. Harbige, L. and Sharief, M. (2007) 'Polyunsaturated fatty acids in the pathogenesis and treatment of multiple sclerosis.' *British Journal of Nutrition 98*, 1, S46–53.

27. Berquin, I.M., Edwards, I.J. and Chen, Y.Q. (2008) 'Multi-targeted therapy of cancer by omega-3 fatty acids.' *Cancer Letters 269*, 2, 363–77.

28. Hanciles, S. and Pimlott, Z. (2010) 'PUFAs in the Brain.' In L. Nicolle and A. Woodriff Beirne (eds) *Biochemical Imbalances in Disease*. London: Singing Dragon.

29. Calder, P.C. (2006) 'Ω3 Polyunsaturated fatty acids, inflammation, and inflammatory diseases.' *American Journal of Clinical Nutrition 83*, 1505–19S.

30. Calder, P.C. (2007) 'Immunomodulation by omega-3 fatty acids.' *Prostaglandins, Leukotrienes and Essential Fatty Acids 77*, 327–35.

31. Abeywardena, M.Y. and Patten, G.S. (2011) 'Role of omega-3 long chain PUFAs in reducing cardio-metabolic risk factors.' *Endocrine, Metabolic and Immune Disorders – Drug Targets 11*, 3, 232–46.

32. Lee, J.H., O'Keefe, J.H., Lvie, C.J., Marchiolo, R. and Harris, W.S. (2008) 'Omega-3 fatty acids for cardioprotection.' *Mayo Clinic Proceedings 83*, 3, 324–32.

33. Mozaffarian, D. and Wu, J.H. (2011) 'Omega-3 fatty acids and CVD: Effects on risk factors, molecular pathways and clinical events.' *Journal of the American College of Cardiology 58*, 20, 2047–67.

34. Das, U.N. (2003) 'Is there a role for saturated and long-chain fatty acids in multiple sclerosis?' *Nutrition 19*, 163–8.

35. Simopoulos, A.P. (2006) 'Evolutionary aspects of diet, the omega 6/omega 3 ratio and genetic variation: Nutritional implications for chronic disease.' *Biomedicine and Pharmacotherapy 60*, 502–7.

36. Barre, D.E. (2007) 'The role of consumption of alpha-linolenic, EPA and DHA in human metabolic syndrome and type 2 diabetes: A mini-review.' *Journal of Oleo Science 56*, 7, 319–25.

37. Murphy, R.A., Mourtzadis, M., Chu, Q.S., Baracos, V., Reiman, T. and Mazurak, V.C. (2011) 'Nutritional intervention with fish oil provides a benefit over standard of care for weight and skeletal muscle mass in patients with nonsmall cell lung cancer receiving chemotherapy.' *Cancer 117*, 8, 1775–82.

38. Norkvick, I., Myhr, K.M., Nyland, H. and Bjerve, K.S. (2000) 'Effect of dietary advice and Ω supplementation in newly diagnosed MS patients.' *Acta Neurologica Scandinavica 102*, 143–9.

39. Shinto, L., Marracci, G., Baldauf-Wagner, S., Strehlow, A. *et al.* (2009) 'Omega-3 fatty acid supplementation decreases matrix metalloproteinase-9 production in relapsing-remitting multiple sclerosis.' *Prostaglandins, Leukotrienes and Essential Fatty Acids 80*, 2–3, 131–6.

40. Calder, P.C. (2008) 'Session 3: Joint Nutrition Society and Irish Nutrition and Dietetic Institute Symposium on Nutrition and autoimmune disease PFA, inflammatory processes and RA.' *Proceedings of the Nutrition Society 67*, 4, 409–18.

41. Stamp, L.K., James, M.J. and Cleland, L.G. (2005) 'Diet and RA: A review of the literature.' *Seminars in Arthritis and Rheumatism 35*, 2, 77–94.

42. Maggio, M., Artoni, A., Lauretani, F., Borghi, L. *et al.* (2009) 'The impact of omega-3 fatty acids on osteoporosis.' *Current Pharmaceutical Design 15*, 36, 4157–64.

43. Richardson, A.J. and Montgomery, P. (2005) 'The Oxford-Durham Study: A randomized, controlled trial of supplementation with fatty acids in children with developmental coordination disorder.' *Pediatrics 115*, 5, 1360–6.

44. Ross, B.M., Seguin, J. and Sieswerda, L.E. (2007) 'Omega-3 fatty acids as treatments for mental illness: Which disorder and which fatty acid?' *Lipids in Health and Disease 6*, 21.

45. Mazereeuw, G., Lanctôt, K.L., Chau, S.A., Swardfager, W. and Hermann, N. (2012) 'Effects of omega-3 fatty acids on cognitive performance: A meta-analysis.' *Neurobiology of Aging,* Epub ahead of print.

46. Lopez-Miranda, J., Perez-Jimenez, F. and Ros, E. (2010) 'Olive oil and health: Summary of the II international conference on olive oil and health consensus report, Jaen and Cordoba (Spain) 2008.' *Nutrition, Metabolism and Cardiovascular Diseases 20,* 4, 284–94.

47. Konstantididou, V., Covas, M.I., Muñoz-Aguayo, D., Khymenets, O. *et al.* (2010) 'In vivo nutrigenomic effects of virgin olive oil polyphenols within the frame of the Mediterranean diet: A randomized controlled trial.' *Journal of the Federation of American Societies for Experimental Biology 24,* 7, 2546–57.

48. Ottoboni, A. and Ottoboni, F. (2004) 'The food guide pyramid: Will the defects be corrected?' *Journal of American Physicians and Surgeons 9,* 4, 109–13.

49. Willett ,W.C. (2006) 'Ask the doctor. I have heard that coconut is bad for the heart and that it is good for the heart. Which is right?' *Harvard Heart Letter 17,* 1, 8.

50. Feranil, A.B., Duazo, P.L., Kuzawa, C.W. and Adair, L.S. (2011) 'Coconut oil is associated with a beneficial lipid profile in premenopausal women in the Philippines.' *Asia Pacific Journal of Clinical Nutrition 20,* 2, 190–5.

51. Clegg, M.E. (2010) 'Medium-chain triglycerides are advantageous in promoting weight loss although not beneficial to exercise performance.' *International Journal of Food Sciences and Nutrition 61,* 7, 653–79.

52. St-Onge, M.P. (2005) 'Dietary fats, teas, dairy, and nuts: Potential functional foods for weight control?' *American Journal of Clinical Nutrition 81,* 1, 7–15.

53. Bergsson, G., Arnfinnsson, J., Steingrinsson, O. and Thormar, H. (2001) 'In vitro killing of Candida albicans by fatty acids and monoglycerides.' *Antimicrobial Agents and Chemotherapy 5,* 11, 3209–12.

54. Kitahara, T., Koyama, N., Matsuda, J., Aoyama, Y. *et al.* (2004) 'Antimicrobial activity of saturated fatty acids and fatty amines against methicillin-resistant Staphylococcus aureus.' *Biological and Pharmaceutical Bulletin 27,* 9, 1321.

55. Sun, C.Q., O'Connor, C.J. and Roberton, A.M. (2003) 'Antibacterial actions of fatty acids and monoglycerides against Helicobacter pylori.' *FEMS Immunology and Medical Microbiology 15,* 36 (1–2), 9–17.

56. Chàjes, V., Thiébaut, A.C.M., Rovital, M., Gauthier, E. *et al.* (2008) 'Association between serum trans-monounsaturated fatty acids and breast cancer risk in the E3N-EPIC study.' *American Journal of Epidemiology 167,* 11, 1312–20.

57. Ros, E. and Mataix, J. (2006) 'Fatty acids composition of nuts: Implications for cardiovascular health.' *British Journal of Nutrition 96,* S29–35.

58. Mozaffiran, D., Aro, A. and Willet, W.C. (2009) 'Health effects of trans-fatty acids: Experimental and observational evidence.' *European Journal of Clinical Nutrition 63,* Suppl. 2, S5–21.

59. Lopez-Garcia, G., Schulze, M.B., Meigs, J.B., Manson, J.E. *et al.* (2005) 'Consumption of trans fatty acids is related to plasma biomarkers of inflammation and endothelial dysfunction.' *Journal of Nutrition 135,* 3, 562–6.

60. Mozaffarian, D. and Clarke, R. (2009) 'Quantitative effects of CV risk factors and CHD risk of replacing partically hydrogenated vegetable oils with other fats and oils.' *European Journal of Clinical Nutrition 62,* Suppl. 2, S22–33.

61. Gilsing, A.M., Weijenberg, M.P., Goldborhm, R.A., van den Brandt, P.A. and Schouten, L.J. (2011) 'Consumption of dietary fat and meat and risk of ovarian cancer in the Netherlands Cohort Study.' *American Journal of Clinical Nutrition 93,* 1, 118–26.

62. Leth, T., Jensen, H.G., Mikkelsone, A.A. and Bysted, A. (2006) 'The effect of the regulation on trans fatty acid content in Danish food.' *Atherosclerosis Supplements 7,* 2, 53–6.

63. Stender, S., Dyerberg, J., Bysted, A., Leth, T. and Astrup, A. (2006) 'A trans world journey.' *Atherosclerosis Supplements 7,* 2, 47–52.

64. French, P., Stanton, C., Lawless, F., O'Riordan, E.G. *et al.* (2000) 'Fatty acid composition, including conjugated linoleic acid, of intramuscular fat from steers offered grazed grass, grass silage, or concentrate-based diets.' *Journal of Animal Science 78,* 2849–55.

5

Managing Blood Glucose Levels

Glucose is an important sugar because it is the body's primary source of fuel. In optimal health, glucose is transported from the liver to the bloodstream and then into the cells, at a rate that is appropriate to meet the body's energy needs and to keep blood glucose levels stable. Sometimes problems can develop with this physiological process and this is referred to as dysglycaemia.

Dysglycaemia is so common that almost everyone recognises its symptoms, either in themselves or in someone they know. It typically starts with hypoglycaemic episodes (the dark grey curve in Figure 5.1) and can eventually lead to the cells developing a resistance to insulin (the light grey curve in Figure 5.1).

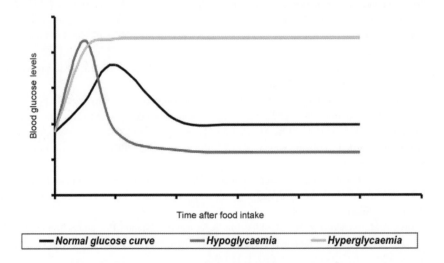

Figure 5.1   Some typical patterns of disrupted post-prandial blood glucose control: hypo- and hyperglycaemia (not to scale)

Sharp rises in blood glucose levels trigger excessive insulin release, leading to plummeting blood glucose levels (hypoglycaemia), unless cells have become insulin-resistant, in which case glucose stays excessively high (hyperglycaemia).

In hyperglycaemia, the low intracellular glucose levels trigger the release of even more insulin from the pancreas, leading eventually to hyperinsulinaemia. The period of time during which cells remain resistant to insulin in such circumstances varies according to the severity of the condition.

Some typical signs and symptoms that could indicate dysglycaemia

- Starch/sugar cravings (reactive hypoglycaemia).

- Pre-menstrual syndrome.

- Night-time waking and alertness (hypoglycaemic episodes trigger the stress-response release of adrenalin and cortisol).

- If a meal is missed, feeling irritable and/or unable to cope with stress, with poor concentration and/or shakiness.

- Regular headaches.

- A waist-to-hip ratio of above 0.8 (for women) and 1 (for men).

- Blood results that show elevated:

    ◦ fasting triglycerides, low-density lipoprotein cholesterol (LDL-c) and/or insulin

    ◦ haemoglobin A1c (Hb A1c): this is the level to which haemoglobin has become 'glycated' (damaged by becoming attached to sugars in the bloodstream – see Chapter 11); it is used as an indicator of long-term hyperglycaemia

    ◦ high-sensitive C-reactive protein (hs CRP), which is a key inflammatory marker.

What health conditions is dysglycaemia linked to in the long term?

- Insulin resistance. It has been suggested that insulin insensitivity may be the single most important underlying metabolic dysfunction related to chronic disease'.[1]

- Polycystic ovarian syndrome. This can include insulin resistance, hirsuitism, male pattern balding, acne vulgaris and infertility.

- Non-alcoholic fatty liver disease.[2, 3]

- Type 2 diabetes. Indefinite hyperglycaemia and often hyperinsulinaemia, although there can eventually be an accompanying failure of the pancreatic beta-cells to continue to produce insulin.

- Diabetic complications, such as retinopathy, neuropathy and renal disease.

- Cardiovascular disease (CVD). The term 'metabolic syndrome' (MetS) refers to a cluster of insulin-resistant-related signs and symptoms (such as hypertension, central obesity and elevated triglycerides) that increase the risk of CVD. The condition is estimated to affect a quarter of all adults in Europe and in the US it is estimated that 40 per cent of the adult population are affected by the age of 60.[3]

- Increased cancer risk.[4]

- Cognitive impairment, including dementia.[5, 6]

There also appears to be an association between MetS and psychological disorders, such as depression.[7]

As insulin resistance is associated with the biochemical imbalances of increased oxidation, inflammation and glycation, it may also be helpful to refer to Chapters 8, 9 and 11, where these are discussed in more detail. Recently, for example, it has been proposed that chronic, low-grade inflammation is key to the pathogenesis of insulin resistance and MetS.[3, 8]

Key nutritional interventions to consider

What to eat and drink

- Choose foods with a low glycaemic load (GL) (see Focus box 5.1), as they slow down the release of glucose into the bloodstream:

  - Proteins: lean meat, poultry, fish and shellfish, eggs, low-fat dairy, nuts and seeds.

  - Foods high in soluble fibre: beans, pulses, turnip, swede (rutabaga), okra, oats, brown rice, xanthum gum and guar gum. Soluble fibre has also been shown to reduce serum lipids.[9, 10] Guar and xanthum gums are commonly used in small amounts in gluten-free baking, pastry fillings and ice creams to combine ingredients, improve texture and add lightness. See, for example, our recipe for *Liquorice Yoghurt Ice* in Chapter 6. (Note that a minority of individuals, including those with coeliac disease or inflammatory bowel disease, appear to be sensitive to xanthum gum.)

- Vegetables in abundance.

- Lower-sugar, deeply and brightly coloured fruits (berries, apples, pears, plums, peaches, cherries, citrus).

- Use olive oil (containing monounsaturated fatty acids) as your main fat, including for cooking with liquids (soups, stews and sauces). Studies have shown olive oil to reduce insulin resistance and markers of CVD risk more than diets high in saturated fats or vegetable oils.[11, 12]

- Eat omega-3 fatty acids for the membrane insulin receptors and for synthesis of eicosonoids (hormone-like chemicals) to help improve the dyslipidaemia and inflammation found in MetS.[13] Eat oily fish (herring, mackerel, salmon, trout and sardines) three times a week. Also eat walnuts, flax (linseeds), hemp, chia and pumpkin seeds and their oils, as these foods contain precursors to the anti-inflammatory fatty acids found in oily fish. See Chapter 4 for more information.

- Include foods containing micronutrients that are cofactors in glucose and/or insulin metabolism.

  - Chromium:[14, 15] good food sources are romaine lettuce, raw onions, ripe tomatoes, brewer's yeast, liver, oysters and wholegrains, especially barley.

  - Magnesium:[16] eat cooked Swiss chard and spinach, kelp, squash, pumpkin seeds, steamed broccoli, halibut and, to a lesser extent, other green vegetables, nuts and seeds.

  - Zinc:[17, 18] eat lean cuts of beef, pork, venison and lamb, crab, poultry, calf's liver, seeds, sea vegetables and wholegrains.

- Eat foods high in antioxidants. Diabetes and pre-diabetic states are characterised by inflammation and oxidative stress, due to a disruption to the normal balance of free radicals and antioxidants.[19, 8] Choose deeply and brightly coloured fruits, vegetables and herbs, and drink green tea. Flavonoids found in berries may help protect against diabetes and complications such as retinopathy.[20] See Chapter 9 for a fuller discussion of antioxidants.

- Special foods to include as often as possible are onions and garlic, cinnamon, gymnema sylvestre (which is easily taken in a tea), fenugreek and bitter melon.[21, 22] Bitter melon, also known as bitter gourd, can be found in Asian stores and is available frozen in some supermarkets. It is commonly used in Thai dishes, stir-fries and curries. Remove the seeds and stem before using. Salting the vegetable for a few minutes and then rinsing before using helps to reduce the bitterness. Try our nutritious stir-fry dish below.

- Drink green tea. While it contains some caffeine, there is preliminary evidence that the catechins in green tea may reduce plasma glucose and insulin levels in healthy and diabetic subjects, increase the hormone adiponectin (which improves insulin sensitivity) and reduce haemoglobin A1c.[23, 24]

- As seen in Chapter 3, recent research indicates that people who drink more coffee may have a lower risk of developing diabetes.[25, 26, 27, 28] Given the paradoxical effect of caffeine on glucose metabolism, the decaffeinated variety would be preferable for individuals who are caffeine-sensitive and/or who have trouble controlling blood glucose levels. Discuss this with your nutrition adviser and agree the type and quality of coffee intake that is right for you.

- Add apple cider vinegar to dressings. Not only does it contain vitamins, minerals and bioflavonoids, but vinegar has been found to lower post-eating blood glucose and insulin levels in healthy individuals[29] and to improve serum lipid profiles (triglycerides, HDL-c and LDL-c) in normal and diabetic rats.[30] See the meal plan below for other ideas for drinks.

What not *to eat and drink*

- Don't eat too much. The amount eaten at any one sitting influences the glycaemic response.[31] What's more, an excessively high-calorie diet is associated with insulin resistance, while calorie restriction (CR) in animal studies has been found to reduce elevated blood glucose and insulin levels, by activating a sirtuin gene called SIRT-1 (see Chapter 11).[10, 8] Studies on diabetic patients have used very low-calorie diets (400–1000kcal per day) with promising results.[32] Other work by the prominent raw foods advocate Dr Gabriel Cousens uses calorie restriction together with green juicing and a nutrient-dense, vegan, low-glycemic diet of living foods over a 21-day period, with positive results.[33] Similar studies together with the use of pancreatic enzymes have also demonstrated positive results.[34, 35] Such a regime should only be undertaken with the close supervision of a suitably qualified healthcare professional.

- Minimise your intake of foods with a high GL, as they cause sharp peaks in blood glucose levels (see Figure 5.1):

  ○ Alcohol. In excess, alcohol not only disrupts blood glucose levels, but also contributes to fatty liver, high cholesterol and weight gain. Such conditions are often found in individuals with dysglycaemia.

- Sugars, including added sucrose, fructose (especially high-fructose corn syrup), glucose and maltose (see Focus box 5.2 for an overview of common sugars and sweetners, and Focus box 5.3 for a list of the many terms used to denote 'sugars' on food labels). As seen in Chapter 4, excessive fructose is converted to fat in the liver and is implicated in elevated serum triglyceride levels, non-alcoholic fatty liver disease,[36] insulin resistance and metabolic syndrome.[37, 38, 39] Although most of the detrimental fructose effects arise from its inclusion in processed foods, it is wise to limit your intake to 2–3 pieces of fruit a day and to choose the lower-fructose varieties, such as berries. Fruit juices are concentrated sources of sugar and are therefore best avoided or used infrequently and sparingly.

- Refined starches, including many commercial breakfast cereals and snack foods.

- Potatoes, although small portions of boiled new potatoes in their skins are generally fine if eaten with a high-quality protein and you are not trying to lose weight.

- No more than a single portion at each meal of grains (which should be wholegrains). A portion size is roughly 2–3 tbsp (50g/1¾oz) or 2 small oat cakes or 1 slice of whole rye bread.

- Steer clear of adrenal gland stimulants, as they encourage the liver to rapidly break down glycogen stores and inject glucose into the bloodstream (via adrenalin and cortisol):

  - Excessive levels of caffeine (in, for example, tea, coffee, colas and chocolate). Green tea is an exception (see above) and coffee may be beneficial if drunk within the individual's caffeine tolerance threshold (see above and Chapter 3). If your tolerance is low, stick to (organic) decaff.

  - Nicotine and other recreational drugs. Smoking also increases oxidative load. As nicotine is so strongly addictive, many people find hypnotherapy and/or psychotherapy helpful.

- Don't eat industrially produced *trans*-fats (found in processed foods), as they lead to unwanted weight gain, insulin resistance, inflammation and an increased risk of diabetes and CVD (see Chapter 4). Also avoid excessive intake of animal fats (no more than 10% of daily calories) and avoid heating vegetable, seed and nut oils, as this increases the body's burden of oxidative stress, which, as seen, is a factor in diabetes and CVD.

Lifestyle

- Stop smoking (see above).

- Take steps to lose weight if you are carrying too much. Excess visceral adipose tissue (the fat which surrounds the internal organs) produces 'adipokines', such as adiponectin, resistin, leptin, tumour necrosis factor-alpha (TNF-α) and interleukin-6 (IL-6). These influence many metabolic processes, including appetite control, insulin resistance and inflammation.[40, 41]

- Manage the stress in your life. Chronic stress is associated with weight gain and increased risk of developing MetS.[42]

- Take regular exercise. This improves insulin sensitivity by reducing stress, promoting weight loss[43] and by other mechanisms, such as by inducing GLUT-4 activity.[44] GLUT-4 is a key glucose transporter, allowing glucose and insulin into the cells.

- Ensure good-quality, and sufficient quantity of, sleep. Recent research has found sleep deficit to affect glucose metabolism and insulin sensitivity.[45, 46] If you have trouble sleeping, make sure your bedroom is completely dark and well-ventilated, switch off all the electrics at the plug sockets and keep the two hours prior to bedtime free of computers, television, intense exercise, caffeine and bright lighting. Relax in a warm bath with chamomile or lavender essential oils added.

How to eat

- Follow the general dietary guidelines in Chapter 1.

- In addition:

  ○ You may find it easier to control your blood glucose levels by eating little and often – that is, five small meals a day, rather than three large ones.

  ○ Take time to eat, as this reduces the body's glycaemic response to the meal.[47]

  ○ Every meal should be mainly vegetables, with some protein and fat. Unless you are trying to gain weight or are doing a lot of exercise, starchy carbohydrates, such as potatoes and grains, are not recommended in a blood sugar balancing programme. Cutting right back has been found to reduce insulin fluctuations, improve markers of CVD risk and MetS and to be as effective for weight loss as low-fat diets.[48] Remember that carbohydrates are still found in vegetables and fruits (limit to 2–3 pieces of fruit a day).

Focus box 5.1   Glycaemic index (GI) and glycaemic load (GL)

The concepts of GI and GL are important to understand if you are aiming to improve your blood glucose control, as eating a high GI and GL diet is associated with an increased risk of diabetes.

GI refers to the extent to which blood glucose rises after eating a food, relative to the reference foods glucose and white bread, both of which are indexed at 100. A food's GI is influenced by its fibre, protein and fat content, as well as by the type of starch it contains (amylose versus amylopectin) and the way in which it has been processed and/or cooked.

Knowing the GL of a food is considered more useful than simply knowing the GI, as the GL takes account of the GI *and* the amount eaten. A food's GL is calculated by multiplying its GI as a decimal by the amount of carbohydrate per serving. A GL equal to or greater than 20 is considered high and equal to or less than 10 is considered low.

Thus, foods comprising a higher proportion of carbohydrate tend to have a higher GL than foods that comprise more protein, fat, fibre or water. For example, a cup of white rice has a similar (high) GI to a cup of watermelon. But, because the rice contains a significantly higher proportion of carbohydrates than does the watermelon (being mainly composed of water), their GLs are significantly different – white rice's being high and watermelon's being relatively low.

Thus, meat, poultry, fish, eggs, beans, pulses, nuts, seeds, dairy, vegetables, fruits, fats and oils have a lower GL than grains. Wholegrains have a lower GL than white starches, sugars and alcohol.

For an extensive table of the GI and GL of more than 750 different types of food, see the free access article Foster-Powell, Holt and Brand-Miller (2002).[49]

Focus box 5.2   Sugar and the role of natural sweeteners

There is no scientific doubt that high-sugar diets are detrimental to health. Sugar naturally occurs in many foods and is added, in one form or another, to most processed foods, making it difficult to avoid altogether. Excess sugar consumption has been associated with conditions such as high blood pressure, high cholesterol, cardiovascular disease, obesity and premature ageing; and restricting sugar intake is recognised as crucial in preventing the development of such chronic diseases.[50]

It is easy to become confused by the various sugars and sweeteners available. Not all sugars are created equal and just because something is termed 'natural' does not mean it is necessarily beneficial to our health. Even healthier sugars and sweeteners should be limited and used sparingly. Here is a summary of the different forms and a guide to some healthier options.

Some widely used sugars

Dextrose, fructose and glucose are all monosaccharides, known as simple sugars. The primary difference between them is the way in which they are metabolised in the body. Fructose, found naturally in fruit, is metabolised in the liver.

Fructose has been marketed as a healthier sugar in MetS and diabetes because it does not cause sharp spikes in blood glucose levels. But recently we have seen that a high intake of *isolated* fructose (as in 'high-fructose corn syrup' – HFCS), may promote overeating and weight gain because, unlike some other sugars, it does not stimulate the satiety hormone *leptin*.[51]

HFCS is 55 per cent fructose and 45 per cent glucose and is now present in many processed foods and drinks. While HFCS contains the same two sugars as sucrose (see below), they are not bound together, as they are in table sugar. This means that they don't need to be broken down in the digestive tract. Instead, they are absorbed so quickly that in high amounts the liver can become overwhelmed, leading to elevated blood levels of triglycerides, very-low-density lipoprotein (VLDL), low-density lipoprotein cholesterol (LDL-c) and decreased high-density lipoprotein cholesterol (HDL-c);[52] and also to alcoholic fatty liver disease and insulin resistance (Chapter 4).

Dextrose, which comes from the hydrolysis of cornflower (cornstarch), is present in many processed foods. Like sucrose, dextrose may deplete the body of valuable vitamins and minerals.

Sucrose, also known as saccharose, is a disaccharide, made up of glucose and fructose. It is present in table sugar, maple syrup and molasses. Raw sugar, Turbinado sugar or natural sugar, although often promoted as being healthier than standard table sugar, has the same effect on the body as sucrose.

Sugar alcohols, such as xylitol, glycerol, sorbitol, maltitol, mannitol and erythritol, are in reality neither sugars nor alcohols and are becoming increasingly popular as sweeteners. They are incompletely absorbed from the gut, meaning that they provide fewer calories than sugar. In some cases, excess can result in symptoms such as bloating, diarrhoea and flatulence.

Artificial sweeteners, including Sucralose (Splenda), aspartame and saccharin, have been linked to a variety of health conditions, despite being low in calories.[53] Overall, the evidence is somewhat contradictory as to their safety and we therefore recommend replacing them with natural sugars.

Agave syrup is made from the juice of the agave cactus. Agave is most commonly available as a highly processed syrup and is usually 70–80 per cent fructose. Raw agave nectar has a lower fructose content and also contains some trace minerals. While agave has a lower GI score than many other sugars, its high fructose content means it should only be used in small quantities.

Some other natural sugars to consider

Fresh and dried fruit make useful sweeteners in sweet and savoury dishes and have the benefit of containing fibre, vitamins and minerals. The fibre helps modulate the blood glucose response. Dates are particularly useful when soaked and blended to thicken and sweeten puddings and sauces, and they also act as a binding agent in cakes and biscuits.

Maple syrup is made from the boiled sap of the maple tree. It contains around 65 per cent sucrose and has a relatively high GI, so should only be used sparingly. It does, however, contain trace amounts of minerals (such as manganese and zinc) and is rich in antioxidants, especially phenolics such as quebecol.[54] Choose an organic maple syrup and avoid forms that are mixed with other syrups, such as corn syrup.

Molasses is made by refining sugar cane and sugar beets. During processing, sugar crystals are extracted leaving a dark, syrupy mixture. Blackstrap molasses generally contains less sugar and a greater concentration of minerals, including iron, calcium and magnesium.

Stevia is a highly sweet herb derived from the leaf of the South American stevia plant. It is safe to consume in its natural form, even for diabetics and people with hypoglycaemia, because it is calorie-free and does not cause spikes in blood glucose levels. Stevia is 200–300 times sweeter than sugar. It is available in both powder and liquid form, at different concentrations.[55, 56]

Lo han (or luohanguo) is a natural sweetener derived from the lo han guo, which is a member of the gourd family. Like stevia, it is 250–400 times sweeter than sugar, contains no calories and is safe for diabetics and hypoglycaemics.[57, 58]

Xylitol is a natural sweetener extracted from birch cellulose. Xylitol has been shown to help fight dental cavities and to facilitate the remineralisation of dental enamel.[59] It tastes similar to sugar and comes in a granular form, making it an easy substitute for sugar in recipes, yet contains 40 per cent fewer calories. It has a low GI score, helpful in a blood glucose balancing diet.

Honey contains around 53 per cent fructose. It may confer some health benefits when used in moderation as it is rich in antioxidants and raw forms possess antimicrobial properties. Manuka honey has been found to be effective against bacterial infections, such as *H. Pylori*.[60] Honey is one-and-a-half times sweeter than sugar, so less is needed in recipes. Honey should not be given to babies under one year old.

Bee pollen is an easy-to-digest natural sweetener that contains a range of nutrients, including enzymes, vitamins, trace minerals, flavonoids and carotenoids. It can be sprinkled over foods and added to drinks, smoothies and ice creams, but it should not be heated. As it is perishable, it is best kept frozen.

Maca powder is derived from a Peruvian root vegetable. The colour and flavour is similar to brown sugar and it can be used to naturally sweeten drinks and desserts. Rich in protein and minerals, including iron and calcium, it is also considered to be a natural hormone balancer and an adaptogen, supporting the adrenal glands and increasing energy levels.[61, 62]

Mesquite is made from the pods of the mesquite tree. It has a mild caramel-like flavour and is delicious in drinks, ice creams, desserts and baked dishes. It has a relatively low GI and contains some protein and minerals, including calcium, magnesium, potassium, iron and zinc. At present mesquite is classed as a 'novel food' in Europe and restrictions are in place regarding its sale.

Yacon syrup is made from an edible tuber from South America. Naturally sweet and low in calories (around 20 calories per tbsp), it has a low GI score and works well as an alternative to syrups and honey in recipes. Yacon contains inulin, a useful prebiotic to support a healthy microbial balance in the gut.

Coconut sugar is derived from the sap of coconut flowers. Coconut sugar is low in calories and has a low GI score (around 35). It contains 70–79 per cent sucrose. It also contains traces of minerals, including potassium, zinc, magnesium and iron. Choose organic coconut sugar to ensure purity.

Focus box 5.3 Some common sugars on labels

When checking food labels, it's worthwhile knowing how to recognise 'sugar'. The terms below are the most commonly used to designate a form of sugar, some of which are described in Focus box 5.2.

Agave nectar	Date sugar	Glucose solids	Molasses
Barbados sugar	Demerara sugar	Golden sugar	Muscovado sugar
Barley malt	Dextrin	Golden syrup	Organic raw sugar
Beet sugar	Dextran	Granulated sugar	Panocha
Blackstrap molasses	Dextrose	Grape sugar	Powdered sugar
Brown sugar	Diastatic malt	Grape juice	Raw sugar
Buttered syrup	Diatase	concentrate	Refiner's syrup
Cane crystals	D-mannose	HFCS	Rice syrup
Cane juice crystals	Evaporated cane	High-fructose corn	Sorbitol
Cane sugar	juice	syrup	Sorghum syrup
Caramel	Ethyl maltol	Honey	Sucrose
Carob syrup	Florida Crystals	Icing sugar	Saccharose
Caster sugar	Free Flowing	Invert sugar	Sugar
Confectioner's	Fructose	Lactose	Syrup
sugar	Fruit juice	Malt syrup	Table sugar
Corn syrup	Fruit juice	Maltodextrin	Treacle
Corn sweetener	concentrate	Maltose	Turbinado sugar
Corn syrup solids	Galactose	Mannitol	Yellow sugar
Crystalline fructose	Glucose	Maple syrup	

Three-day meal plan

Dishes and snacks in italics are supported by recipes in this chapter or other chapters as indicated.

Day 1

Breakfast: *Fresh Berries with Cinnamon Nut Cream*, 4 tbsp full-fat natural yoghurt or *Chicken Liver Pate* (Chapter 6) with vegetable sticks

Snack: Carrot sticks and low-fat cottage cheese or *Avocado Spiced Hummus* (Chapter 11)

Lunch: *Stir-Fried Bitter Melon with Egg* and a mixed salad or *Raw Vegetable Spaghetti with Cashew Nut Cream Sauce* (accompany with some sprouted beans or a hard-boiled egg for additional protein)

Snack: Small handful of almonds and mixed seeds

Dinner: *Loin of Venison with Blackberry/Blueberry and Juniper Sauce* and steamed greens, kale or cabbage

Day 2

Breakfast: 1–2 poached eggs with wilted spinach and chopped tomatoes

Snack: Small handful of walnut halves (7–8)

Lunch: *Griddled Squid with Pepper and Fennel Salad*

Snack: *Hemp Milkshake* (Chapter 4) or *Supergreens Berry Smoothie* (Chapter 3)

Dinner: *Fenugreek Bean Curry* with steamed greens or mixed salad

Day 3

Breakfast: *Avocado Cacao Smoothie*

Snack: Hard-boiled egg and cherry tomatoes

Lunch: *Fattoush with Chickpeas*

Snack: *Sesame Tamari Dip* and carrot sticks

Dinner: *Lemon and Pumpkin Seed Crusted Halibut with a Caper Dressing* with a salad of mixed leaves and herbs

Drinks

- Fresh filtered water and herbal teas, drunk either hot or cold. Herbal teas can be chilled and drunk like a punch (that is, with soaked fruit and ice). Some teas to try: green tea, white tea, red bush, gymnema sylvestre, cinnamon and any of the teas in Chapter 6.

- Also consider drinking a good-quality aloe vera juice, either as a shot, or diluted in water, or by adding it to a smoothie (such as the *Avocado Cacao Smoothie*, *Hemp Milkshake* in Chapter 4 or *Supergreens Berry Smoothie* in Chapter 3). Although trials are required to establish its true clinical efficacy, preliminary research indicates that aloe vera may help to improve glucose control.[63, 64]

Recipes

Breakfast

Fresh Berries with Cinnamon Nut Cream

A delicious bowl of antioxidant-rich berries served with a protein-rich nut cream makes the perfect snack, dessert or breakfast option. Berries are lower in sugar than other types of fruit and blackberries and raspberries are particularly low in fructose. Nuts contain protein and fat, both of which help to stabilise blood sugar, keeping you fuller for longer. Cinnamon is a useful spice for helping to improve glucose metabolism and makes a perfect accompaniment to the fruit. This nut cream would be equally delicious with stewed apple or pears.

- SERVES 4

300g/10½oz mixed berries

Cream
125g/4½oz almonds
1 tsp ground cinnamon
100ml/3½fl oz orange juice
Few drops vanilla extract
2 nectarines, peeled and sliced
Water to thin as needed

Divide the berries between four bowls.

Place all the ingredients for the cream into a blender and blend until very smooth. Add a little water if needed to blend to the desired consistency. Spoon the nut cream over the berries to serve.

Nutritional information per serving
Calories 245kcal
Protein 8.7g
Carbohydrates 12.8g of which sugars 12.3g
Total fat 17.8g of which saturates 1.5g

Avocado Cacao Smoothie

Using avocado in a smoothie may seem a little unusual but it creates a lovely creamy texture, as well as providing plenty of healthy monounsaturated fat, vitamins and minerals. It also contains the antioxidant and liver-supportive polypeptide glutathione. Raw cacao is rich in antioxidants, while the addition of flaxseed boosts the intake of fibre and omega-3 fats. Almond milk is a dairy-free, protein-rich milk, but coconut milk would work equally well. The addition of coconut water provides electrolytes (especially potassium, phosphorous and magnesium) for effective hydration.

- SERVES 4

1 ripe avocado, peeled and stoned
500ml/17fl oz/2 cups almond milk
   or coconut milk (check the label
   for sugar-free versions)
250ml/8fl oz/1 cup coconut water
1–2 tbsp raw cacao powder to taste
1 tsp vanilla extract
1 tbsp ground flaxseed
1 tsp cinnamon
250g/9oz fresh or frozen raspberries

Simply place all the ingredients in a high-speed blender and process until smooth. Best served immediately.

Nutritional information per serving
Calories 136kcal
Protein 3.4g
Carbohydrates 13.9g of which sugars 8.8g
Total fat 7.5g of which saturates 1.8g

Lunch

Stir-Fried Bitter Melon with Egg

Although it may be an acquired taste, bitter melon is useful in its ability to help stabilise blood sugar levels and improve insulin function. This is a simple dish with egg, flavoured with tamari soy sauce and xylitol, for a hint of tangy sweet and sour. This can be served as a light lunch with steamed greens. If you wish to remove some of the bitterness, you can salt the bitter melon for 30 minutes or place in salted water; rinse before using.

• SERVES 2

1 large bitter melon (300g/10½oz),
   peeled, seeded and sliced
   (available fresh in Asian stores or
   frozen in many supermarkets)
Sea salt
1 tbsp coconut oil
3 cloves garlic, peeled and crushed
1 small red onion, finely chopped
3 eggs, beaten
2 tbsp tamari soy sauce
2 tsp xylitol
125ml/4fl oz/½ cup vegetable or
   chicken stock

Cut the bitter melon vertically in half. Take out hard seeds, if any, and discard. Slice the bitter melon, and put the slices on to kitchen paper. Sprinkle sea salt over the bitter melon slices, and wrap them tightly in the kitchen paper. Leave for 30 minutes, then rinse. Alternatively, place in salted water for 15–20 minutes, then rinse.

Heat a wok and melt the coconut oil. Stir-fry the garlic and onion for 1 minute. Mix the egg with the tamari and xylitol and add to the pan. Stir for a few times and after a minute stir in the bitter melon. Stir again for a further minute.

Pour in the vegetable stock and cook for 2–3 minutes until the bitter melon is just cooked.

Nutritional information per serving
Calories 187kcal
Protein 11g
Carbohydrates 7.3g of which sugars 3.8g
Total fat 13.2g of which saturates 6.3g

Raw Vegetable Spaghetti with Cashew Nut Cream Sauce

A delicious low-carbohydrate dish, using long strips of courgettes (zucchini) and butternut squash to create vegetable 'pasta'. You can use a spiraliser to create very thin spaghetti-like strands, or, alternatively, a vegetable peeler to create long ribbons. Instead of butternut squash, you could use carrots. Toss in the dressing just before serving.

▪ SERVES 4

2 medium courgettes (zucchini)
½ small butternut squash or 2 carrots
1 medium red pepper
12 asparagus tips
1 tbsp olive oil
Pinch of sea salt

Cream sauce
60g/2oz/½ cup cashew nuts
1 tbsp nutritional yeast flakes
1 garlic clove, crushed
1 red pepper, deseeded and cored
1 tbsp lemon juice
Black pepper
Rocket leaves (arugula) to serve

Peel the courgette, carrots or butternut squash and discard the ends. Using a spiraliser or vegetable peeler, slice the vegetables into long ribbons. Discard the seeded centre of the courgette. Cut the red pepper into thin julienne strips.

Place all the vegetables in a large bowl and massage the oil and sea salt by hand.

For the dressing, place all the ingredients in a blender and process until thick and creamy.

Combine the cream sauce with the vegetables. Season with black pepper.

Serve on a bed of rocket and eat immediately.

Nutritional information per serving
Calories 159kcal
Protein 5.8g
Carbohydrates 10.5g of which sugars 8.3g
Total fat 10.3g of which saturates 1.9g

Griddled Squid with Pepper and Fennel Salad

A summery, Mediterranean-inspired dish, rich in protein and antioxidants, which serves well as a light lunch or a quick after-work dish. Using flaxseed oil in the lemon dressing is an easy way to increase your intake of the omega-3 fat alpha-linolenic acid (ALA). Prawns or crab could be used in place of the squid. You could also replace the peppers with a jar of roasted red peppers to save time.

▪ SERVES 4

Dressing
Juice of 1 lemon
Grated zest of 1 lemon
3 tbsp flaxseed oil
2 tbsp extra virgin olive oil
Sea salt and freshly ground black pepper
2 tsp chopped fresh parsley
2 tsp chopped fresh mint

Make up the dressing by simply combining all the ingredients together.

Turn the grill on to high. Place the peppers on a baking sheet cut side down and grill until the skin is blackened. Remove and place in a bowl. Cover with cling film and allow to cool. Once cool enough to handle, remove the skin and cut the peppers into thick strips. Place in a bowl. Alternatively, use roasted peppers from a jar.

1 red pepper, halved
1 orange pepper, halved
1 fennel bulb, trimmed and sliced
   lengthways thinly
A little melted coconut oil or olive oil for
   brushing
115g/4oz sun-dried tomatoes in oil,
   drained
3 squid, cleaned
2 tbsp melted coconut oil or olive oil
1 tbsp lemon juice
1 red chilli, deseeded and diced
250g/9oz bag of leafy green salad leaves
   (e.g. rocket/arugula, spinach, lamb's
   lettuce)

Brush the fennel with a little melted coconut oil or olive oil. Heat a griddle pan and add the fennel. Cook for 1 minute on each side until softened, then remove from the heat. Place in the bowl with the peppers and add the sun-dried tomatoes. Drizzle over a little of the dressing and set aside.

Prepare the squid: slice open each squid lengthways, score a criss-cross pattern on the inside and cut each into three pieces.

Mix the squid pieces with the coconut oil, lemon juice and chilli and leave to marinate for 10 minutes.

Heat the griddle pan and cook the squid pieces for 1 minute only on each side. Toss lightly with the fennel and peppers.

Place the salad leaves in a bowl and lightly dress with the vinaigrette.

To serve, place the salad leaves in the centre of each plate, top with the squid and vegetables. Season with a little extra black pepper.

Nutritional information per serving (with 1 tbsp dressing)

Calories 356kcal
Protein 15.6g
Carbohydrates 7.5g of which sugars 5.9g
Total fat 28.9g of which saturates 7.2g

Fattoush with Chickpeas

This Lebanese-inspired salad is lightly spiced with sumac and dressed with a pomegranate walnut dressing. Romaine lettuce, onion and tomatoes are good sources of chromium, while the chickpeas provide protein and magnesium. The dressing can be prepared ahead and stored chilled for 2–3 days.

▪ SERVES 4

Dressing
Juice and zest of 1 lemon
3 tbsp pomegranate molasses (available
   from some supermarkets, Middle
   Eastern food stores and online)
3 tbsp walnut oil
3 tbsp extra virgin olive oil
Sea salt and freshly ground black pepper

Whisk all the ingredients for the dressing together. Chill until needed.

Combine all the salad ingredients together in a large bowl and mix lightly.

Just before serving, pour a little of the dressing over the salad and toss.

2 tsp sumac or to taste (find sumac in the spice section)

....

1 romaine lettuce, cut into thin strips
200g/7oz cherry tomatoes, halved
½ red onion, diced
½ cucumber, peeled and deseeded and cut into chunks
½ red pepper, deseeded and cut into dice
½ green pepper, deseeded and cut into dice
1 tbsp fresh mint leaves, chopped
4 radishes, thinly sliced
2 x 400g/14oz cans chickpeas, drained and rinsed
1 slice of lightly toasted pumpernickel (optional), cut into small pieces

Nutritional information per serving (with 1 tbsp dressing)

Calories 207kcal
Protein 9.5g
Carbohdyrates 24.3g of which sugars 6.9g
Total fat 9.6g of which saturates 1.1g

Dinner

Loin of Venison with Blackberry/Blueberry and Juniper Sauce

Berries are delicious in savoury sauces and blackberries and blueberries are well matched to the rich flavour of venison. This mouth-watering dish provides protein to help stabilise blood sugar levels and it also includes protective antioxidants, while being low in saturated fat. Venison is a source of B vitamins, including B12, and the minerals iron, selenium, zinc and copper. Good accompaniments are celeriac mash and lightly steamed vegetables.

▪ SERVES 4

450g/1lb venison loin
2 tbsp juniper berries
1 tsp black peppercorns
2 tbsp olive oil
1 tbsp coconut oil
200ml/7fl oz/generous ¾ cup organic beef or lamb stock
1 tbsp bramble jelly or redcurrant jelly (no added sugar)
200g/7oz blackberries or blueberries fresh or frozen and defrosted
1 square of dark chocolate (75% cocoa solids)
Sea salt and freshly ground black pepper

Preheat the oven to 180°C/350°F, gas mark 4.

For the venison, crush 1 tbsp juniper berries and the peppercorns using a pestle and mortar. Mix in the olive oil and then rub the mixture all over the venison fillet. Allow to marinate for 10–15 minutes.

Heat the coconut oil in a large frying pan and sear the venison on all sides for 1 minute only.

Place the venison in the oven (if the frying pan is not ovenproof, transfer to an ovenproof dish) and cook for 8–10 minutes until cooked but still a little pink in the centre. Remove the venison from the pan. Place the venison on a plate and cover with foil to keep warm.

For the sauce, add the stock to a pan with the venison juices and remaining juniper berries, crushed. Simmer for about 5 minutes until the volume of stock has reduced slightly.

Strain the sauce and return it to the pan, then add the bramble jelly and blackberries. Cook for about 4 minutes or until the blackberries are softened, then crush them slightly. Add the chocolate and stir until melted. Season with sea salt and freshly ground black pepper.

Cut the venison into slices and serve with the blackberry sauce.

Nutritional information per serving

Calories 218kcal
Protein 25.8g
Carbohydrates 5.3g of which sugars 3.1g
Total fat 10.7g of which saturates 2.4g

Fenugreek Bean Curry

Fenugreek seeds are aromatic, with a slightly bitter taste, and are typically roasted and ground to be used in curries. The leaves from the plant (often sold as methi) can be used in salads and sprinkled over stews and curries. The combination of the fenugreek seeds and the soluble fibre from the beans helps to support healthy blood sugar levels. Bitter melon could also be added. Accompany with some steamed leafy greens or a mixed salad.

- SERVES 4

2 tsp cumin seeds
2 tsp coriander seeds
1 tsp fennel seeds
1 tsp black mustard seeds
1 tsp fenugreek seeds
1 tbsp coconut oil
1 medium onion, finely chopped
2 cloves garlic, peeled and crushed
2cm/1in piece fresh ginger, grated
400g/14oz can kidney beans,
    drained and rinsed
400g/14oz can borlotti beans,
    drained and rinsed
Pinch of crushed chilli flakes
400g/14oz can chopped tomatoes

Place the cumin, coriander, fennel, mustard seeds and fenugreek seeds in a small frying pan. Roast on a medium heat, stirring until the spices turn golden and become aromatic.

Grind the spices into a fine powder in a coffee grinder or mini food processor.

Heat the coconut oil in a large pan over medium heat. Add the onion, garlic, ginger and spices and cook for 1–2 minutes.

Stir in the canned beans, chilli flakes, tomatoes and stock. Bring to the boil.

Turn the heat to low, cover and simmer for 10 minutes. Add the green beans and cook for a further 5 minutes.

200ml/7fl oz/scant 1 cup vegetable stock

200g/7oz green beans, halved

1 tbsp fresh coriander leaves (cilantro), chopped

1 tbsp fenugreek leaves (optional)

2 tbsp unsweetened coconut flakes (available from health food shops)

Top with coriander leaves, fenugreek leaves (if using) and coconut flakes to serve.

Nutritional information per serving

Calories 178kcal
Protein 10.8g
Carbohydrates 24.4g of which sugars 8.6g
Total fat 4.9g of which saturates 2.8g

Lemon and Pumpkin Seed Crusted Halibut with a Caper Dressing

This speedy magnesium-rich dish combines the delicate flavour of halibut with a crispy oat and seed crumb. Pumpkin seeds provide protein, healthy fats (omegas 6 and 9) and a range of vitamins and minerals (including iron, zinc, potassium and magnesium). The crispy crumb topping keeps the fish beautifully moist while cooking and adds a nutty, crunchy texture. The crust is also delicious sprinkled over scallops or prawns before baking in the oven, or as a gratin topping for vegetable bakes. Halibut is source of magnesium, omega-3 fats, protein and B vitamins. However, other fish, such as turbot, brill or plaice, could be used instead. The caper dressing is packed with omega-rich oils. It can be drizzled over salads or steamed vegetables and is particularly good with lamb dishes.

▪ SERVES 4

Topping

150g/5oz/1½ cup oat flakes (use gluten-free oats or buckwheat flakes if needed, or ground almonds for a grain-free option)

2 tbsp fresh parsley

4 tbsp pumpkin seeds

Zest of 1 lemon

1 egg, beaten

4 halibut fillets (125g/4½oz each) with skin

1 tbsp coconut oil

Dressing

2 tbsp capers, finely chopped

1 anchovy, finely chopped

1 garlic clove, crushed

Pinch of dried chilli flakes (optional)

1 tbsp mint leaves, chopped

Place the oats, parsley, pumpkin seeds and lemon zest in a food processor and process to form fine crumbs.

Place on a plate and season.

Beat the egg and place on a separate plate. Dip the halibut fillets, flesh side only, into the egg then press flesh side on to the oat crumb mixture. Ensure the flesh side of the fish is thoroughly coated with the crumbs.

Heat the coconut oil in a frying pan. Place the fish skin side down and cook for 2–3 minutes until the skin is lightly golden. Place the pan under a hot grill for 2 minutes only (until the topping begins to turn colour but is not yet browned).

Make up the dressing by mixing all the ingredients together.

Place a handful of salad leaves in a bowl and toss with a little of the dressing.

Serve the halibut with the salad leaves. Drizzle a little of the dressing over the fish to serve.

1 tbsp coriander leaves (cilantro), chopped
1 tbsp parsley leaves, chopped
3 tbsp apple cider vinegar
3 tbsp flaxseed oil
4 tbsp olive oil
Sea salt and freshly ground black pepper

....

Mixed leafy green and herb salad to serve

Nutritional information per serving (with 1 tbsp dressing)
Calories 463kcal
Protein 31.1g
Carbohydrates 25.5g of which sugars 0.2g
Total fat 25.6g of which saturates 4.9g

Snack

Sesame Tamari Dip

This dip works well with all types of vegetable crudités and is a good source of zinc, calcium and magnesium. You can also thin it a little with some extra yoghurt and use it as a creamy dressing, spooned over vegetables or new potatoes. For a vegan option, use either silken tofu or, for a soy-free version, a blend of oat cream and cashew nuts.

- SERVES 4

25g/1oz sesame seeds, lightly toasted but not browned
2 tbsp tamari soy sauce
1 tbsp tahini
60g/2oz crème fraiche
60g/2oz thick Greek yoghurt

Simply combine all the ingredients together and chill until required.

Nutritional information per tbsp
Calories 46kcal
Protein 1.4g
Carbohydrates 0.5g of which sugars 0.4g
Total fat 4.2g of which saturates 1.2g

References

1. Lukaczer, D. (2005) 'The Epidemic of Insulin Insensitivity.' In D.S. Jones (ed.) *The Textbook of Functional Medicine.* Gig Harbor, WA: Institute for Functional Medicine. Page 245.
2. Smith, B.W. and Adams, L.A. (2011) 'Non-alcoholic fatty liver disease.' *Critical Reviews in Clinical Laboratory Sciences 48*, 3, 97–113.
3. Cho, L.W. (2011) 'Metabolic Syndrome.' *Singapore Medical Journal 52*, 11, 779–85.
4. Doyle, S.L., Donohoe, C.L., Lysaght , J. and Reynolds, J.V. (2012) 'Visceral obesity, metabolic syndrome, insulin resistance and cancer.' *Proceedings of the Nutrition Society 71*, 1, 181–9.

5. Panza, F., Frisardi, V., Capurso, C., Imbimbo, B.P. *et al.* (2010) 'Metabolic syndrome and cognitive impairment: Current epidemiology and possible underlying mechanisms.' *Journal of Alzheimer's Disease 21*, 3, 691–724.

6. Kroner, Z. (2009) 'The relationship between AD and diabetes: Type 3 diabetes?' *Alternative Medicine Review 14*, 4, 373–9.

7. Kozumplik, O. and Uzun, S. (2011) 'Metabolic syndrome in patients with depressive disorder: Features of comorbidity.' *Psychiatria Danubina 23*, 1, 84–8.

8. Willcox, D.C., Willcox, B.J., Todoriki, H. and Suzuki, M. (2009) 'The Okinawan diet: Health implications of a low-calorie, nutrient-dense, antioxidant-rich dietary pattern low in glycemic load.' *Journal of the American College of Nutrition 28*, Suppl., 500–16S.

9. Butt, M.S., Shahzadi, N.M., Sarif, M.K. and Nasir, M. (2007) 'Guar gum: A miracle therapy for hypercholesterolemia, hyperglycemia and obesity.' *Critical Reviews in Food Science and Nutrition 47*, 4, 389–96.

10. Gunness, P. and Gidley, M.J. (2010) 'Mechanisms underlying the cholesterol-lowering properties of soluble dietary fibre polysaccharides.' *Food and Function 1*, 2, 149–55.

11. Culp, M. (2010) 'The Metabolic Syndrome.' In L. Nicolle and A. Woodriff Beirne (eds) *Biochemical Imbalances in Disease*. London: Singing Dragon.

12. Lopez-Miranda , J., Perez-Jimenez, F. and Ros, E. (2010) 'Olive oil and health: Summary of the II international conference on olive oil and health consensus report, Jaen and Cordoba (Spain) 2008.' *Nutrition, Metabolism and Cardiovascular Diseases 20*, 4, 284–94.

13. Nicolle, L. and Hallam, A. (2010) 'PUFA Imbalances.' In L. Nicolle and A. Woodriff Beirne (eds) *Biochemical Imbalances in Disease*. London: Singing Dragon. Page 111.

14. Wang, Z.Q. and Cefalu, W.T. (2010) 'Current concepts about chromium supplementation in type 2 diabetes and insulin resistance.' *Current Diabetes Reports 10*, 2, 145–51.

15. Anderson, R.A. (2008) 'Chromium and polyphenols from cinnamon improve insulin sensitivity.' *Proceedings of the Nutrition Society 67*, 1, 48–53.

16. Barbagallo, M. and Dominquez, L.J. (2007) 'Magnesium metabolism in type 2 diabetes mellitus, metabolic syndrome and insulin resistance.' *Archives of Biochemistry and Biophysics 458*, 1, 40–7.

17. Foster, M. and Samman, S. (2010) 'Zinc and redox signalling: Perturbations associated with cardiovascular disease and diabetes mellitus.' *Antioxidants and Redox Signaling 13*, 10, 1549–73.

18. Chausmer, A.B. (1998) 'Zinc, insulin and diabetes.' *Journal of the American College of Nutrition 17*, 2, 109–15.

19. Wiernsperger, N. and Rapin, J.R. (2010) 'Trace elements in glucometabolic disorders: An update.' *Diabetology and Metabolic Syndrome 2*, 70, 1–9.

20. Knecht, P., Kumpulainen, J., Järvinen, R., Rissanen, H. *et al.* (2002) 'Flavonoid intake and risk of chronic diseases.' *American Journal of Clinical Nutrition 76*, 560–8.

21. Culp, M. (2010) 'The Metabolic Syndrome.' In L. Nicolle and A. Woodriff Beirne (eds) *Biochemical Imbalances in Disease*. London: Singing Dragon.

22. Dey, L., Attele, A. and Yuan, C.S. (2001) 'Alternative therapies for type 2 diabetes.' *Alternative Medicine Review 7*, 1, 45–58.

23. Wolfram, S. (2007) 'Effects of green tea and EGCG on cardiovascular and metabolic health.' *Journal of the American College of Nutrition 26*, 4, 373–88S.

24. Thielecke, F. and Boschmann, M. (2009) 'The potential role of green tea catechins in the prevention of the metabolic syndrome: A review.' *Phytochemistry 70*, 1, 11–24.

25. Huxley, R., Lee, C.M., Timmermeister, L., Czernichow, M.D. *et al.* (2009) 'Coffee, decaffeinated coffee and tea consumption in relation to incident type 2 diabetes mellitus: A systematic review with meta-analysis.' *Archives of Internal Medicine 169*, 22, 2053–63.

26. Zhang, Y., Lee, E.T. and Cowan, L.D. (2011) 'Coffee consumption and the incidence of type 2 diabetes in men and women with normal glucose tolerance: the Strong Heart Study.' *Nutrition, Metabolism, and Cardiovascular Diseases* 21, 6, 418–23.

27. Muley, A., Muley, P. and Shah, M. (2012) 'Coffee to reduce risk of type 2 diabetes? A systematic review.' *Current Diabetes Reviews.*

28. Natella, F. and Scaccini, C. (2012) 'Role of coffee in modulation of diabetes risk.' *Nutrition Reviews* 70, 4, 207–17.

29. Ostman, E., Granfeldt, Y., Persson, L. and Bjorck, I. (2005) 'Vinegar supplementation lowers glucose and insulin responses and increases satiety after a bread meal in healthy subjects.' *European Journal of Clinical Nutrition 59*, 9, 983–8.

30. Hishehbor, F., Mansoori, A., Sarkaki, A.R. and Jalali, M.T. (2008) 'Apple cider vinegar attenuates lipid profile in normal and diabetic rats.' *Pakistan Journal of Biological Sciences 11*, 23, 2634–8.

31. Venn, B.J. and Green, T.J. (2007) 'Glycemic index and glycemic load: Measurement issues that their effect on diet-disease relationships.' *European Journal of Clinical Nutrition 61*, Suppl. 1, S122–31.

32. Wing, R.R., Blair, E.H., Bononi, P., Marcus, M.D., Watanabe, R. and Bergman, R.N. (1994) 'Caloric restriction per se is a significant factor in improvements in glycemic control and insulin sensitivity during weight loss in obese NIDDM patients.' *Diabetes Care 17*, 1, 30–36.

33. Cousens, G. (2008) *There Is a Cure for Diabetes: The Tree of Life 21-day+ Program.* Berkeley, CA: North Atlantic Books.

34. Wing, R.R., Blair, E.H., Bononi, P., Marcus, M.D., Watanabe. R. and Bergman, R.N. (1994) 'Caloric Restriction Per Se Is a Significant Factor in Improvements in Glycemic Control and Insulin Sensitivity During Weight Loss in Obese NIDDM Patients.' *Diabetes Care 17*, 1, 30–36.

35. Banting, F.G., Best, C.H., Collip, J.B., Campbell, W.R. and Fletcher, A.A. (1991) 'Pancreatic extracts in the treatment of diabetes mellitus.' *Canadian Medical Association Journal 145*, 10, 1281–6.

36. Gaby, R. (2005) 'Adverse effects of dietary fructose.' *Alternative Medicine Review 10*, 4, 294–306.

37. Samual, V.T. (2011) 'Fructose induced lipogenesis: from sugar to fat to insulin resistance.' *Trends in Endonocrinology and Metabolism 22*, 2, 60–5.

38. Dekker, M.J., Su, Q., Baker, C. *et al.* (2010) 'Fructose: a highly lipogenic nutrient implicated in insulin resistance, hepatic steatosis, and the metabolic syndrome.' *American Journal of Physiology, Endocrinology and Metabolism 299*, 5, E685–94.

39. Seneff, S., Wainwright, G. and Mascitelli, L. (2011) 'Is the metabolic syndrome caused by a high fructose, and relatively low fat, low cholesterol diet?' *Archives of Medical Science 7*, 1, 8–20.

40. Harwood, H.J. Jr (2011) 'The adipocyte as an endocrine organ in the regulation of metabolic homeostasis.' *Neuropharmacology*, Epub ahead of print.

41. Scotece, M., Conde, J., Gómez, R., López, V. *et al.* (2011) 'Beyond fat mass: Exploring the role of adipokines in rheumatic diseases.' *Scientific World Journal 11*, 1932–47.

42. Tamashiro, K.L., Sadai, R.R., Shively, C.A., Karatsoreos, I.N. and Reagan, L.P. (2011) 'Chronic stress, metabolism and metabolic syndrome.' *Stress 14*, 5, 468–74.

43. Ryan, A.S. (2000) 'Insulin resistance with aging: Effects of diet and exercise.' *Sports Medicine 30*, 5, 327–46.

44. MacLean, P.S., Zheng, D., Jones, J.P., Olson, A.L. and Dohm, G.L. (2002) 'Exercise-induced transcription of the muscle glucose transporter (GLUT 4) gene.' *Biochemical and Biophysical Research Communications 292*, 2, 409–14.

45. Martins, R.C., Andersen, M.L. and Tufik, S. (2008) 'The reciprocal interaction between sleep and type 2 diabetes mellitus: Facts and perspectives.' *Brazilian Journal of Medical and Biological Research 41*, 3, 180–7.

46. Miller, M.A. and Cappuccio, F.P. (2007) 'Inflammation, sleep, obesity and cardiovascular disease.' *Current Vascular Pharmacology 5*, 2, 93–102.

47. Culp, M. (2010) 'The Metabolic Syndrome.' In L. Nicolle and A. Woodriff Beirne (eds) *Biochemical Imbalances in Disease*. London: Singing Dragon. Page 158.

48. Accurso, A., Bernstein, R., Dahlqvist, A., Drazhin, B. *et al.* (2008) 'Dietary carbohydrate restriction in type 2 diabetes mellitus and metabolic syndrome: Time for a critical appraisal.' *Nutrition and Metabolism 5*, 9.

49. Foster-Powell, K., Holt, S. and Brand-Miller, J. (2002) 'International table of GI and GL values.' *American Journal of Clinical Nutrition 76*, 1, 5–56.

50. Misra, A., Sharma, R., Gulati, S., Joshi, S.R. *et al.* (2011) 'Consensus dietary guidelines for healthy living and prevention of obesity, the metabolic syndrome, diabetes, and related disorders in Asian Indians.' *Diabetes Technology and Therapeutics 13*, 6, 683–94.

51. Shapiro, A., Mu, W., Roncal, C., Cheng, K.Y., Johnson, R.J. and Scarpace, P.J. (2008) 'Fructose-induced leptin resistance exacerbates weight gain in response to subsequent high fat feeding.' *American Journal of Physiology, Regulatory, Integrative and Comparative Physiology 295*, 5, 1370–5.

52. Bantle, J., Raatz, S., Thomas, W. and Georgopoulos, A. (2000) 'Effects of dietary fructose on plasma lipids in healthy subjects.' *American Journal of Clinical Nutrition 72*, 1128–34.

53. Lim, U., Subar, A.F., Mouw, T., Hartge, P. *et al.* (2006) 'Consumption of aspartame-containing beverages and incidence of hematopoietic and brain malignancies.' *Cancer Epidemiology, Biomarkers and Prevention 15*, 9, 1654–9.

54. Li, L. and Seeram, N. (2011) 'Quebecol, a novel phenolic compound isolated from Canadian maple syrup.' *Journal of Functional Foods 3*, 2, 125–8.

55. Carakostas, , M.C., Curry, L.L., Boileau, A.C. and Brusick, D.J. (2008) 'Overview: The history, technical function and safety of rebaudioside A, a naturally occurring steviol glycoside, for use in food and beverages.' *Food and Chemical Toxicology 46*, 7, Suppl., S1–10.

56. Ferri, L.A., Alves-Do-Prado, W., Yamada, S.S., Gazola, S., Batista, M.R. and Bazotte, R.B. (2006) 'Investigation of the antihypertensive effect of oral crude stevioside in patients with mild essential hypertension.' *Phytotherapy Research 20*, 9, 732–6.

57. Qin, X., Xiaojian, S., Ronggan, L., Yuxian, W. *et al.* (2006) 'Subchronic 90-day oral (Gavage) toxicity study of a Luo Han Guo mogroside extract in dogs.' *Food and Chemical Toxicology 44*, 12, 2106–9.

58. Suzuki, Y.A., Inui, H., Sugiura, M. and Nakano, Y. (2005) 'Triterpene glycosides of Siraitia grosvenori inhibit rat intestinal maltase and suppress the rise in blood glucose level after a single oral administration of maltose in rats.' *Journal of Agricultural and Food Chemistry 53*, 8, 2941–6.

59. Burt, J. (2006) 'The use of sorbitol- and xylitol-sweetened chewing gum in caries control.' *Journal of the American Dental Association 137*, 2, 190–6.

60. al Somal, N., Koley, K.E., Molan, P.C. and Hancock, B.M. (1994) 'Susceptibility of Helicobacter pylori to the antibacterial activity of manuka honey.' *Journal of the Royal Society of Medicine 87*, 1, 9–12.

61. Gonzales, G.F., Córdova, A., Vega, K., Chung, A., Villena, A. and Góñez, C. (2003) 'Effect of Lepidium meyenii (Maca), a root with aphrodisiac and fertility-enhancing properties, on serum reproductive hormone levels in adult healthy men.' *Journal of Endocrinology 76*, 1, 163–8.

62. Balick, M.J. and Lee, R. (2001) 'Maca: From traditional food crop to energy and libido stimulant.' *Alternative Therapies in Health and Medicine 8*, 96–8.

63. Yeh, G.Y., Eisenberg, D.M., Kaptchuk, T.J. and Phillips, R.S. (2003) 'Systematic review of herbs and dietary supplements for glycemic control in diabetes.' *Diabetes Care 26*, 4, 1277–94.

64. Vogler, B.K. and Ernst, E. (1999) 'Aloe vera: A systematic review of its clinical effectiveness.' *British Journal of General Practice 49*, 4447, 823–8.

6

Supporting Adrenal and Thyroid Function

The adrenal and thyroid glands function as part of the hypothalamus–pituitary–adrenal (HPA) axis and the hypothalamus–pituitary–thyroid (HPT) axis, respectively. The adrenal glands control our response to stressors, while the thyroid gland regulates our metabolic rate.

These systems share a chapter because they so closely modulate each other's function. An excessive output of the adrenal hormone cortisol, for example, leads to functional hypothyroidism. This is because it blocks the conversion of the thyroid pre-hormone T4 to the active hormone T3, and instead promotes T4's conversion to the inactive form of T3 (reverse T3, or rT3),[1] slowing the metabolism.

It is also important to remember that the HPA and HPT axes communicate closely with other endocrine pathways (and neuro–endocrine–immune pathways). Hormones balance each other to create homeostasis. Thus, if the output of one hormone is disrupted, the whole 'symphony' becomes imbalanced.

Sub-optimal adrenal function refers to a situation where the adrenal glands' hormonal output is disrupted, particularly with regard to cortisol and dehydroepiandrosterone (DHEA). Cortisol triggers physiological changes that enable the body to better deal with the immediate stressor, while DHEA helps to counteract some of the negative side effects of excess cortisol. A disrupted pattern of their output may manifest as overproduction (a hyperactive HPA axis), underproduction (a hypoactive HPA axis, classed in its more severe form as 'adrenal fatigue'), or a combination of the two states.

Sub-optimal thyroid function occurs where there is either too much or, more commonly, too little functional thyroid hormone. The latter case is characterised by too little T3 being in circulation and/or the T3 not being as effective as it should be. This can be due to competitive inhibition by 'reverse' T3, brought on by stress. This leads to a slowing of the metabolism and many debilitating signs and symptoms.

Note that a functional *over*active thyroid situation is far less common and will therefore not be covered here. For patients with hyperthyroidism, the medical intervention should be complemented with a consideration for optimal intakes of protein and higher than average intakes of antioxidant-rich whole foods (see Chapter 9) to help counteract the free radicals produced by the increased rate of metabolism. Calcium- and phosphorous-rich foods are also important, due to the increased risk of bone loss in hyperthyroid patients.[2]

Some typical signs and symptoms that could indicate adrenal and/or thyroid dysfunction

Be aware that symptoms may overlap, so it is important to look for clusters and, where possible, undertake laboratory testing to elucidate the extent of the imbalance.

- Long-term high cortisol:
  - 'tired but wired'
  - anxiety
  - negativity and depression
  - poor sleep
  - shakiness between meals, cravings for sugars and starchy foods
  - irritability, on a 'short fuse'
  - unable to deal with stressful situations
  - exhaustion on waking
  - weight gain around the abdomen.
- Adrenal fatigue:
  - excessive sleep
  - fatigue, apathy, but often feeling better after 9pm
  - depression, tearfulness, seasonal affective disorder (SAD)
  - muscle and/or joint pains
  - poor memory, concentration and motivation.
- Sluggish thyroid:
  - weight gain (but in many patients there is no weight gain)
  - fatigue, especially on waking
  - morning stiffness, Raynaud's-type symptoms

- slow cognition, poor memory
- low mood
- sluggish bowels, constipation
- cold hands and feet
- low sex drive
- infertility
- hair loss
- dry skin
- loss of the outer third of the eyebrows
- low heart rate and basal body temperature.

Laboratory tests may include the following:

- Adrenals:
  - abnormal urinary metabolites of adrenal hormones
  - low serum cortisol output following a CRH (corticotropin-releasing hormone) challenge
  - abnormal salivary diurnal variation in cortisol output, using four saliva samples spread over the course of the day
  - abnormal cortisol awakening response, which measures the reactive capacity of the HPA axis, by plotting the pattern of salivary cortisol within the first hour after waking
  - abnormal salivary levels of DHEA.
- Thyroid:
  - raised LDL-cholesterol
  - raised levels of thyroid antibodies
  - abnormal blood levels of TSH (thyroid-stimulating hormone), T4, T3, rT3 and the T3:rT3 ratio. It is important to remember that the laboratory reference ranges for thyroid hormones are wide and that what may be an optimal level for one individual may not be enough to produce homeostasis in another.[3] For more a detailed discussion on interpreting thyroid tests, please refer to Weatherby and Ferguson (2002).[4]

What health conditions are adrenal and thyroid imbalances linked to in the long term?

One of the earliest researchers to link chronic adrenal activation with an increased risk of degenerative diseases was the Canadian endocrinologist Hans Selye. He was the first to observe the pattern of adrenal hormone output that we now call the 'stress response' and he claimed that 'Every stress leaves an indelible scar, and the organism pays for its survival after a stressful situation by becoming a little older.'[5]

- Chronically elevated cortisol (that is, from a hyperactive HPA axis):
  - affects the availability of thyroid hormone (see above)
  - suppresses the immune system
  - contributes to digestive problems (see Chapter 2)
  - is an independent predictor of fracture risk[6]
  - is implicated in the development of obesity, metabolic syndrome and type 2 diabetes;[7, 8] and depression[9, 10]
  - is associated with impaired cognitive function in ageing[11]
  - may diminish the synthesis of sex hormones, by sequestering the precursor hormone (pregnenolone)[12]
  - eventually leads to 'adrenal fatigue', characterised by insufficient functional adrenal hormones. (This should not be confused with Addison's disease, which is a medical condition in which cortisol cannot be produced.)

- A depressed HPA axis ('adrenal fatigue'):
  - is associated with autoimmune inflammatory diseases, such as rheumatoid arthritis and polymyalgia rheumatica[13, 14]
  - is a factor in chronic fatigue syndrome,[15] 'atypical' depression, including SAD,[16] and fibromyalgia[17, 18]
  - contributes to low thyroid function, as cortisol is required for the conversion of T4 to T3.[2]

Thus, stress creates changes in the way the brain works and in a number of different functional body systems.

- Low thyroid function (subclinical hypothyroidism):
  - can progress to overt autoimmune thyroiditis
  - is now becoming recognised as a causative factor in cardiovascular problems,[19, 20, 21] poor pregnancy outcomes and increased mortality in

the long term.[20] For example, it is linked with increased levels of LDL-cholesterol, which often return to normal levels following thyroid hormone treatment.[21]

Key nutritional interventions to consider

Aims of the dietary programme

- To reduce inflammation, as this disrupts cortisol secretion[22] and the conversion of T4 to T3.[1] Moreover, poor immune 'tolerance' (see Chapter 8) increases the risk of developing autoimmune conditions of the adrenals and/or thyroid.

- To improve stress management.

- To encourage the loss of excess weight.

- To optimise nutrients for adrenal and thyroid hormone synthesis.

- To optimise nutrient cofactors for the conversion of pre-hormones to active hormones.

- To support cell membrane health to improve hormone sensitivity.

- To reduce toxicants that may interfere with hormone metabolism.

- To promote optimal detoxification of hormones (see Chapter 3).

What to eat and drink

- Eat foods with a low glycaemic load (GL) (see Chapter 5 for advice on avoiding hypoglycaemia). In the hypoglycaemic state, the body is effectively energy-starved. The adrenal glands are triggered to release adrenalin and then cortisol to help deal with the stress of the starvation. The cortisol induces glycogen break-down in the liver, so that the bloodstream is replenished with glucose to restore homeostasis. Thus hypoglycaemia is a significant physiological stressor.

- Regular protein is essential, especially foods that contain tyrosine, which is a building block for T4. (Tyrosine is also the precursor to adrenalin and noradrenalin produced by the adrenal glands.) Good food sources are sesame, sunflower and pumpkin seeds, dairy products, fish and egg white.

- Include minerals in your diet. The adrenals and/or thyroid glands will not function properly if you are deficient in any of the following:

- ◦ Magnesium. Deficiency causes HPA axis dysregulation and anxiety.[23] Eat lightly cooked Swiss chard and spinach, kelp, squash, pumpkin seeds, steamed broccoli, halibut and, to a lesser extent, other green vegetables, nuts and seeds.

- ◦ Iodine. This is a key component of T4 and T3 and deficiency has long been known to cause thyroid problems.[1, 24, 25] Good sources of iodine are sea fish, shellfish and seaweeds, and there is also some in eggs, meat and milk. Iodised salt is also available.

- ◦ Iron. This is required in the synthesis of T4 (for the haem-dependent enzyme thyroid peroxidise). Greater improvements in thyroid function are seen when correcting deficiencies not only of iodine, but also of iron.[24, 25] The most bioavailable iron is haem iron from lean red meat, especially liver and the darker meat from game, poultry and oily fish, as well as eggs. Vegetarian iron, which is less bioavailable, is found in beans, pulses, dark green leafy vegetables and dried fruit. It is better absorbed when eaten with foods rich in vitamin C, such as fruit and raw or lightly cooked vegetables. (As seen in Chapter 3, some green leaves contain oxalic acid, which can impair mineral absorption. Boiling and steaming may somewhat reduce the oxalate load.)

- ◦ Zinc. This is involved in thyroid function and the T3 receptors.[1, 25, 26, 27] Eat lean cuts of beef, pork, venison and lamb, crab, poultry, calf's liver, seeds, sea vegetables and wholegrains.

- ◦ Selenium. This is a cofactor for thyroid function enzymes, including 5'-deiodinase that converts T4 to active T3.[1, 25, 26, 27] Selenium is found in brazil nuts, meat, poultry, fish and wholegrains.

- Choose foods high in B vitamins, which are cofactors in adrenal and thyroid hormone production. In particular, pantothenic acid (vitamin B5) is necessary for adrenal hormone synthesis.[28, 29] Eat the protein foods mentioned above, as well as nuts, seeds, wholegrains and leafy greens.

- Eat vitamin C-rich foods. Vitamin C is present in high concentrations in the adrenal glands and its deficiency is a significant stressor to the body.[3, 28] Good sources are salad greens, broccoli, bell peppers and fresh fruits, especially strawberries and citrus fruits.

- Opt for foods that contain vitamin A (liver, eggs and dairy products), which is a crucial cofactor in thyroid function.[24]

- Make sure you consume a good balance of essential fatty acids (EFAs), from oily fish, nuts, seeds and their (cold-pressed) oils. See Chapter 4 for more information on these fats. EFAs help improve the health of cell membranes, in which are seated the receptors for thyroid and adrenal hormones.

- Include maca (*Lepidium peruvianum*) in your diet. This is a Peruvian root that can be bought in powdered form from health food shops and online. It has long been used traditionally to support the body in times of stress and can easily be added to smoothies and desserts and used in baking. An animal study of an extract of maca found it to attenuate stress-induced raised cortisol and reduce stress-related ulcers, as well as improve other markers of stress.[30]

- Note that isothiocyanates (chemicals that are produced with the consumption of cruciferous vegetables) have in the past been said to interfere with iodine uptake[2] (cruciferous vegetables include broccoli, cauliflower, cabbage, Brussels sprouts, kale, rocket/arugula and watercress). However, this view does not seem to be evident from the scientific studies.[31] Thus, we suggest that, even if you have a sluggish thyroid, you include lightly cooked (but not raw) cruciferous vegetables in your diet, as they have been found to support liver detoxification and reduce the risk of cancer (see Chapter 3).

What not to eat and drink

- Avoid adrenal stimulants: sugars, refined carbohydrates, alcohol and excessive levels of caffeinated drinks (tea, coffee, cola) and foods (chocolate). Despite the wealth of evidence for the benefits of tea and coffee (as outlined in Chapter 3), be aware that excessive caffeine intake can be particularly detrimental to individuals with compromised adrenal function. Decaffeinated beverages may be a better option in such cases. However, caffeine tolerance varies considerably between individuals, so you should discuss this issue with your nutrition practitioner. In addition, chronic alcohol intake may reduce the synthesis of the active thyroid hormone T3.[1]

- Don't eat any foods to which you are sensitive or allergic, as this causes inflammation. Inflammation is a stressor and can also directly affect the conversion of T4 to T3.[3]

- Cut out processed foods, especially those with added sugar and *trans-*, hydrogenated or oxidised fats, as these can be inflammatory (see Chapter 8).

- There is an association between coeliac disease and autoimmune thyroid disease.[32] While not everyone with low thyroid function is affected by gluten, given that gluten is implicated in the development of intestinal permeability (see Chapter 2), you could experiment with avoiding it for a few weeks and monitoring your symptoms. Gluten is found naturally in wheat, rye and barley. See Chapter 2 for the many gluten-free alternatives to use.

- There has been concern that isoflavones in soy foods may disrupt thyroid function. While the evidence for this in adults appears contradictory and is overall rather weak,[33, 34] soy may reduce the absorption of thyroid medication and it may also hamper thyroid function in cases of iodine depletion.[35] We recommend ensuring that iodine intake is sufficient and that if soy foods are to be eaten they are to be used occasionally, to add variety, rather than as a staple. (Leave at least three hours from taking thyroid medication.)

How to eat

- Follow the general dietary guidelines in Chapter 1 and also in Chapter 5.

- Do not under- or overeat, as both these states cause physiological stress. In addition, although calorie restriction (CR) and intermittent fasting have been found to improve insulin sensitivity and other markers of healthy ageing (see Chpater 11), these practices are not recommended if you have sub-optimal thyroid function, as they lead to reduced T3 production and increased rT3.[1, 36]

Lifestyle – the central role of stress

Stress is at the centre of adrenal hormone disruption, and often thyroid hormone disruption too. (Stress activates the sympathetic nervous system, increasing adrenalin and noradrenalin, and then the HPA axis, raising cortisol levels. As seen, prolonged activation is potentially harmful.) While dietary changes are important, any improvements in health will be limited unless you also take steps to identify and address the mental, emotional and psychological sources of stress in your life.

Stress is cumulative and research shows that it is relatively common for an individual's current state of health to be affected by stressors that occurred at a previous point in his/her life history, even in the early years.[37, 38, 39] The concept of 'allostatic load' provides a useful way of looking at this idea (see Focus box 6.1). By looking back over your life history, perhaps with a psychotherapist or other health professional, you may be able to identify some of the earlier life stressors, and then consider whether and how to address them or come to terms with them.

Other lifestyle changes that may help to reduce stress include:

- Appropriate exercise.[40] Exercise also promotes thyroid function and thyroid hormone sensitivity.[2] However, the amount and type of exercise needs to be carefully monitored, as too much can have a detrimental effect, especially in individuals with adrenal fatigue (see Focus box 6.2).

- Getting enough sleep. Sleep deprivation is associated with high cortisol levels. This, in turn, leads to disruptions in immune system control (leading to inflammation) and in the hormonal control of appetite and insulin sensitivity.[40, 41] The average number of hours' sleep per night has reduced from 9 in the year 1910 to 6.8 in 2005.[41] If you have trouble sleeping, make sure your bedroom is completely dark and well-ventilated, switch off all the electrics at the plug sockets and keep the two hours prior to bedtime free of computers, television, intense exercise, caffeine and bright lighting. Relax in a warm bath with chamomile or lavender essential oils added.

- Being part of a good social support network.[40] You can make a start by doing your best to connect with, and be good to, those around you.

- Being mindful that chronic stress makes us more open to using addictive substances, such as alcohol, sugar, cigarettes and drugs, to help us to manage the stress in the short term.

You should also assess your exposure to environmental toxins (see Chapter 3), as these can affect the thyroid and adrenal glands. Mercury from dental amalgam, for example, may be a risk factor for autoimmune thyroiditis in some individuals;[42] the removal of the amalgam may reduce levels of thyroid-related antibodies in individuals with mercury sensitivity.[43] Cadmium from smoking antagonises essential minerals such as zinc and may also affect adrenal- and thyroid-related pituitary hormones.[44] High exposure to cadmium, mercury and lead has also been associated with poor conversion of T4 to T3.[1]

Focus box 6.1   Stress and allostatic load

As we go through life, the set-points of all our body systems naturally shift slightly up and down, adapting to the current environment. This has been termed 'allostasis'.[45] 'Allostatic load' is used to describe situations where, due to long-term accumulated stress, cortisol's 'resting' set-point has been altered – it has been reset at too high a level (or, eventually, too low a level), leading to damage to body systems and tissues.[40] Allostatic load is therefore 'the price the body pays for being forced to adapt to various psychosocial challenges and adverse environments'.[46]

An increased allostatic load can affect the set-point of many physiological process, such as blood glucose and insulin control, blood pressure levels and the rate of metabolism. With regard to the latter, we have already seen that long-term high cortisol levels lead to reduced T3 and increased rT3.[1] While the consequent slower metabolism may be useful in cases of severe injury or illness, problems start to arise if this adaptation to a lower thyroid function remains in the long term. Such a 'maladaptive' response, seen in people suffering from chronic stress, causes symptoms of functional hypothyroidism.[47]

The concept of allostatic load is important in a personalised approach to healthcare because it reinforces the value of reflecting on your life history, in order to better identify particular causes of stress (and ill health). For a more detailed discussion, see the free access article McEwan (2006).[48]

Focus box 6.2   **Train not drain – physical exercise to support the thyroid and adrenals**

As the 'no pain, no gain' mantra implies, most people think that exercise requires physical strain to get results. But many experts are now saying otherwise. They say that, in order to benefit the most, you should train within your limits, feeling comfortable and in control and avoiding excessive strain.[49, 50, 51, 52, 53]

Here are three tips to help create a balanced exercise programme:

1. Learn to breathe

We take on average 26,000 breaths a day. Yet one of the side effects of our sedentary lifestyles is less effective breathing.[50, 52, 54, 55] With long-term incorrect breathing, the ribcage and spine become locked, restricting the normal functioning of the respiratory system, meaning any exercise we perform will not give optimal benefits.[50, 54, 55]

We come into this world as 'obligate nose breathers' – that is, without the voluntary ability to breathe through our mouths. Mouth breathing is a learned response triggered by emergency stress.[50] Yet, breathing through the nose, making full use of the diaphragm, as certain Eastern traditions have done for centuries, creates far better conditions for optimal health and fitness.[56, 57]

Once nose breathing is relearned, the heart rate will be around 10–20 beats lower during exercise than when breathing inefficiently. This is due to the abdominal contractions during exhalation, pushing on the diaphragm and heart. This pressure stimulates the vagus nerve to activate the parasympathetic nervous system, lowering heart rate and producing a calming effect. Thus every breath becomes rejuvenating and invigorating.[50, 55]

2. Balance 'internal' and 'external' exercise

When exercise is mentioned, most people think of activities such as running, weight training, aerobics and cycling. These are sometimes referred to as 'external exercises'. It is important to balance these activities with 'internal exercises', such as gentle walking, qigong, yoga and taiji. These cultivate more energy than they expend, leaving enough energy to stimulate and fortify the body's healing processes.[54, 56, 58, 59]

Any standard gym routine can be turned into an internal exercise, by performing it slowly, with deep breathing and a relaxed mind. (You should pick a familiar exercise, in which little or no thinking is required.) The combination of low-intensity movement and proper breathing with a quiet mind stimulates digestion and elimination, as well as promoting a reduction in cortisol and an elevation in sex, growth and repair hormones.[54, 58]

If you are feeling particularly low in energy and vitality, a fast-paced exercise routine may do more harm than good. In such situations, internal exercises are often a better choice. After a short time, you are likely to find that you have increased your energy and can begin to add some external exercises to the programme.[54, 58]

Many of the symptoms that have been discussed in this chapter are a consequence of sympathetic nervous system dominance, an overly stressful and/or inactive lifestyle. This problem could also arise in an athlete who overtrains or is affected by other sources of stress.[54, 56, 57, 58] Internal exercises switch the sympathetic nervous system off and trigger the parasympathetic nervous system to allow rest and recovery.[54, 56, 57, 58]

Indicators of sympathetic dominance include:

- increased resting and exercise heart rate and blood pressure

- slow heart-rate recovery and general recovery from exercise

- irritability and mood swings

- menstrual irregularities

- poor digestion and decreased salivation

- constipation

- sleep disruption

- anxiety, nervousness

- increased muscle tension

- increased inflammatory conditions

- increased susceptibility to infection.[54, 59]

At the other end of the scale, a parasympathetic-dominant person, who might be described as a 'couch potato' type, must be guided into exercise very slowly, as they may not have the conditioning to deal with much physical activity. So, paradoxically, they should also begin with internal exercises to prepare them for external exercise when they are conditioned to do so.[54] With both the sympathetic dominant and parasympathetic dominant cases, the goal is to bring about balance.[54, 56]

Indicators of the rarer case of (excessive) parasympathetic dominance include:

- low normal resting and exercise heart rate and blood pressure

- fast heart-rate recovery after exercise

- strong or excessive digestion

- hyperactive bowel

- decreased respiratory rate

- decreased perspiration

- poor-quality sleep

- mucous secretions

- lethargy, depression

- hands warm and dry

- an increase in white blood cell count, causing an increase in allergies.[54, 59]

3. Avoid excessive fatigue

When you train in a way that avoids excessive fatigue, strength training and aerobic exercise are great ways to achieve a fit and healthy body. Strength training studies show that you can gain strength and power without going to fatigue or muscular failure. The results from an eight-week study in 2006,[61] for example, showed that strength training that avoided going to muscular failure, resulted not only in better muscle mass and strength, but also in lower resting cortisol levels and higher resting testosterone. Conversely, training to failure may make you more prone to overuse injuries.[60]

Even when performing aerobic exercise, such as running and cycling, fatigue should not be a factor.[52, 53] The goal should be to end a workout feeling stronger and more energised than when you started. This applies to beginner exercisers and professional athletes alike.[51, 52, 53]

The majority of elite athletes stick to training within their limits. The Olympic weight lifter may be lifting 200kg, the runner may doing five-minute miles and the cyclist tough hill climb intervals, but the training is comfortable to them, due to the many years of conditioning. While it is true that athletes may push to the limits when 'peaking' for competition, fatigue is always carefully monitored.[51, 52, 53] Working within your limits should not be confused with not progressing; the goal is to improve (lifting a heavier weight, running a greater distance, etc.) with each training session.

Avoiding excessive fatigue also helps to make physical activity more enjoyable. After all, the best exercise plan is one that you love to do!

Source: Mark Lawrence, Personal Trainer

Three-day meal plan

Dishes and snacks in italics are supported by recipes in this chapter or other chapters as indicated.

Day 1

Breakfast: *Maca Strawberry Milkshake*

Snack: One oat cake with pumpkin seed butter or tahini

Lunch: *Prawn, Enoki and Alfalfa Hand Rolls*

Snack: Handful of raw, mixed seeds

Dinner: *Moroccan Lamb Tagine* with a green leaf salad and a little brown basmati rice (optional)

Day 2

Breakfast: *Chicken Liver Pate* spread on a slice of *Buckwheat and Almond Bread* (Chapter 11) or served with vegetable sticks or *Supergreens Berry Smoothie* (Chapter 3)

Snack: *Alkaline Detox Broth* (Chapter 3)

Lunch: *Asparagus and Broad Bean Frittata* with a mixed salad

Snack: *Oat, Apricot and Brazil Nut Fruit Bars*

Dinner: *Sea Vegetable Salad with Japanese Dressing* with some steamed or baked salmon (steam for 15 minutes or until cooked through, or bake in parchment with lemon juice for 15–20 minutes)

Day 3

Breakfast: *Homemade Yoghurt* (Chapter 1) with 1 tbsp mixed ground seeds and a small handful of fresh or frozen berries (add a teaspoon of maca if desired) or *Fresh Berries with Cinnamon Nut Cream* (Chapter 5)

Snack: *Speedy Mushroom Miso Soup*

Lunch: *Roasted Vegetable and White Bean Salad* or *Thai Squash Soup.* Optional dessert: *Liquorice Yoghurt Ice*

Snack: Handful of Brazil nuts

Dinner: *Quick and Easy Seafood Salad with Lime Vinaigrette*

Drinks

- Herbal teas of ginseng and/or liquorice for low HPA function. Liquorice helps to keep cortisol in circulation by inhibiting the enzyme that metabolises it.[62] It makes a deliciously sweet tea for those with sugar cravings – see our recipe for *Ginger Liquorice Tea* (not to be drunk heavily in cases of hypertension).

- Green tea is also recommended, in moderation, because it contains L-theanine, which is thought to have a calming effect on the nervous system (see Chapter 10). Chamomile and lemon balm are also good choices if you are feeling stressed and 'wired'.

Recipes

Breakfast

Maca Strawberry Milkshake

Made with maca, cacao powder and nuts, this rich, creamy milkshake will energise you without causing a sudden crash in blood glucose levels a few hours later. A well-known adaptogen, maca is one of nature's powerful superfoods to help the adrenals – a little bit goes a long way in recipes.

- SERVES 2

60g/2oz almonds
400ml/14fl oz/scant 1⅔ cup
    coconut water or water
1–2 tsp maca powder to taste
1 tbsp cacao powder
½ tsp ground cinnamon
250g/9oz strawberries

Place the almonds and coconut water in a high-speed blender and process until smooth. Add the remaining ingredients and blend to form a creamy smoothie.

Pour into glasses and serve immediately.

Nutritional information per serving

Calories 304kcal
Protein 10.8g
Carbohydrates 25.6g of which sugars 10.2g
Total fat 17.9g of which saturates 1.7g

Chicken Liver Pate

This healthy chicken pate is packed full of nutrients, including protein, zinc, iron, folate and vitamins B12, B6 and A, to nourish and energise the body. It is delicious spread on oat cakes, crackers or toast for breakfast. It also makes a mid-afternoon snack with some raw vegetable sticks. Use organic chicken livers and organic butter if possible.

- SERVES 4

2 tbsp organic butter
1 tbsp olive oil
1 onion, chopped
4 brown mushrooms, chopped
3 cloves garlic, chopped
250g/9oz organic chicken livers
2 tbsp white wine
1 tsp tamari soy sauce
2 tsp fresh thyme, chopped
2 tsp fresh parsley, chopped
Freshly ground black pepper and
    pinch of sea salt to taste

Heat the butter and oil in a pan over a low heat and cook the chopped onion, mushrooms and garlic for 3–4 minutes until lightly brown.

Add the chicken livers, white wine, tamari, thyme and parsley. Cook the chicken livers for 5 minutes, turning them frequently to ensure they are cooked through.

Spoon the mixture into a food processor and blend till smooth. Season to taste.

Transfer to a glass container and refrigerate.

Nutritional information per serving

Calories 151kcal
Protein 11.5g
Carbohydrates 1.5g of which sugars 1g
Total fat 10.5g of which saturates 4.8g

Lunch

Prawn, Enoki and Alfalfa Hand Rolls

If you love sushi but feel daunted by making your own, these hand rolls are a great alternative. Sea vegetables are a useful source of iodine, an important nutrient for thyroid function. Rather than rice, these rolls contain soft rice noodles, combined with prawns to provide protein, omega-3 fats and minerals (selenium, zinc, copper and iron) for thyroid function. Serve with a little tamari soy sauce, chilli dipping or plum sauce if desired. For a vegetarian option, use sliced avocado instead of prawns.

- SERVES 2–4

30g/1oz vermicelli rice noodles
Handful of enoki mushrooms
2 tsp rice vinegar
1 tbsp tamari soy sauce
1 tbsp wasabi paste
4 nori sheets, quartered
Handful of alfalfa sprouts
100g/3½oz small cooked prawns (shrimp)

Place the rice noodles in a bowl and pour boiling water over them. Leave them to stand for 5 minutes until soft. Drain and rinse under cold water.

Place in a bowl with the enoki, rice vinegar and tamari.

To make the rolls, brush a little wasabi diagonally down the centre of each nori square. Top with a few rice noodles and enoki. Place on top some of the alfalfa sprouts and prawns. Wet the edge of the nori then roll into a cone shape. Repeat to make 15 more cones.

Nutritional information per roll

Calories 113kcal
Protein 13.4g
Carbohydrates 12g of which sugars 0.6g
Total fat 0.6g of which saturates 0.1g

Asparagus and Broad Bean Frittata

A simple lunch or supper dish, this is just as delicious served cold in wedges. Broad beans are a good source of protein and soluble fibre to support blood sugar control, and eggs contain minerals that act as cofactors in thyroid function.

- SERVES 4

100g/3½oz small broad beans, pods removed (podded weight)
6 spears of asparagus, cut into 1cm/0.5in lengths
2 tbsp coconut oil
1 small red onion, peeled and chopped
Sea salt and freshly ground black pepper
6 large organic eggs

Cook the broad beans and asparagus in a pan of boiling for 2 minutes until just tender. Drain well, then refresh in cold water.

When the beans are cool enough to handle, peel away the outer membranes.

Heat the oil in a small ovenproof frying pan over a low heat. Add the onion and season. Fry over a low heat for 5 minutes until softened.

Preheat the grill to high.

100g/3½oz feta cheese, crumbled
1 tbsp chopped mint leaves

Whisk the eggs until well combined, then season to taste.

Increase the heat to medium and pour in the beaten eggs. Sprinkle over the crumbled feta, mint, asparagus and broad beans. Cook for 2–3 minutes, or until the underside of the egg mixture is pale golden-brown.

Place the pan under the grill and cook for a further 2–3 minutes, or until the top side of the egg mixture is firm and pale golden-brown.

Place a large plate upside down over the pan, then turn the pan over so that the frittata falls on to the plate. Cut into wedges to serve.

Nutritional information per serving

Calories 250kcal
Protein 15.4g
Carbohydrates 3.5g of which sugars 1.8g
Total fat 19.3g of which saturates 10.6g

Roasted Vegetable and White Bean Salad

This simple warm salad is packed full of antioxidant-rich vegetables, including beta-carotene, which is the precursor to vitamin A. Sprinkle with some iodine-rich seaweed flakes just before serving. For additional protein, add one hard-boiled egg per serving.

▪ SERVES 4

Marinade oil
2 tbsp coconut oil
2 garlic cloves, crushed
½ tsp ground cumin
Zest and juice of ½ lemon
2 tsp honey
Sea salt and freshly ground black
    pepper

....

450g/1lb butternut squash, peeled
    and cut into 2cm/1in cubes
1 sweet potato, peeled and cut into
    chunks
2 red onions, cut into wedges
2 red peppers, cut into large chunks
2 yellow peppers, cut into large
    chunks
2 courgettes (zucchini), cut into thick
    slices on the diagonal

Heat the coconut oil in a pan and stir in the remaining ingredients to make the marinade.

Heat the oven to 200°C/400°F, gas mark 6.

Place the vegetables in a roasting dish and drizzle over the marinade. Season with sea salt and black pepper.

Bake in the oven for 30 minutes. Remove the dish from the oven then stir in the beans. Return to the oven for 10 minutes until the vegetables are golden.

Sprinkle over the nori or sea vegetable flakes, fresh mint leaves and pine nuts.

Nutritional information per serving

Calories 360kcal
Protein 12.7g
Carbohydrates 45.4g of which sugars 19.9g
Total fat 14.1g of which saturates 7.1g

2 x 400g/14oz cans cannellini
   beans, drained and rinsed
1 nori sheet, crumbled, or sea
   vegetable flakes
2 tbsp chopped fresh mint to serve
4 tbsp pine nuts to serve

Thai Squash Soup

This lightly spiced soup, with a hint of ginger, chilli and lemongrass, is wonderfully creamy with the addition of coconut milk. Squashes and pumpkins are rich in carotenoids, vitamin C and soluble fibre. Sprinkle some toasted seeds on the top of your soup for additional flavour and nutrients.

▪ SERVES 4

¼ tsp cumin seeds
¼ tsp coriander seeds
600g/1lb 5oz butternut squash,
   peeled, deseeded and cut into
   chunks
½ small onion peeled, cut in half
1 tbsp coconut oil
¼ red chilli, deseeded
1cm/0.5in piece fresh ginger, peeled
½ lemongrass stalk, finely chopped
1 garlic clove, peeled and chopped
400ml/14fl oz/scant 1⅔ cups
   coconut milk
200ml/7fl oz/generous ¾ cup hot
   vegetable stock
1 tsp xylitol
1 tbsp tamari soy sauce
1 tbsp fresh lime juice
4 tbsp toasted pumpkin seeds to
   garnish

Heat a heavy-based frying pan over a low heat. Add the cumin seeds and coriander seeds and dry-fry for 2–3 minutes until they start to turn golden. Set aside.

Preheat the oven to 190°C/375°F, gas mark 5.

Place the squash and onion in a baking tray and dot with coconut oil.

Bake in the oven until tender, about 20–30 minutes.

Place all the ingredients in a large saucepan and simmer for 10 minutes. Blitz in a blender until smooth and creamy. Taste and adjust seasoning if necessary.

Ladle into bowls and sprinkle over a few toasted pumpkin seeds to serve.

Nutritional information per serving
Calories 193kcal
Protein 6.4g
Carbohydrates 20.5g of which sugars 13.1g
Total fat 10.1g of which saturates 3.2g

Dinner

Moroccan Lamb Tagine

This hearty, warming dish benefits from being cooked in advance, making it a perfect get-ahead meal. It also requires very little preparation. As it will serve 8 people, you can halve the ingredients if needed or make a large batch to cover a couple of meals. Serve with a leafy green salad.

▪ SERVES 8

2 tbsp coconut oil
2 onions, chopped
1 tsp ground cumin
1 tsp ground ginger
1 tsp turmeric
½ tsp cinnamon
1kg/2lb 3oz boneless leg of lamb,
    chopped into bite-sized pieces
4 whole garlic cloves, peeled
400g/14oz can pitted black olives in
    brine, rinsed and drained to give
    150g/5oz drained weight
400g/14oz can chickpeas, drained
    and rinsed
Handful of pitted dates
250ml/8fl oz pomegranate juice
250ml/8fl oz chicken or beef stock

Preheat the oven to 150°C/300°F, gas mark 2.

Heat the coconut oil in a large lidded casserole and sauté the onion and spices for 1 minute. Add the lamb and stir until lightly golden. Add the rest of the ingredients and stir well.

Bring to the boil. Place the lid on the casserole and transfer to the oven. Cook for at least 2 hours, or until the lamb is very tender.

Nutritional information per serving

Calories 311kcal
Protein 28.3g
Carbohydrates 11.6g of which sugars 6.7g
Total fat 16.9g of which saturates 7.3g

Sea Vegetable Salad with Japanese Dressing

This is an easy-to-assemble salad, rich in iodine and trace minerals to support the thyroid gland. The dressing can be prepared in advance and kept in the fridge for 3–4 days. It is also delicious drizzled over steamed vegetables.

▪ SERVES 4

Dressing
1 tbsp extra virgin olive oil
1 tsp sesame oil
1 tbsp flaxseed oil
1 tbsp rice vinegar
1 tbsp rice wine
1 tbsp fresh orange juice
1 tbsp white miso

Mix all the dressing ingredients together.

Soak the sea vegetables in water for 5 minutes, then drain.

Blanch the green beans in boiling water for 2 minutes. Drain and rinse under cold water.

Combine all the salad ingredients together and drizzle over the dressing. Toss to coat and serve.

30g/1oz mixed sea vegetables, such
    as dulse, arame, nori, sea lettuce
    and wakame
150g/5oz green beans, halved
225g/8oz bag of mixed leafy greens
6 cherry tomatoes, halved
Handful of black olives, pitted and
    halved

Nutritional information per serving

Calories 125kcal
Protein 3.7g
Carbohydrates 2.3g of which sugars 1.8g
Total fat 11.1g of which saturates 1.5g

Quick and Easy Seafood Salad with Lime Vinaigrette

This is an easy, substantial salad for those days when there is limited time to cook or when your energy levels are low. Prepared mixed seafood is readily available from delis at the supermarket.

▪ SERVES 4

Dressing
Zest of 2 limes
Juice of 1 lime
Pinch of xylitol
1 roasted chilli in olive oil, drained and chopped
2 tbsp apple cider vinegar
3 tbsp flaxseed oil
3 tbsp olive oil
Sea salt and freshly ground black pepper

. . . .

1 tbsp coconut oil
1 garlic clove, crushed
1 raddichio or chicory (endive), shredded
400g/14oz prepared cooked mixed seafood
400g/14oz can chickpeas, drained and rinsed
100g/3½oz cherry tomatoes, halved
Handful of fresh parsley, chopped

Mix all the dressing ingredients together and chill until needed.

Heat the coconut oil in a pan and toss in the garlic and seafood salad. Stir to heat through, then add the chickpeas and cherry tomatoes.

Take off the heat and drizzle over a little of the dressing and the chopped parsley.

Arrange the salad leaves on a platter and spoon the seafood salad on top. Serve with the remaining dressing.

Nutritional information per serving
Calories 368kcal
Protein 24.9g
Carbohydrates 12.6g of which sugars 1.9g
Total fat 24g of which saturates 4.5g

Drinks and snacks

Ginger Liquorice Tea

This is a refreshing tea that is delicious hot or cold. Sip it throughout the day but avoid drinking it in the afternoon if you have difficulty sleeping, as liquorice can be stimulating.

▪ SERVES 4

1 litre/2 pints water
2–3 liquorice tea bags to taste
1 finger's length fresh ginger, sliced

Fill a saucepan with water.

Add the liquorice tea bags and fresh ginger.

Bring to a boil, then reduce heat and simmer for 10 minutes.

Strain and serve hot in mugs or allow to cool and drink as an iced tea.

Oat, Apricot and Brazil Nut Fruit Bars

This is a really easy raw protein bar and so much healthier than many shop-bought versions. Rich in thyroid-supporting minerals, such as selenium and iron, this bar is perfect when you are short of time and need something to support your blood sugar levels. A great healthy breakfast option or snack. These can be frozen in batches for up to 1 month.

• MAKES 12

200g/7oz/1½ cups Brazil nuts
60g/2oz gluten-free oats or
    buckwheat flakes
30g/1oz ground chia seeds
250g/9oz ready to eat apricots,
    chopped
3 heaped tbsp protein powder plain
    or vanilla flavour
Zest of 1 orange
Pinch of sea salt

Place the nuts and oats in a food processor and process until fine. Add the rest of the ingredients and pulse until the mixture comes together to form a firm dough. This may take a few minutes.

Press the mixture into a 20cm/8in square pan lined with baking parchment and freeze for at least one hour. When frozen, cut into 12 bars.

Store in the fridge or freezer until needed.

Nutritional information per bar
Calories 195kcal
Protein 5.6g
Carbohydrates 13.4g of which sugars 8.4g
Total fat 13.2g of which saturates 3.1g

Speedy Mushroom Miso Soup

Miso soup is quick and easy to assemble, making it ideal for a speedy warming drink. You can make it more substantial by adding some shredded greens and beansprouts.

• SERVES 4

1 litre/2 pints vegetable stock
4 shiitake mushrooms, thinly sliced
100g/3½oz firm tofu, diced
2 spring onions (scallions), finely
    sliced
Handful of frozen peas

Bring the vegetable stock to the boil in a saucepan.

Add the mushrooms, tofu, spring onions, peas and nori and simmer for 2–3 minutes.

Stir in the miso paste and tamari and cook for a further minute.

2 sheets of nori, cut into small
squares
4 tbsp white miso paste
1 tbsp tamari soy sauce

Pour into bowls and serve.

Nutritional information per serving
Calories 69kcal
Protein 6.2g
Carbohydrate 5.3g of which sugars 0.9g
Total fat 2.4g of which saturates 0.2g

Liquorice Yoghurt Ice

This is a cooling and soothing treat. Adding a scoop of protein powder will provide extra nutritional benefit. We have added a pinch of stevia to sweeten the ice cream but this could be omitted or replaced with a teaspoon of raw honey, according to taste.

▪ SERVES 4

175g/6oz low-fat Greek yoghurt
1 tbsp liquorice solid extract
(available from health food stores
or online)
Pinch of stevia (¼ tsp) or 1 tsp raw
honey (optional)
30g/1oz vanilla protein powder
(optional)
3 bananas, chopped and frozen

Simply place all the ingredients in a food processor and blend until smooth and creamy. This will create a soft-scoop ice cream which can be eaten straight away or you can transfer to a container and freeze until firm.

Take out 20 minutes before you wish to serve it to allow it to soften slightly.

Nutritional information per serving
Calories 128kcal
Protein 6g
Carbohydrates 21.9g of which sugars 18.8g
Total fat 1.7g of which saturates 0.6g

References

1. Kelly, G.S. (2000) 'Peripheral metabolism of thyroid hormones: A review.' *Alternative Medicine Review* 5, 4, 306–33.
2. Nodder, J. (2010) 'Compromised Thyroid and Adrenal Function.' In L. Nicolle and A. Woodriff Beirne (eds) *Biochemical Imbalances in Disease*. London: Singing Dragon.
3. Hanaway, P. (2011) *Assessment and Treatment of Adrenal and Thyroid Disorders*. Presentation given at the Advanced Functional Medicine in Clinical Practice (AFMCP) symposium, October 2011. London: IFM.
4. Weatherby, R. and Ferguson, S. (2002) *Blood Chemistry and CBC Analysis*. Jacksonville, OR: Bear Mountain Publishing.
5. Selye, H. (1956) *The Stress of Life*. New York, NY: McGraw Hill.
6. Greendale, G.A., Unger, J.B., Rowe, J.W. and Seeman, T.E. (1999) 'The relation between cortisol excretion and fractures in healthy older people: Results from the MacArthur studies-Mac.' *Journal of the American Geriatrics Society 47*, 7, 799–803.

7.   Rosmond, R. (2003) 'Stress induced disturbances of the HPA axis: A pathway to type 2 diabetes?' *Medical Science Monitor 9*, 2, RA35–9.

8.   Pasquali, R., Vicennati, V., Cacciari, M. and Pagotto, U. (2006) 'The HPA axis activity in obesity and the metabolic syndrome.' *Annals of the New York Academy of Science 1083*, 111–28.

9.   Swaab, D.F., Bao, A.M. and Lucassen, P.J. (2005) 'The stress system in the human brain in depression and neurodegeneration.' *Ageing Research Reviews 4*, 2, 141–94.

10.   McEwan, B.S. (2006) 'Protective and damaging effects of stress mediators: Central role of the brain.' *Dialogues in Clinical Neuroscience 8*, 4, 367–81.

11.   Lupien, S.J., Schwartz, G., Ng, Y.K., Fiocco, A. *et al.* (2005) 'The Douglas Hospital longitudinal study of normal and pathological aging: Summary of findings.' *Journal of Psychiatry and Neuroscience 30*, 5, 328–34.

12.   Parker, L.N., Levin, E.R. and Lifrak, E.T. (1985) 'Evidence for adrenaocortical adaptation to severe illness.' *Journal of Clinical Endocrinology and Metabolism 60*, 5, 947–52.

13.   Cutolo, M., Foppiani, L. and Minuto, F. (2002) 'Hypothalamic-pituitary-adrenal axis impairment in the pathogenesis of rheumatoid arthritis and polymyalgia rheumatica.' *Journal of Endocrinological Investigation 25*, 10, Suppl., 19–23.

14.   Cutolo, M., Sulli, A., Pizzorni, C., Craviotto, C. and Straub, R.N. (2003) 'Hypothalamic-pituitary-adrenocortical and gonadal functions in RA.' *Annals of the New York Academy of Sciences 992*, 107–17.

15.   Van Houdenhove, B., Van Den Eede, F. and Luyten, P. (2009) 'Does hypothalamic-pituitary-adrenal axis hypofunction in chronic fatigue syndrome reflect a "crash" in the stress system?' *Medical Hypotheses 72*, 6, 701–5.

16.   Juruena, M.F. and Cleare, A.J. (2007. 'Overlap between atypical depression, seasonal affective disorder and chronic fatigue syndrome.' *Revista Brasileira de Psiquiatria 29*, Suppl. 1, S19–25.

17.   Egle, U.T., Ecker-Egle , M.L., Nickel, R. and Van Houdenhove, B. (2004) 'Fibromyalgia as a dysfunction of the central pain and stress response.' *Psychotherapie Psychosomatik, Medizinische Psychologie 54*, 3–4, 137–47.

18.   Van Houdenhove, B. and Egle, U.T. (2004) 'Fibromyalgia: A stress disorder? Piecing the biopsychosocial puzzle together.' *Psychotherapy and Psychosomatics 73*, 5, 267–75.

19.   Biondi, B. and Cooper, D.S. (2008) 'The clinical significance of subclinical thyroid dysfunction.' *Endocrine Reviews 29*, 1, 76–131.

20.   Wartofsky, L., Van Nostrand, D. and Burman, K.D. (2006) 'Overt and "subclinical" hypothyroidism in women.' *Obstetrical and Gynecological Survey 61*, 8, 535–42.

21.   Ito, M., Arishima, T., Kudo, T. Nishihara, E. *et al.* (2007) 'Effect of levo-thyroxine replacement on non-high-density lipoprotein cholesterol in hypothyroid patients.' *Journal of Clinical Endocrinology and Metabolism 92*, 2, 608–11.

22.   Straub, R.H., Schölmerich, J. and Zietz, B. (2000) 'Replacement therapy with DHEA plus corticosteroids in patients with chronic inflammatory diseases: Substitutes of adrenal and sex hormones. *Zeitschrift für Rheumatologie 59*, Suppl. 2, 108–18.

23.   Sartori, S.B., Whittle, N., Hetzenauer, A. and Singewald, N. (2012) 'Magnesium deficiency induces anxiety and HPA axis dysregulation: Modulation by therapeutic drug treatment.' *Neuropharmacology 62*, 1, 304–12.

24.   Hess, S.Y. (2010) 'The impact of common micronutrient deficiencies on iodine and thyroid metabolism: The evidence from human studies.' *Best Practice and Research: Clinical Endocrinology and Metabolism 24*, 1, 117–32.

25.   Zimmerman, M.B. and Köhrle, J. (2002) 'The impact of iron and selenium deficiencies on iodine and thyroid metabolism: Biochemistry and relevance to public health.' *Thyroid 12*, 10, 867–78.

26.   Arthur, J.R. and Beckett, G.J. (1999) 'Thyroid function.' *British Medical Bulletin 55*, 3, 658–68.

27. Olivieri, O., Girelli, D., Stanzial, A.M., Rossi, L., Bassi, A. and Corrocher, R. (1996) 'Selenium, zinc and thyroid hormones in healthy subjects: Low T3/T4 ratio in the elderly is related to impaired selenium status.' *Biological Trace Element Research 51*, 1, 31–41.

28. Eisenstein, A.B. (1957) 'Effects of dietary factors on production of adrenal steroid hormones.' *American Journal of Clinical Nutrition 5*, 4, 369–76.

29. Jaroenporn, S., Yamamoto, T., Itabashi, A., Nazamura, K. *et al.* (2008) 'Effects of pantothenic acid supplementation on adrenal steroid secretion from mail rats.' *Biological and Pharmaceutical Bulletin 31*, 6, 1205–8.

30. Lopez-Fando, A., Gomez-Serranillos, M.P., Iglesias, I., Lock, O., Upamayta, U.P. and Carretero, M.E. (2004) 'Lepidium peruvianum chacon restores homeostasis impaired by restraint stress.' *Phytotherapy Research 18*, 6, 471–4.

31. Shapiro, T.A., Fahey, J.W., Dinkova-Kostova, A.T., Holtzclaw, W.D. *et al.* (2006) 'Safety, tolerance and metabolism of broccoli sprout glucosinolates and isothiocyanantes: A clinical phase 1 study.' *Nutrition and Cancer 55*, 1, 53–62.

32. Sategna-Guidetti, C., Volta, U., Ciacci, C., Usai, P. *et al.* (2001) 'Prevalence of thyroid disorders in untreated adult celiac disease patients and effect of gluten withdrawal: An Italian multicenter study.' *American Journal of Gastroenterology 96*, 3, 751–7.

33. de Souza Dos Santos, M.C., Goncalves, C.F., Vaisman, M., Ferreira, A.C. and de Carvalho, D.P. (2011) 'Impact of flavonoids on thryoid function.' *Food and Chemical Toxicology 49*, 10, 2495–502.

34. Mittal, N., Hota, D. and Dutta, P. (2011) 'Evaluation of effect of isoflavone on thyroid economy and autoimmunity in ovariectomised women: A randomised, double-blind, placebo-controlled trial.' *Indian Journal of Medical Research 133*, 6, 633–40.

35. Messinea, M. and Redmond, G. (2006) 'Effects of soy protein and soybean isoflavones on thyroid function in healthy adults and hypothyroid patients: A review of the relevant literature.' *Thyroid 16*, 3, 249–58.

36. Roti, E., Minelli, R. and Salvi, M. (2000) 'Thyroid hormone metabolism in obesity.' *International Journal of Obesity and Related Metabolic Disorders 24*, Suppl. 2, S113–5.

37. Swaab, D.F., Bao, A.M. and Lucassen, P.J. (2005) 'The stress system in the human brain in depression and neurodegeneration.' *Ageing Research Reviews 4*, 2, 141–94.

38. Egle, U.T., Ecker-Egle, M.L., Nickel, R. and Van Houdenhove, B. (2004) 'Fibromyalgia as a dysfunction of the central pain and stress response.' *Psychotherapie Psychosomatik, Medizinische Psychologie 54*, 3–4, 137–47.

39. Halligan, S.L., Herbert, J., Goodyer, I.M. and Murray, L. (2004) 'Exposure to postnatal depression predicts elevated cortisol in adolescent offspring.' *Biological Psychiatry 55*, 4, 376–81.

40. McEwan, B.S. (2008) 'Central effects of stress hormones in health and disease: Understanding the protective and damaging effects of stress and stress mediators.' *European Journal of Pharmacology 583*, 2–3, 174–85.

41. Miller, M. and Cappuccino, F. (2007) 'Inflammation, sleep, obesity and cardiovascular disease.' *Current Vascular Pharmacology 5*, 93–102.

42. Bártová, J., Procházkková, J., Krátká, Z., Benetková, K, Venclikvá, Z and Sterzl, L. (2003) 'Dental amalgam as one of the risk factors in autoimmune diseases.' *Neuroendocrinology Letters 24*, 1–2, 65–7.

43. Sterzl, I., Prochazkova, J., Hrda, P., Matucha, P., Bartova, J. and Stejska, V. (2006) 'Removal of dental amalgam decreases anti-TPO and anti-Tg autoantibodies in patients with autoimmuen thyroiditis.' *Neuroendocrinology Letters 27*, Suppl. 1, 25–30.

44. Lafuente, A., Cano, P. and Esquifino, A. (2003) 'Are cadmium effects on plasma gonadotrophins, prolactin, ACTH, GH and TSH levels, dose-dependent?' *Biometals 16*, 2, 243–50.

45. Sterling, P. and Eyer, J. (1988) 'Allostasis: A New Paradigm to Explain Arousal Pathology.' In S. Fisher and J. Reason (eds) *Handbook of Life Stress, Cognition and Health*. New York, NY: John Wiley and Sons.

46. McEwan, B.S. and Seeman, T. (1999) 'Protective and damaging effects of mediators of stress: Elaborating and testing the concepts of allostasis and allostatic load.' *Annals of the New York Academy of Sciences 896*, 1, 30–47.

47. Lukaczer, D. (2011) *Hormonal Regulation, Adrenal Fatigue, Insulin Resistance and Thyroid*. Presentation given at the Advance Functional Medicine in Clinical Practice (AFMCP) symposium, October 2011. London: IFM.

48. McEwan, B.S. (2006) 'Protective and damaging effects of stress mediators: Central role of the brain.' *Dialogues in Clinical Neuroscience 8*, 4, 367–81.

49. Chek, P. (2001) *Movement that Matters*. Vista, CA: CHEK Institute.

50. Douillard, J. (2001) *Body, Mind and Sport*. New York, NY: Three Rivers Press.

51. Kramer, W.J. and Zatsiorsky, V.M. (2006) *Science and Practice of Strength Training*, Second Edition. Champaign, IL: Human Kinetics.

52. Maffetone, P. (2012) *The Big Book of Health and Fitness*. New York, NY: Skyhorse Publishing.

53. Maffetone, P. (2010) *The Big Book of Endurance Training and Racing*. New York, NY: Skyhorse Publishing.

54. Chek, P. (2011) *Movement as Medicine Webinar Part 1 and 2*. Vista, CA: CHEK Institute.

55. Farhi, D. (1996) *The Breathing Book*. New York, NY: Henry Holt and Company.

56. Yan Lei, S. (2009) *Qi Gong Workout for Longevity*. China: Yan Lei Press.

57. Chang, E.C. (2000) *Knocking at the Gate of Life: Healing Exercises from the Official Manual of the People's Republic of China*. Dublin, Eire: Newleaf.

58. Chek, P. (2005) *The Last 4 Doctors You'll Ever Need: How To Get Healthy Now!* Mulitmedia e-book, available from www.ppssuccess.com/ProductsPrograms/TheLast4DoctorsYoullEverNeedOnlineeBook/tabid/320/Default.aspx.

59. Chek, P. (2004/2009*) How to Eat, Move and Be Healthy*. Vista, CA: CHEK Institute.

60. Willardson, J.M. (2007) 'The application of training to failure in periodized multiple-set resistance exercise programs.' *Journal of Strength and Conditioning Research 21*, 2, 628–31.

61. Izquierdo, M. (2006) 'Differential effects of strength training leading to failure versus not to failure on hormonal responses, strength, and muscle power gains.' *Journal of Applied Physiology 100*, 5, 1647–56.

62. Armanini, D., Mattarello, M.J., Fiore, C., Bonanni, G. *et al.* (2004) 'Licorice reduces serum testosterone in healthy women.' *Steroids 69*, 11–12, 763–6.

7

Supporting Sex Hormone Function

In this chapter we are focusing on some of the more common problems that occur with female sex hormone disruption. The key female sex hormones are the steroids oestrogen, testosterone and progesterone, and the pituitary hormones follicle stimulating hormone, luteinising hormone and prolactin.

The focus of this chapter is the functioning of the hypothalamic–pituitary–ovarian (HPO) axis. But it is important to note that the functioning of the HPO axis is influenced by other physiological processes, hormonal and non-hormonal. For example:

- A hyperactive hypothalamus–pituitary–adrenal (HPA) axis (see Chapter 6) can diminish the synthesis of sex hormones, by sequestering the precursor hormone (pregnenolone).[1] Moreover, the severity of menopausal symptoms is partly determined by cortisol levels, worsening when cortisol is chronically high.[2]

- Chronically elevated insulin increases the synthesis of androgen hormones, such as dihydrotestosterone (DHT).

- Sub-optimal detoxification can lead to a build up of oestrogen and harmful oestrogen metabolites.

- Gastro-intestinal dysbiosis can contribute to 'oestrogen dominance' (see below) through the bacterially produced enzyme beta-glucuronidase.

Thus, it is important to consider imbalances in these other body systems and in particular the HPA axis. We recommend reading Chapter 6 and any other relevant chapters before you follow the guidance in this one.

Conversely, the relative levels of the sex hormones, including oestrogens and their metabolites, affect the functional levels of many other hormones, neurotransmitters and immune system cytokines. Both excessive and insufficient levels of oestrogen can trigger an inflammatory response. We see this in, for example, post-menopausal osteoporosis, where the sharp fall in oestrogen triggers a rise in the inflammatory cytokines interleukin-1 (IL-1), IL-6 and tumour necrosis factor-alpha (TNF-a), which, in turn, leads to osteoclast proliferation and reduced bone density.[3]

In optimising the function of the sex hormones, we need to consider their synthesis, conversion to and from other hormones, transport around the body, receptor-binding ability, detoxification (both phases 1 and 2) and elimination. Signs and symptoms of ill health will soon occur if any of these links in the chain are weak, or if the ratios between individual hormones become imbalanced.

Types of hormone imbalance

One of the most commonly described sex hormone imbalances is that of 'oestrogen dominance', in which there is excessive oestrogen relative to progesterone.[4] Such a situation is often found during peri-menopause[5] and also in many female health problems, such as fibroids, endometriosis, some types of PMS and some types of breast, uterine and ovarian cancers.[5, 6]

Imbalances of oestrogen *metabolites* also affect health. For example, phase 1 detoxification enzymes (see Chapter 3) produce both weak-acting (cancer-protective) oestrogen metabolites (called 2-hydroxy-oestrogens, or 2-OH oestrogens) and more potent metabolites (called 4-hydroxy- and 16-alpha-hydroxy-oestrogens, or 4-OH and 16-a-OH oestrogens). The balance of these is crucial because it may help predict oestrogen-driven cancer risk.[7]

Symptoms can also arise due to a sudden drop in oestrogen levels – for example, during the menopause and at some points during peri-menopause (where hormone levels are subject to significant fluctuations).

There are, of course, many other types of hormonal imbalance, but these are the ones we will focus on here. For a more in-depth discussion of the biochemical pathways involved, see Neil (2010).[6]

Some typical signs and symptoms of sex hormone imbalances

- Heavy, painful and/or irregular periods.
- Breast tenderness.
- Peri-menopausal hot flushes, night sweats.
- Monthly irritability, mood swings and/or carbohydrate cravings.
- Headaches.
- Fatigue, slow cognition, poor memory.
- Depression and anxiety.

- Low libido, vaginal dryness.

  - Insomnia.

  - Male pattern hair loss.

  - Hirsuitism.

  - Acne.

  - Unexplained weight gain.

As mentioned, the sex hormones are affected by other biochemical pathways – thus, the symptoms listed here are rarely due entirely to oestrogen, progesterone or testosterone imbalances. So it is important to consider the HPA and any other imbalances first.

Potentially useful laboratory tests include saliva, blood and/or urine tests that indicate:

- the balance of female hormones at particular times of the month or, alternatively, on various days over the entire course of the month (note that the test results of symptomatic patients are sometimes within the normal range, which is another reason to identify possible imbalances in other body systems first)

- the ratios of phase 1 oestrogen metabolites (see above)

- levels of organic acids that are related to methyl cycle function and nutrient cofactor availability for hormone synthesis and metabolism

- homocysteine status, which indicates the efficiency of the phase 2 methylation detoxification pathway (see Figure 7.1) and also whether there may be problems with glutathione and sulphate synthesis.

  It is useful to know about methylation function because this is the pathway through which the potentially damaging oestrogen metabolites (4-OH and 16-a-OH oestrogens – see above) are neutralised. In cases of poor methylation, these metabolites are converted into quinones, which can damage DNA.

  Glutathione is crucial in helping to disable quinones. (In addition, the alternative phase 2 conjugation pathways glucuronidation and sulphation can step in for the methylation pathway if necessary, so these also need to be functioning well – see Chapter 3 for more information on the detoxification pathways.)

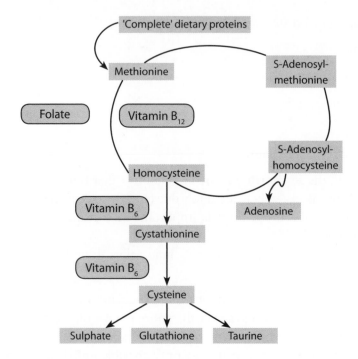

Figure 7.1 *Simplified schematic of the methyl cycle, showing the requirement of dietary protein and the methyl donors folate and vitamin B12*

In addition, the cofactor vitamin B6 is required for the metabolism of homocysteine to cysteine and then to glutathione, sulphate and taurine. Methylation is required for hormone detoxification, healthy cell replication, neurotransmitter synthesis and other body processes.

What health conditions are sex hormone imbalances linked to in the long term?

- Oestrogen dominance is a well-established factor in many common female hormone conditions, such as fibroids and endometriosis. But the fact that elevated oestrogen causes inflammation[8] means that this imbalance may increase the risk of almost all chronic diseases, as they inevitably carry an inflammatory component (see Chapter 8).

- Oestrogen and progesterone affect brain neurochemistry. Excessive oestrogen causes neuronal excitability,[9] which can lead to anxiety and some types of pre-menstrual syndrome, while progesterone has an inhibitory affect on the brain.

- Fluctuations in oestrogen levels are associated with migraine at peri-menopause[10] and at other times of life.[11]

- As seen, the ratio of phase 1 oestrogen metabolites produced in the liver affects breast cancer risk,[7] as does the efficiency of the phase 2 processes in disabling these metabolites.[12]

- The ratio of the oestrogen metabolites also affects the symptoms of the autoimmune condition systemic lupus erythematosus (SLE). (A lower 2:16 alpha-hydroxyestrone ratio is thought to increase disease activity.)[13]

There are, of course, a great many more pathologies associated with female sex hormone imbalances, including polycystic ovarian syndrome (PCOS), in which chronically elevated insulin levels stimulate excessive production of androgen hormones, such as dihydrotestosterone (DHT); and cardiovascular disease and osteoporosis, which are exacerbated by a sudden drop in oestrogen levels. Whatever hormonal condition is present, the objective is to encourage the various sex hormones back into the appropriate *balance*.

Key nutritional interventions to consider

Aims of the dietary plan

- To prevent the enzyme aromatase rising to excessive levels. Aromatase converts androgens to oestrogens, thus increasing the risk for oestrogen dominance.

- To normalise levels of sex hormone binding globulin (SHBG) (see Focus box 7.1).

- To reduce inflammation. Inflammation stimulates aromatase and is found in many hormonal conditions, fibroids and endometriosis.[14]

- To stabilise insulin output.

- To ensure healthy gut microflora balance. Problematic bacteria in the gut can produce the enzyme beta-glucuronidase. This breaks apart the glucuronide complexes within which oestrogens are bound for excretion. In turn, this increases the levels of free oestrogens in the gut, which can be reabsorbed into the bloodstream, increasing the systemic oestrogen load.

- To reduce oxidative load, including by supporting the detoxification pathways.

- To reduce stress and normalise cortisol output.

- To support the health of the membrane hormone receptors.

What to eat and drink

Follow the healthy eating guidelines in Chapter 1, as well as the recommendations in Chapters 3, 6 and any others relevant to the individual case. In particular, pay attention to the following:

- Eat a low glycaemic load diet (see Chapter 5). Not only is poor glucose control a significant stressor to the body, but chronically high blood glucose and/or insulin levels directly affect hormones by:

  ○ increasing aromatase activity

  ○ stimulating the production of androgen hormones, such as dihydrotestosterone (DHT), that contribute to the development of polycystic ovarian syndrome (PCOS)

  ○ suppressing levels of the oestrogen and testosterone binder SHBG.

  In addition, post-menopausal women who have metabolic syndrome are more likely to experience hot flushes and sweating,[15] and even in healthy menopausal women hot flushes seem to occur more when blood glucose falls between meals.[16]

- Eat high-quality protein on a daily basis, for the transporters and enzymes required for hormone metabolism. Eating organic or wild fish, poultry, eggs, low-fat dairy and a little lean meat will provide not only high-quality protein (including the sulphur amino acids methionine and cysteine) but also vitamins B6 and B12. These are all crucial for the hormone detoxification pathways. B6 has also been found helpful in PMS symptoms.[17] These amino acids and vitamin B6 are also found in sesame seeds, brazil nuts and corn. And some sulphur is found in garlic, onions, leeks, chives and cruciferous vegetables. But B12 is not found in plant foods, so vegans may want to undertake a blood test for B12 status.

- Green leafy vegetables should be eaten in abundance, as they contain folic acid, another important cofactor for the methylation and other phase 2 detoxification pathways. (Note that some green leaves contain oxalic acid, which can impair mineral absorption – see Chapter 3. Boiling and steaming reduces the oxalate load.)

- Consume onions, garlic and cruciferous vegetables such as broccoli, cauliflower, Brussels sprouts, kale, rocket (arugula) and watercress, which help to optimise both phases 1 and 2 of oestrogen detoxification (see Chapter 3).

- Eat oats, brown rice, pulses, vegetables and flaxseeds, as they contain soluble fibre and lignans. High-fibre diets may help to prevent free oestrogens from being reabsorbed from the gut into the bloodstream,[18] by binding them and increasing faecal excretion.

- Eat oily fish, such as sardines, mackerel, herring, trout and salmon. They contain the omega-3 fat eicosapentaenoic acid (EPA), which may help increase the beneficial 2-OH oestrogen metabolites and reduce the harmful 16-a-OH metabolites.[6, 14] Omega-3 fatty acids also help to keep cell membranes healthy, which is important because this is where the hormone receptors are found.

  Moreover, EPA reduces the inflammatory prostaglandin PGE2. PGE2 increases the risk of oestrogen dominance by stimulating aromatase. Avoid the largest species of oily fish (shark, tuna and marlin), as these are more likely to be polluted, and keep your intake of oily fish to no more than twice a week if you are pregnant or breastfeeding.

- Include foods that contain phytoestrogens: soy (for its isoflavones), such as tempeh, miso, tofu and natto, as well as other sources, such as linseeds (for the lignans) and pulses. (Note that flax lignans are phytoestrogens, while flax lignin is a type of soluble fibre.) See Focus box 7.1 for more information on phytoestrogens.

- Sage is a useful culinary herb in menopause and peri-menopause, as it has been found to reduce hot flushes.[19]

- Eat foods containing friendly bacteria (*Homemade Yoghurt*, *Homemade Kefir* and *Homemade Sauerkraut* in Chapter 1) and prebiotics (Jerusalem artichokes, asparagus, leeks, onion, garlic). A healthy gastro-intestinal flora is required for phytoestrogen activation and also to control levels of the beta-glucuronidase enzyme that can contribute to oestrogen dominance. If you are unused to eating these types of foods, increase them very gradually, as they may cause transient wind and bloating if dysbiosis is present.

- Include calcium-rich foods (cruciferous vegetables, beans, pulses, nuts and seeds; low-fat dairy if you tolerate it well). A 2009 systematic review of trials of 62 herbs, vitamins and minerals found that calcium had the most evidence for being helpful in PMS.[20] Calcium and other minerals are also crucial for maintaining bone density during the menopause.

- Eat magnesium-rich foods. Good sources are cooked Swiss chard and spinach, kelp, squash, pumpkin seeds, steamed broccoli, halibut and, to a lesser extent, other green vegetables, nuts and seeds. Magnesium is a cofactor in the methylation detoxification pathway for oestrogen. The body also uses magnesium to make glutathione, a crucial antioxidant molecule for disabling harmful oestrogen metabolites. What's more, magnesium has been found to work with B6 to help reduce PMS symptoms.[17]

- Include foods high in zinc, such as lean cuts of beef, venison and lamb, crab, poultry, calf's liver, seeds, sea vegetables and wholegrains. Together with magnesium and B6, zinc is required for reproductive functions. PMS sufferers have been found to be zinc-deficient, compared to non-sufferers.[21]

- Increase your intake of antioxidants, as these help prevent the oxidation of 2-OH and 4-OH oestrogen metabolites to the reactive quinone molecules that damage DNA.[22] This means increasing your fruit and vegetable intake so that you are eating some at every meal and, where possible, snack.

What not *to eat and drink*

- Don't eat overcooked meat (browned or blackened), as this contains chemicals (polycyclic aromatic hydrocarbons – PAHs) that encourage the production of more potentially carcinogenic 4-hydroxy-oestrogen metabolites.[6, 22] For the same reason, avoid exhaust fumes as far as possible, and do not smoke.

- Avoid intensively farmed full-fat dairy products and meat. These are high in arachidonic acid, which increases levels of the inflammatory chemical PGE2. Chronically high PGE2 levels also lead to oestrogen dominance, by up-regulating the aromatase enzyme. Many oestrogen-related diseases have an inflammatory component, such as fibroids, endometriosis and breast cancer.

- *Trans-*, oxidised and hydrogenated fats, found in mass-produced cooking oils, margarines and processed foods, should be avoided. Sex hormones need to bind to receptors in order to have an effect. These receptors are situated in the membrane of the cell. Damaged fats prevent the cell membrane from functioning well. Some simple changes to make include avoiding processed foods, using olive, seed and vegetable oils only if they are cold-pressed and avoiding heating them to high temperatures. Coconut fat is a more stable oil for cooking. See Chapter 4 for a fuller discussion.

- Minimise your intake of sugars, including refined starches, excessive amounts of fruit and/or fruit juices (2–3 pieces a day is ideal) and any foods with added sugar – see Focus box 5.3 for a list of the many terms used to denote 'sugars' on food labels. Excess sugar intake leads to elevated blood levels of sugar and insulin. This, in turn, disrupts hormones in a number of different ways (see the points made above in the section on eating a low GL diet).

- If you are oestrogen-dominant, watch your intake of foods that contain biogenic amines. Eating too much of these can make you more prone to the effects of high adrenalin and noradrenalin, such as anxiety, headache, migraine and hypertension. Biogenic amines are found in many fermented foods, such as red wine, beer, aged cheeses/meats, yeast extracts, vinegar and pickles, as well as some fruits (raspberries, plums, bananas, tomatoes, avocados and aubergine/eggplant), chocolate (cocoa) and chicken liver.

- Reduce or avoid adrenal stimulants (cigarettes, alcohol and caffeine) because adrenal stress is such a significant factor in hormone-related issues. Alcohol also reduces the liver's ability to detoxify hormones and it depletes B vitamins required for the main oestrogen detoxification pathway (methylation).

Lifestyle

- At the centre of the lifestyle approach lies the need to manage stress. Chronically raised adrenalin and cortisol levels affect sex hormones and many symptoms of sex hormone imbalance (see above). Stress reduction strategies include improving relationships and getting regular exercise, relaxation and high-quality sleep (see Chapter 6).

- Take weight-bearing exercise for 30 minutes a day, even if this is simply a brisk walk in the park. Physically active people tend to have lower rates of breast and other cancers and improved cancer outcomes; and exercise has been shown to modulate various blood markers of cancer risk.[23] A 2011 review of studies found a 25 per cent reduced risk of breast cancer among physically active women compared to the least active women.[24] Regular weight-bearing exercise is also important in helping to reduce the risk of post-menopausal osteoporosis.[25]

- Minimise your exposure to environmental toxins (see Chapter 3). Cocktails of endocrine-disrupting pollutants may contribute to the risk of oestrogen-driven breast cancers.[26] Toxic metals, pesticides, PAHs (see above) and a variety of chemicals, such as phthalates from PVC products and cosmetics, may disrupt hormone balance.[6] Simple changes you can make include:

  ○ switching your brands of personal care products and cosmetics to those that are chemical-free (there are now many on the market)

  ○ binning your Teflon and using uncoated cook- and bakeware

  ○ avoiding plastics for use in the microwave

  ○ ensuring that containers used for food storage and smoothie shakers are free from bisphenol A (BPA)

  ○ using greaseproof paper in place of cling film or foil for wrapping food

  ○ using white vinegar, bicarbonate of soda and other natural household cleaning agents

   ◦   taking physical exercise in zones that are relatively traffic-free.

See Focus box 10.2 for more suggestions.

- Take action to reach a healthy weight. Being underweight pre-menopausally can inhibit ovulation; and post-menopausally it can lead to oestrogen levels that are too low for wellbeing. This is because much of the oestrogen production after the menopause is undertaken within the fat cells, using precursor hormones produced in the ovaries and adrenals.[5]

  However, carrying excessive fat around the abdomen can lead to oestrogen dominance and the consequent health problems – the more excess fat you are carrying, the more oestrogen you will produce.

- Steroid hormones are synthesised from cholesterol – thus, blood levels of cholesterol need to be within the normal range and not too low. If you are taking cholesterol-lowering medication, it would be wise to periodically monitor your blood levels.[14]

Focus box 7.1   Phytoestrogen-rich foods

Phytoestrogens have oestrogenic activity that is many hundreds of times weaker than endogenous oestrogen. By latching on to the body's oestrogen receptor sites, phytoestrogens can increase functional oestrogen levels when endogenous levels are low, such as during the menopause. Conversely, by the same mechanism, they can reduce overall levels in cases of oestrogen dominance.

Phytoestrogens also have a number of other oestrogen-modulating mechanisms: they disrupt aromatase function, increase sex hormone binding globulin (SHBG)[27] and shift oestrogen metabolism away from the production of potentially carcinogenic metabolites (16-a-OH) to those that are more benign (2-OH).[22]

Studies have shown phytoestrogens may help reduce some symptoms of pre-menstrual syndrome,[28, 29] as well as menopausal hot flushes[30] and osteoporosis.[27] However, trial results have not consistently shown such effects. This may be partly because phytoestrogens' effects depend on their metabolism by the gastro-intestinal microbiota, the composition of which varies between individuals. Thus, it is important to address any gut microflora imbalance to get the most benefit from phytoestrogen-rich foods.

If you have a personal or family history of oestrogen-related cancer, it would be best to seek advice from your health adviser before you decide to regularly eat phytoestrogen foods more than three times a week. This is because, although there are many studies on phytoestrogens and breast cancer, the results have been somewhat contradictory and there is still a lack of consensus as to whether they have a beneficial or negative effect on risk.[27, 31]

Some food sources of phytoestrogens are listed below. Such minimally processed soy foods are advocated over the more highly processed forms found in supermarket fast foods.[32]

Table 7.1 Sources of phytoestrogens

Food	Phytoestrogen content (μg/100g)	Food	Phytoestrogen content (μg/100g)
Flaxseed	379,380.0	Pistachios	382.5
Soy bean	103,920.0	Dried dates	329.5
Tofu	27,150.1	Sunflower seeds	216.0
Soy yoghurt	10,275.0	Chestnuts	210.2
Multi grain bread	4,798.7	Dried prunes	183.5
Natto	5,893.0	Olive oil	180.7
Tempeh	4,352.0	Walnuts	139.5
Soy milk	2,957.2	Almonds	131.1
Hummus	993.0	Cashew nuts	121.9
Garlic	603.6	Winter squash	113.7
Mung bean sprouts	495.1	Green beans	105.8
Dried apricots	444.5	Onion	32.0
Alfalfa sprouts	441.4	Blueberries	17.5

Three-day meal plan

Dishes and snacks in italics are supported by recipes in this chapter or other chapters as indicated.

To increase the phytoestrogen content, you could replace one of these meals with the *Natto Fried Rice* (Chapter 11).

Day 1

Breakfast: Porridge/oatmeal made with 2 dessertspoons of oats, soya milk and a handful of berries (fresh or frozen); once cooked, stir in a tablespoon each of ground flaxseeds and ground chia seeds

Snack: *Tangy Kale Crisps*

Lunch: *Poached Egg with Asparagus and Cashew Nut Butter Sauce* and a bitter green salad (e.g. rocket/arugula and/or watercress)

Snack: *Coconut Chocolate Mousse*

Dinner: *Creamed Brussels and Chestnuts with Sage* accompanied with some additional protein, such as canned aduki beans (or sprouted beans) or shredded cooked chicken

Day 2

Breakfast: *Creamy Tropical Smoothie* (Chapter 8)

Snack: One slice of lightly toasted *Buckwheat and Almond Bread* (Chapter 11) with almond butter

Lunch: *Roasted Tempeh Skewers with Plum Sauce and Pak Choi*

Snack: *Liquorice Yoghurt Ice* (Chapter 6)

Dinner: *Pomegranate and Chickpea Pilaf*

Day 3

Breakfast: *Homemade Yoghurt* (Chapter 1) with a handful of berries and seeds or *Maca Strawberry Milkshake* (Chapter 6)

Snack: *Simple Nut Cheese* (Chapter 1) spread on one slice of pumpernickel or an oat cake

Lunch: *Aduki Bean Chilli Soup with Coriander Yoghurt*

Snack: *Mango and Ginger Sorbet*

Dinner: *Almond-Crusted Trout with Wilted Peas and Beans* and a small baked sweet potato if desired

Drinks

- Herbal teas include red raspberry leaf, used traditionally for hormonal balance and pre-conception, and green tea, high in antioxidants to help counter the free radicals produced in from the phase 1 oestrogen metabolites. Other useful herbal teas include sage, Dong quai, liquorice, ginseng and liver supportive herbs, such as dandelion and nettle.

- If you are having problems sleeping, you might want to try a relaxing tea, such as chamomile, valerian, hops, wild lettuce, lemon balm or passion flower.

Recipes

Lunch

Poached Egg with Asparagus and Cashew Nut Butter Sauce

This is an easy breakfast dish but equally delicious as a lunch served with a leafy green salad. The sauce can be made in advance and served hot or cold. Asparagus is a good source of folate and B vitamins, important for methylation, while the eggs provide plenty of essential amino acids.

- SERVES 4

Sauce

2 tbsp cashew nut butter

2–3 tbsp water

Pinch of xylitol (optional)

3 tbsp lemon juice and zest from 1 lemon

1 tbsp fresh tarragon or parsley, chopped

Sea salt and freshly ground black pepper

....

Splash of white wine vinegar

4 organic eggs at room temperature

2 bunches (about 20 spears) asparagus

For the sauce, place the nut butter, water, xylitol (if using) and lemon juice and zest in a blender and process until smooth. Add a little more water to thin the sauce as needed. Stir in the herbs. Season with sea salt and black pepper.

Bring a pan of water to the boil and add the vinegar. Crack the eggs into the pan and cook for 3 minutes. Remove with a slotted spoon and keep warm.

In the same water blanch the asparagus for 2–3 minutes until just tender. Remove from the pan.

Divide the asparagus spears between 4 plates. Top with a poached egg and drizzle over the nut butter sauce to serve.

Nutritional information per serving
Calories 136kcal
Protein 9.6g
Carbohydrates 2.1g of which sugars 1.6g
Total fat 9.9g of which saturates 2.6g

Roasted Tempeh Skewers with Plum Sauce and Pak Choi

This is a delicious way of serving tempeh, which is a fermented form of soy. If this is hard to get hold of, use firm tofu instead. Although it is rather bland on its own, it soaks up the tangy flavours of the plum sauce. Instead of pak choi, you could use little gem lettuce or tenderstem broccoli.

▪ SERVES 4

1 tbsp coconut oil

1 shallot, finely chopped

2 star anise

1 cinnamon stick

Freshly ground black pepper

450g/1lb plums, stoned and quartered

4 tbsp rice wine vinegar

2 tbsp xylitol

1 tbsp olive oil

2 tbsp tamari soy sauce

450g/1lb tempeh, cut in 2cm/1in cubes

2 pak choi, halved

2cm/1in piece of ginger, cut into thin strips

350–400g/12–14oz steamed greens

Heat the coconut oil in a frying pan and sauté the shallot for 1 minute, then add the spices and pepper. Stir-fry for 1 minute, then tip in the plums and cook for a further minute. Pour over the rice wine vinegar and xylitol and cook over a low heat for 3–4 minutes until the plums have softened. Spoon out the star anise and cinnamon stick. Purée the sauce in a blender until smooth. Allow to cool.

Mix half of the plum sauce with the olive oil and 1 tbsp tamari. Pour over the tempeh and allow to marinate for 1 hour.

Preheat the grill to high.

Thread the tempeh cubes on skewers. If you are using wooden skewers, soak them for 1 hour in cold water before using to stop them burning. Place on a baking tray. Grill on each side for 6–7 minutes until the tempeh is golden brown.

Meanwhile, place the pak choi in a steamer with the ginger and pour over the remaining tamari. Steam for 3–4 minutes until just tender. Serve the skewers with the remaining plum sauce and steamed greens.

Nutritional information per serving
Calories 328kcal
Protein 27.7g
Carbohydrates 25.8g of which sugars 19.4g
Total fat 13g of which saturates 2.4g

Aduki Bean Chilli Soup with Coriander Yoghurt

This warming soup is rich in soluble fibre and antioxidants and makes an ideal lunch or snack. The beans also contain phytoestrogens. Accompany with a little pumpernickel bread or a couple of oat cakes if desired.

■ SERVES 4

1 tbsp coconut oil
1 red onion, chopped
2 garlic cloves, crushed
2 sticks celery, sliced
1 carrot, cut into small dice
pinch chilli flakes
½ tsp ground cumin
400g/14oz can chopped tomatoes
400ml/14fl oz/scant 1⅔ cups
    vegetable stock
400g/14oz can aduki or kidney
    beans, rinsed and drained
150g/5oz natural live yoghurt
Handful of coriander leaves
    (cilantro), chopped
Sea salt and freshly ground black
    pepper

Heat the coconut oil in a pan and sauté the onion, garlic, celery and carrot for 3–4 minutes until softened. Add the chilli flakes and cumin and cook for a minute. Pour in the tomatoes, stock and beans, then simmer for 15–20 minutes, until the vegetables are tender.

Mix together the yoghurt and coriander and season with sea salt and black pepper.

Spoon the soup into bowls, then top with the yoghurt to serve.

Nutritional information per serving
Calories 136kcal
Protein 7.5g
Carbohydrates 18.6g of which sugars 10.2g
Total fat 3.4g of which saturates 2.3g

Dinner

Creamed Brussels and Chestnuts with Sage

This is a tasty way of serving Brussels sprouts, even if you're not a great fan. The inclusion of sage may help to reduce menopausal hot flushes (see text). Serve this as a side dish to meat or fish or add some beans, tempeh or tofu for a vegetarian option.

▪ SERVES 4

1 tbsp coconut oil
2 shallots, finely chopped
2 garlic cloves, finely chopped
280g/10oz Brussels sprouts, finely
    sliced
100ml/3½fl oz/scant ½ cup chicken
    or vegetable stock
Handful of sage leaves, finely sliced
150ml/5fl oz/scant ⅔ cup soy cream
150g/5oz cooked chestnuts, roughly
    chopped
Freshly ground black pepper
Handful of fresh flat leaf parsley,
    chopped

Heat the coconut oil in a frying pan. Add the shallots and garlic and sauté for 2–3 minutes until soft.

Add the Brussels sprouts and stir-fry for 1 minute. Pour in the stock and sage leaves and simmer for 2–3 minutes to allow the liquid to reduce down. Pour in the soy cream and chestnuts and cook for a further 2–3 minutes to thicken the sauce.

Season with black pepper and toss in the parsley leaves to serve.

Nutritional information per serving

Calories 195kcal
Protein 4.8g
Carbohydrates 17.6g of which sugars 6.2g
Total fat 11.6g of which saturates 6.9g

Pomegranate and Chickpea Pilaf

Pomegranate adds a wonderful sweetness to this rice dish. The chickpeas provide protein, fibre and phytoestrogens. You could also use puy lentils or other beans instead of chickpeas.

▪ SERVES 4

1 tsp cumin seeds
1 tsp coriander seeds
1 tbsp coconut oil
1 white onion, finely chopped
1 tsp ground turmeric
175g/6oz brown basmati rice
375ml/13fl oz/1½ cup vegetable
    stock
1 red onion, sliced
30g/1oz dried cherries
1 tbsp pomegranate molasses
Sea salt and freshly ground black
    pepper

Heat a dry frying pan and add the cumin and coriander seeds. Fry over a medium heat for 2–3 minutes, or until aromatic and lightly browned. Transfer to a mortar and grind with a pestle.

Heat half the coconut oil in a pan and fry the white onion over a medium-low heat for 4 minutes, or until softened. Add the ground toasted spices, ground turmeric and rice and cook for 2–3 minutes.

Pour in the stock, cover the pan with a lid and cook over a low heat for 12–15 minutes, or until the rice is tender.

Meanwhile, in a frying pan heat the remaining coconut oil and fry the red onion for 2–3 minutes until soft.

2 x 400g/14oz cans chickpeas, drained
Handful each of fresh mint and parsley, chopped
3 tbsp pomegranate seeds

Add the dried cherries, pomegranate molasses and chickpeas and cook for a minute to combine. Add this mixture to the cooked rice and season.

Toss in the herbs and pomegranate seeds just before serving.

Nutritional information per serving
Calories 345kcal
Protein 12g
Carbohydrates 60.9g of which sugars 10.6g
Total fat 5.9g of which saturates 2.5g

Almond-Crusted Trout with Wilted Greens and Peas

Trout is a good source of omega-3 fatty acids and protein. This delicious dish is simple and easy to assemble, making it suitable for a quick after-work meal. Instead of spinach, shredded spring greens or kale could be used. Use gluten-free breadcrumbs if desired.

▪ SERVES 4

150g/5oz wholemeal breadcrumbs or gluten-free breadcrumbs
150g/5oz almonds, toasted, finely crushed
Sea salt and freshly ground black pepper
4 trout fillets, skin on
2 tsp Dijon mustard
2 tbsp coconut oil
8 spring onions (scallions), thinly sliced
75g/2¾oz frozen peas
150ml/5fl oz/scant ⅔ cup vegetable stock
350g/12oz baby spinach leaves

Preheat the oven to 180°C/350°F, gas mark 4.

Mix the breadcrumbs and almonds together in a bowl and season, to taste, with sea salt and freshly ground black pepper.

Brush the flesh side of the trout fillets with a little mustard, then press on the nut mixture to coat the flesh.

Heat 1 tbsp of the coconut oil in an ovenproof frying pan and fry the trout fillets, crumb-side down, for 1–2 minutes, or until crisp. Transfer to the oven to roast for 8 minutes, or until the fish is cooked through.

Heat the remaining coconut oil in a frying pan and sauté the spring onions for 2 minutes.

Add the peas and stock and cook for another 2 minutes. Drop in handfuls of spinach and stir into the pea mixture until the spinach has wilted. Season to taste. Serve alongside the trout fillets.

Nutritional information per serving
Calories 553kcal
Protein 36g
Carbohydrates 33.1g of which sugars 4.7g
Total fat 30.6g of which saturates 5g

Snacks

Tangy Kale Crisps

These make a super-healthy alternative to crisps and chips. If you have a dehydrator, you can dry the kale overnight to create crunchy crisps. Alternatively, they can be baked in the oven.

- SERVES 4

1 tbsp tahini
60g/2oz/½ cup cashew nuts
2 tbsp nutritional yeast flakes
2 tbsp lemon juice
1 tsp spirulina powder (optional)
1 tsp garlic salt
200g/7oz/1 large head kale,
    chopped into 5cm/2in pieces

Preheat the oven to 150°C/300°F, gas mark 2. Alternatively, set the dehydrator to 45°C/115°F.

Blend the tahini, cashew nuts, nutritional yeast flakes, lemon juice, spirulina powder (if using), garlic salt and 2–3 tbsp water to create a thick sauce.

Put the kale in a large bowl and pour over the tahini mixture. Massage the sauce into the kale using your hands – the kale will start to wilt. Make sure all the kale is thoroughly coated with the tahini sauce.

Grease a baking sheet with coconut oil, arrange the kale in a single layer and bake in the oven for about 15 minutes. Use a fork or spatula to carefully flip the kale chips over and bake for 5–10 more minutes, until they are crisp but not burnt. They should be crunchy. Alternatively, if you have a dehydrator spread the kale onto two teflex-lined trays and dehydrate for 8 hours until dry and crisp.

Allow to cool and store in an airtight container.

Nutritional information per serving

Calories 125kcal
Protein 4.2g
Carbohydrates 1.2g of which sugars 1.1g
Total fat 11.5g of which saturates 1g

Coconut Chocolate Mousse

This creamy chocolate pot includes silken tofu, which is a good source of protein and phytoestrogens. Use dark chocolate (at least 70% cocoa solids) to create an indulgent, yet antioxidant-rich, dessert – great for satisfying those chocolate cravings. Serve in small shot glasses.

▪ SERVES 6

200g/7oz dark chocolate, broken into pieces
350g/12oz silken tofu
1 tbsp vanilla extract
50g/1¾oz/½ cup desiccated coconut
Handful of toasted coconut flakes to garnish

Place the chocolate in a bowl over a pan of simmering water. Stir until melted then allow to cool slightly. Place in a food processor with the rest of the ingredients. Process until smooth and creamy.

Spoon into small shot glasses and decorate with the toasted coconut flakes. Chill in the fridge until needed.

Nutritional information per serving
Calories 263kcal
Protein 6.9g
Carbohydrates 20.6g of which sugars 20.5g
Total fat 16.9g of which saturates 10.3g

Mango and Ginger Sorbet

This is a refreshing tropical sorbet that combines healthy probiotic yoghurt with ripe mango and chunks of stem ginger. Creamy-tasting yet wonderfully light – delicious served on its own or as an accompaniment to fresh or poached fruit.

▪ SERVES 6

1 large ripe mango, peeled and chopped
Zest of 1 lime
200g/7oz organic thick Greek yoghurt
2 pieces of stem ginger, finely chopped

Put the mango in a food processor and process to form a smooth purée. Add the lime zest and yoghurt and blend until smooth.

Stir in chopped ginger. Pour into an ice cream maker and churn until thick. Alternatively, pour the mixture into a shallow freezer-proof container and freeze for 3–4 hours until firm. To serve, remove the sorbet from the freezer and place in the fridge for 20 minutes to soften.

Nutritional information per serving
Calories 71kcal
Protein 2.6g
Carbohydrates 5.5g of which sugars 5.4g
Total fat 4.3g of which saturates 2.8g

References

1. Parker, L.N., Levin, E.R. and Lifrak, E.T. (1985) 'Evidence for adrenocortical adaptation to severe illness.' *Journal of Clinical Endocrinology and Metabolism 60*, 5, 947–52.

2. Cagnacci, A., Cannoletta, M., Caretto, S., Zanin, R., Xholli, A. and Volpe, A. (2009) 'Increased cortisol level: A possible link between climacteric symptoms and cardiovascular risk factors.' *Menopause 18*, 3, 273–8.

3. McCormick, K. (2007) 'Ostoeporosis: Biomarkers and other diagnostic correlates into the management of bone fragility.' *Alternative Medicine Review 12*, 2, 113–45.

4. Lee, J. (1993) *Natural Progesterone: The Multiple Roles of a Remarkable Hormone.* Sebastopol, CA: BLL Publishing.

5. Hays, B. (2011) *Sex Hormones, Signalling and the Menopausal Transition.* Presentation given at the Advance Functional Medicine in Clinical Practice (AFMCP) symposium, October 2011. London: IFM.

6. Neil, K. (2010) 'Sex Hormone Imbalances.' In L. Nicolle and A. Woodriff Beirne (eds) *Biochemical Imbalances in Disease.* London: Singing Dragon.

7. Bolton, J.L. and Thatcher, G.R. (2008) 'Potential mechanisms of oestrogen quinone carcinogenesis.' *Chemical Research in Toxicology 21*, 1, 93–101.

8. Bulun, S.E., Zeitoun, K., Takayama, K., Noble, L. *et al.* (1999) 'Estrogen production in endometriosis and use of aromatase inhibitors to treat endometriosis.' *Endocrine-Related Cancer 6*, 2, 293–301.

9. Finocchi, C. and Ferrari, M. (2011) 'Female reproductive steroids and neuronal excitability.' *Journal of the Neurological Sciences 32*, Suppl. 1, S31–5.

10. MacGregor, E.A. (2012) 'Perimenopausal migraine in women with vasomotor symptoms.' *Maturitas 71*, 1, 79–82.

11. Silberstein, S.D. (2000) 'Sex hormones and headache.' *Revue Neurologique 156*, Suppl. 4, S30–41.

12. Fuhrman, B.J., Schairer, C., Gail, M.H., Boyd-Morin, J. *et al.* (2012) 'Estrogen metabolism and risk of breast cancer in postmenopausal women.' *Journal of the National Cancer Institute 104*, 4, 326–39.

13. McAlindon, T.E., Gulin, J., Chen, T., Klug, T., Lahita, R. and Nuite, M. (2001) 'Indole-3-carbinol in women with SLE: Effect on estrogen metabolism and disease activity.' *Lupus 10*, 11, 779–83.

14. Hays, B. (2011) *Practical Workup and Treatment of Women in Peri-Menopause and Menopause.* Presentation given at the Advance Functional Medicine in Clinical Practice (AFMCP) symposium, October 2011. London: IFM.

15. Lee, S.W., Jo, H.H., Kim, M.R., Kwon, D.J., You, Y.O. and Kim, J.H. (2012) 'Association between menopausal symptoms and metabolic syndrome in postmenopausal women.' *Archives of Gynecology and Obstetrics 285*, 2, 541–8.

16. Dormire, S. and Howham, C. (2007) 'The effect of dietary intake on hot flashes in menopausal women.' *Journal of Obstetric, Gynecologic and Neonatal Nursing 36*, 3, 255–62.

17. Fathizadeh, N., Ebrahimi, E. and Valiani, M. (2010) 'Evaluating the effect of magnesium and magnesium plus vitamin B6 supplement on the severity of premenstrual syndrome.' *Iranian Journal of Nursing and Midwifery Research 15*, Suppl. 1, 401–5.

18. Sher, A. and Rahman, A. (1994) 'Role of diet on the enterohepatic recycling of estrogen in women taking contraceptive pills.' *Journal of the Pakistan Medical Association 44*, 9, 213–5.

19. Bommer, S., Klein, P. and Suter, A. (2011) 'First time proof of sage's tolerability and efficacy in menopausal women with hot flushes.' *Advances in Therapy 28*, 6, 490–500.

20. Whelan, A.M., Jurgens, T.M. and Naylor, H. (2009) 'Herbs, vitamins and minerals in the treatment of PMS: A systematic review.' *Canadian Journal of Clinical Pharmacology 16*, 3, e407–29.

21. Chuong, C.J. and Dawson, E.B. (1994) 'Zinc and copper levels in premenstrual syndrome.' *Fertility and Sterility 62*, 2, 313–20.

22. Hays, B. (2005) 'Female Hormones: The Dance of Hormones, Part 1.' In D.S. Jones (ed.) *The Textbook of Functional Medicine*. Gig Harbor, WA: Institute for Functional Medicine.

23. Winzer, B.M., Whiteman, D.C., Reeves, M.M. and Paratz, J.D. (2011) 'Physical activity and cancer prevention: A systematic review of clinical trials.' *Cancer Causes and Control 22*, 6, 811–26.

24. Fridenreich, C.M. (2011).'Physical activity and breast cancer: Review of the epidemiologic evidence and biologic mechanisms.' *Recent Results in Cancer Research 188*, 125–39.

25. ESHRE Capri Workshop Group (2011) 'Perimenopausal risk factors and future health.' *Human Reproduction Update 17*, 5, 706–17.

26. Kortenkamp, A. (2006) 'Breast cancer, oestrogens and environmental pollutants: A re-evaluation from a mixture perspective.' *International Journal of Andrology 29*, 1, 193–8.

27. Patisaul, H.B. and Jefferson, W. (2010) 'The pros and cons of phytoestrogens.' *Frontiers in Neuroendocrinology 31*, 4, 400–19

28. Bryant, M., Cassidy, A., Hill, C., Powell, J., Talbot, D. and Dye, L. (2005) 'Effect of consumption of soy isoflavones on behavioural, somatic and affective symptoms in women with premenstrual syndrome.' *British Journal of Nutrition 93*, 5, 731–9.

29. Kim, H.W., Kwon, M.K., Kim, N.S. and Reame, N.E. (2006) 'Intake of dietary soy isoflavones in relation to perimenstrual symptoms of Korean women living in the USA.' *Nursing and Health Sciences 8*, 2, 108–13.

30. Kurzer, M.S. (2008) 'Soy consumption for reduction of menopausal symptoms.' *Inflammopharmacology 16*, 5, 227–9.

31. Tomar, R.S. and Shiao, R. (2008) 'Early life and adult exposure to isoflavones and breast cancer risk.' *Journal of Environmental Science and Health, Part C Environmental Carcinogenesis and Ecotoxicology Reviews 26*, 2, 113–73.

32. Messina, M. (2010) 'Insights gained from 20 years of soy research.' *The Journal of Nutrition 140*, 12, 22895–22955.

8

Immune Modulation

Anti-Inflammatory Support

This chapter focuses on facilitating an appropriate immune response and preventing chronic inflammation.

Inflammation is the body's initial healing response to trauma from an invader, such as an infection or injury, which damages tissues. Processes of vasodilation, vascular leakiness and chemotaxis enable leukocytes (first neutrophils and then macrophages) and large protein molecules, such as antibodies and fibrinogen, to get quickly to the affected site. Here, they undertake the important roles of phagocytosis and then walling off the inflamed area and/or binding the edges of the wound.

Inflammation is necessary for survival. But the process becomes damaging if it turns chronic, continuing for weeks, months or indefinitely. For chronic inflammation to occur, genetic and/or epigenetic antecedents need to be present, in combination with a trigger. In most cases, intestinal hyperpermeability (otherwise known as a leaky gut) also plays a key role (see below and Focus box 2.1).

Examples of inflammatory triggers include:

- Mechanical injury.

- Environmental toxins:

  - synthetic: cleaning chemicals, pollution, cigarette smoke, food additives (e.g. sulphates), pesticides (e.g. organophosphates), dioxins (from industrial combustion processes) and medications

  - natural: alkaloids, metals such as aluminium, lead and arsenic, polycyclic aromatic hydrocarbons, irritant materials such as wood splinters, radiation, high-fat/high-sugar diets, microbial pathogens (bacterial, viral, fungal, parasitic) and their products/metabolites (often referred to as lipopolysaccharides, or LPSs).

- Endotoxins:
  - secondary bile acids, hydrogen sulphide and other gastro-intestinal gases from dysbiosis and/or leaky gut, nitrosamines, homocysteine, tissue acidosis, psychological stress.

- Allergies and sensitivities:
  - ingested, inhaled and/or skin contact allergens
  - sensitivities to common foods, such as gluten grains.[1]

These trigger nuclear factor kappa B (NF-κB) (see Focus box 8.1), which sets off the inflammatory cascade.

Examples of physiological imbalances that may prolong inflammation include excessive oxidative load, gastro-intestinal problems, poor detoxification function, imbalanced eicosonoid production, dysglycaemia, glycosylation and obesity, sex hormone imbalances and stress and adrenal fatigue. Any of these issues can promote and fuel the fire of inflammation, and vice versa.

The importance of immune tolerance

Chronic inflammation is characterised by a loss of 'immune tolerance'. When the body has a good level of immune tolerance, it mounts effective reactions to invaders when it is necessary, but it is also able to swiftly deactivate the immune response as soon as the goal has been met, and suppress reactions to foreign molecules that are not in themselves harmful to the body. Thus, most of the time, the role of the immune system is *not* to respond to things.

The development and maintenance of immune tolerance depends on many different factors of innate and adaptive immunity, both humoral and cell-mediated, but there is increasing evidence that the starting point is the health of the gastro-intestinal tract. 'Immune tolerance is the essence of good health. An intolerant immune system will lead to a wide range of illnesses, and the gut is where many people first lose immune tolerance.'[2]

Following on from this idea, it is thought that potential exists for arresting autoimmune inflammatory processes by re-establishing intestinal barrier function, as this would inhibit potential inflammatory triggers (of the like listed above) from reaching the body's adaptive immune system.[3] Supporting a healthy GI microbial balance is one of the key points of leverage in improving barrier function. See Focus box 2.1 in Chapter 2 for a fuller discussion.

For more information on the various components of the immune system and their role in immune tolerance see Ash (2010).[4]

Signs and symptoms

Classic signs of inflammation are redness (rubor), swelling (tumour), pain (dolor) and heat (calor). There are a great many 'itis' conditions that are associated with these symptoms, from arthritis to sinusitis.

However, chronic, low-grade inflammation is now thought to be at the root of almost all chronic diseases, including those that do not exhibit these classic inflammatory symptoms (see below). Thus, anyone with a degenerative condition (or a pre-disease condition, such as obesity) will be in an inflammatory state.

Other signs and symptoms may include a history of functional gastro-intestinal disorders (see Chapter 2), increased sensitivity reactions to foods or inhalants, aches and pains in the joints or muscles, skin problems and chronic fatigue.

Relevant laboratory tests include:

- Blood tests for:
  - erythrocyte sedimentation rate (ESR)
  - high-sensitive C-reactive protein (hs CRP), an abnormal glycoprotein produced in the liver in response to inflammation
  - antibodies to self (the type tested for will depend on the symptoms experienced and the pathology suspected).

- Urine, saliva or stool testing for:
  - intestinal permeability (leaky gut), calprotectin, secretory IgA status and dysbiosis
  - any other inflammatory-promoting imbalances that may be suspected – see the relevant chapters. (A urinary organic acids test is a broad-based indicator of a range of possible imbalances.)

What health conditions is inflammation linked to in the long term?

There exists a strong body of evidence for inflammation as a key factor in the development of many chronic diseases,[5] including autoimmune conditions such as rheumatoid arthritis, coeliac disease and inflammatory bowel disease, cardiovasular disease,[6] cancer,[7] diabetes,[8, 9] Alzheimer's disease,[9] osteoporosis[9, 10] and many others.

Key nutritional interventions to consider

What to eat and drink

- Perhaps the most important recommendation is to focus on foods that may help to address any gastro-intestinal imbalances, including dysbiosis, and to heal a leaky gut.

    In particular, eat foods that contain probiotics (*Homemade Yoghurt, Homemade Kefir* and *Homemade Sauerkraut* in Chapter 1) and prebiotics (Jerusalem artichokes, asparagus, leeks, onions and garlic). (Note that prebiotics are best consumed once any microbial balance has been resolved.)

    Recent studies propose that re-establishing intestinal barrier function may arrest the inflammatory autoimmune process in certain conditions.[3] See Focus box 2.1 and follow the recommendations in Chapter 2, including the advice to eat collagen-rich foods, such as chicken soup and meat broths.

- Eat foods rich in vitamin A, such as organic liver and eggs. Due to genetic variations, up to 45 per cent of the population cannot adequately convert beta-carotene to vitamin A,[11] yet this vitamin is crucial for the health of the gastro-intestinal mucous membranes and in improving immune tolerance.[2, 12, 13, 14]

- Eat foods rich in vitamin D: oily fish, shellfish, egg yolk, mushrooms and fortified foods (these vary between countries).

    Vitamin D is thought to have a key role in improving immune tolerance,[14] by enhancing the production of T-regulatory cells (see Focus box 2.1), leading to a reduction in pro-inflammatory cytokines.[15] There is preliminary evidence that vitamin D may have the potential to help in inflammatory autoimmune conditions, such as rheumatoid arthritis, psoriasis, type 1 diabetes, Crohn's, multiple sclerosis and autoimmune hypothyroidism.[15, 16, 17, 18] Randomised controlled trials are now needed.

    Sub-optimal vitamin D levels have also been associated with other chronic conditions with an inflammatory component, such as cardiovascular disease[16] and Alzheimer's.[19, 20, 21] See Focus box 11.2 for more on vitamin D.

- Choose mainly foods with a low glycaemic load (GL) to help control insulin levels (see Chapter 5). High insulin may aggravate the inflammatory cascade by up-regulating the delta-5-desaturase (D5D) enzyme that converts omega-6 fatty acids into inflammatory metabolites.[22] Low-glycaemic index diets have been shown to reduce the inflammatory marker CRP.[23]

- Ensure you eat a good balance of omega-6 and omega-3 fats, as the balance of fatty acids in the cell membranes influences the extent to which the body produces inflammatory versus anti-inflammatory eicosonoids.[13] Experts suggest an optimal omega-6:omega-3 balance for health may be about 3:1 or 4:1 (see Chapter 4), but if your dietary history is light on oily fish and/ or flaxseeds, you are likely to need a lot more omega-3 fats initially. See Chapter 4 for more information on how to balance fatty acids.

Oily fish is also one of the best food sources of vitamin D (see above) and high-quality protein, needed for making immune chemicals. Wild game and lean, grass-fed meats are also acceptable, as they contain higher proportions of essential fatty acids than do meat and poultry from intensively farmed livestock.

- Eat as wide a range of antioxidants as possible, in the form of fresh, brightly coloured fruits and vegetables, including some raw. Antioxidants help to 'mop up' the damaging 'free radical' molecules that are produced by phagocytes (such as macrophages) during an inflammatory episode. Excessive levels of free radicals activate NF-$\varkappa$B (see Focus box 8.1). For more on antioxidants see Chapter 9.

  In particular, enrich your diet with the following plant foods, all of which have been shown to modulate inflammatory processes:

  ○ Orange and dark green vegetables, for their beta-carotene.[4]

  ○ Ginger.[4]

  ○ Green tea, containing epigallocatechin gallate.[4]

  ○ Pineapple, which contains the anti-inflammatory enzyme bromelain.[24]

  ○ Rosemary, for its carnasol.[25]

  ○ Propolis (honeybee resin), a source of caffeic acid phenethyl ester (CAPE), which has been found to inhibit NF-$\varkappa$B.[26] Propolis can be added to many of the raw dishes in this book, such as the smoothies, juices or the raw cacao bar. It has a pleasant taste, so can also be eaten off the spoon.

  ○ Apples, onions, berries, brassicas and capers, for quercetin. This flavonoid may help to inhibit histamine release, having an anti-allergy effect.[27]

  ○ Blueberries, which contain pterostillbene.[28]

  ○ Turmeric, for curcumin. This yellow pigment partially inhibits the activation of NF-$\varkappa$B (see Focus box 8.1) and reduces proinflammatory eicosonoids and cytokines.[5, 29, 30] Adding curcumin to conventional therapies for inflammatory bowel disease has been found to improve symptoms and enable a decrease in the dosage of the medications used.[29]

It has also been shown to exhibit therapeutic potential in many other inflammatory conditions, including Alzheimer's disease, Parkinson's disease, multiple sclerosis, epilepsy, cardiovascular disease, cancer, allergy, asthma, bronchitis, colitis, rheumatoid arthritis, psoriasis, diabetes and depression.[30]

What not to eat and drink

- Experiment with avoiding food groups that may cause inflammatory reactions. Everyone is affected differently, so you won't know until you try. The most common inflammatory groups are listed here – do not avoid all these groups at the same time, or your diet will become extremely restricted. Work with your nutrition consultant to find an elimination trial that is right for you.

  - Histamine-rich foods (red wine and beer, fermented cheese, shellfish, fish, tomatoes, chicken, spinach, cured sausage, chocolate, fermented vegetables (sauerkraut) and soy sauce). This may help if you are prone to itching, sneezing and wheezing, as you may be low in the enzyme that breaks down histamine in foods.[31]

  - Tyramine-rich foods (cheese, beer, wine, bananas, yeast extract, avocados, tinned fish, raspberries, tomatoes, red plums, soy, vinegar and pickles). Avoidance may be helpful particularly if you are a migraine sufferer.

  - Solanine-containing foods (primarily potatoes – especially if green – but also possibly other members of the 'nightshade' family, such as tomatoes and aubergines/eggplants).

  - Excessive intakes of lectin-rich foods, such as beans, pulses, grains and peanuts, especially if improperly cooked. In particular, soybean agglutinin and wheatgerm agglutinin are able to bind with brush border surfaces in the small intestine, increasing the risk of developing intestinal hyperpermeability, or leaky gut (see Focus box 2.1).[32, 33, 34] Wheatgerm agglutinin may also inhibit the actions of anti-inflammatory vitamin D.[35]

  - Dairy products. Some people are unable to digest these, due to a lack of the lactase enzyme and/or an immune reaction to one or more of the dairy proteins. Undigested proteins can lead to a microbial imbalance in the gut and eventually to leaky gut (see Focus box 2.1).

- Avoid sources of toxic metals (such as tuna, marlin or shark), artificial food additives (processed foods) and *trans-* and oxidised fats (all processed foods, including breads, margarines, biscuits, salad dressings and vegeburgers, and any unsaturated oils that have not been cold-pressed). Many of these food components are not recognised by the body and can therefore trigger an immune reaction.

- Limit your intake of red meat and dairy products, as they contain arachidonic acid, which the body can use to make inflammatory eicosonoids (see Chapter 4).

- Avoiding wheat, rye and barley for a few weeks is recommended if you have any inflammatory condition, as gluten can cause zonulin dysregulation.[36] Zonulin is a protein within the tight junctions of the gut mucosa. When it fails to work properly, the integrity of the gut lining is breeched, leading to leaky gut. Leaky gut is considered a key factor in the development of inflammatory conditions (see above and Focus box 2.1). It is now recognised that gluten sensitivity can exist separately from coeliac disease.[37]

- Pulling together the above two points, research indicates that vegan diets free of gluten may improve the signs and symptoms of rheumatoid arthritis.[38, 39] If you are sensitive to gluten be mindful that cross-reactivity to other grains, such as maize, is common. Discuss this with your nutrition adviser.

- Avoid simple sugars because of their insulin-spiking effect (see Chapter 5), as well as the effect that blood glucose problems can have on adrenal gland function.

Lifestyle

- Stop smoking (excessive oxidation causes inflammation). As nicotine is so strongly addictive, many people find hypnotherapy and/or psychotherapy helpful.

- Take steps to lose weight if you are carrying too much. White adipose tissue has in recent years been recognised as a powerful endocrine organ, producing proinflammatory 'adipocytokines',[40] including tumour necrosis factor-alpha (TNF-α) and interleukin 6 (IL-6).[41]

- Improve your response to stress (see Chapter 6), including by controlling blood sugar levels (see Chapter 5). Psychological stress has long been thought to contribute to chronic inflammatory diseases, and recent research has revealed correlations between biomarkers of stress (disrupted cortisol patterns) and inflammation.[42] Stress is one of the main causes of leaky gut.

- For valuable vitamin D, expose your skin to sunlight in the middle of the day, every day from April to September, without sunscreen. Start with

2–3 minutes only and build up gradually to a maximum of 30 minutes, taking care not to burn.

- Avoid sources of toxins as much as possible (see Focus box 10.2).

- Pay attention to oral hygiene, brushing and flossing correctly twice a day. Have regular dental check-ups and professional cleans – agree the frequency with your dentist.

Focus box 8.1   Nuclear factor kappa B (NF-κB) and inflammatory cytokines

NF-κB has become known as the key driver of the inflammatory response. Hence it's worth knowing a bit about it. NF-κB is a transcription factor that induces genes involved in inflammation to produce a range of inflammatory chemicals. These include COX enzymes (leading to the production of inflammatory eicosonoids – see Chapter 4), C-reactive protein, nitric oxide and other reactive oxygen species ('free radicals'), the proinflammatory catabolic enzymes matrix metalloproteinases and a range of cytokines.

Cytokines work by transmitting messages between cells and some are inflammatory (such as TNF-α, IL-1 and IL-6), while others are anti-inflammatory (e.g. IL-10 and TGF-beta). In this way, a healthy inflammatory response is controlled by a *coordinated balance* of cytokines. Up-regulated NF-κB activation can cause cytokine dysregulation, leading to chronic inflammation.

Activated NF-κB is found in inflammatory conditions such as rheumatoid arthritis, inflammatory bowel disease, multiple sclerosis, psoriasis and asthma. In normal conditions it is located in the cytosol of the cell, where it is inhibited by a molecule called inhibitory kappa B alpha (IκB-α). But inflammatory 'triggers' split IκB-a from NF-κB, allowing NF-κB to translocate to the nucleus of the cell, where it binds to DNA, causing inflammatory gene expression.

Examples of NF-κB (inflammatory) triggers are listed at the beginning of this chapter. There is a considerable current research focus on identifying agents that may inhibit NF-κB.

Three-day meal plan

Dishes and snacks in italics are supported by recipes in this chapter or other chapters as indicated.

Day 1

Breakfast: *Creamy Tropical Smoothie*

Snack: Vegetable sticks with *Dill Ranch Nut Dip* (Chapter 1) or *Simple Nut Cheese* (Chapter 1)

Lunch: *Vietnamese Tempeh or Tofu Platter*

Snack: *Strawberry Coconut Ice Cream*

Dinner: Oven baked trout or salmon using the *Mirin and Lemon Baked Salmon or Tofu* recipe (Chapter 9)

Day 2

Breakfast: *Indian Spiced Scrambled Eggs*: heat 1 tsp mustard seeds until they pop, add a little coconut oil and scramble 2 eggs with 1 tsp turmeric. Toss in a few chopped tomatoes while cooking

Snack: *Alkaline Detox Broth* (Chapter 3) or *Speedy Mushroom Miso Soup* (Chapter 6)

Lunch: *Nutrient-Packed Salad* (Chapter 1) with handful of sprouted beans

Snack: Celery sticks with *Avocado Spiced Hummus* (Chapter 11)

Dinner: *Pomegranate Glazed Turkey with Butternut Squash and Leaf Salad.* Optional dessert: *Apple and Berry Spiced Compote with Crispy Almond Topping*

Day 3

Breakfast: *Homemade Yoghurt* (Chapter 1) with a handful of mixed berries (fresh or frozen)

Snack: *Green Olive and Shallot Tapenade* with vegetable crudités

Lunch: *Wild Mushroom and Butterbean Soup* with a side salad

Snack: Small handful of raw mixed nuts and seeds (not peanuts)

Dinner: *Indian Spiced Mackerel with Curried Red Lentils and Coriander Yoghurt Sauce*

Drinks

- Fresh, unfiltered water, herbal teas: ginger, green (especially the matcha green tea, which is very high in antioxidants), Echinacea tea, rooibos.[43]

Recipes

Breakfast

Creamy Tropical Smoothie

This creamy smoothie is a good example of just how easy it is to pack more nutritious greens into your diet. We've used rocket (arugula) leaves, but other greens, such as spinach, kale, beet greens, collards, parsley, coriander (cilantro) and/or romaine lettuce, can be used. The combination of sesame seeds and cashew nuts adds creaminess, protein and monounsaturated and polyunsaturated fats. A little green superfood powder provides additional nutrients and the flaxseed oil is a good source of omega-3 and omega-6 fatty acids. This makes a speedy breakfast option or healthy snack.

- SERVES 2–4

1 tbsp ground flaxseeds
30g/1oz sesame seeds
30g/1oz/¼ cup cashew nuts, soaked in water for at least an hour, then drained (discard the water)
300ml/10½fl oz water or coconut water to thin
1 fresh mango, peeled and diced
1 small banana, chopped and frozen
Large handful of rocket (arugula) leaves
1 tsp green superfood powder (optional – available from health food stores and online)
1 tsp flaxseed oil (optional)

Place the seeds and cashew nuts in a blender with the water and process to break up the nuts and seeds.

Add the remaining ingredients and blend until smooth. Add additional water to obtain the desired consistency.

Nutritional information per serving (2 servings)

Calories 331kcal
Protein 9.1g
Carbohydrates 24g of which sugars 19.5g
Total fat 22.2g of which saturates 3.7g

Lunch

Vietnamese Tempeh or Tofu Platter

This light, flavoursome salad is full of Asian spices and herbs. Tempeh is a fermented soy product available in health shops and Asian stores. Alternatively, you could use large prawns or tofu. The dressing includes plenty of anti-inflammatory garlic and ginger, as well as flaxseed oil, which provides a source of omega-3 fatty acids. The red onion in the salad is a useful source of the antioxidant quercetin.

- SERVES 4

Dressing
2 garlic cloves, crushed
1 red chilli, deseeded and chopped
1 lemongrass stalk (bulb end only), thinly
     sliced
1 tsp grated ginger
2 tbsp Thai fish sauce
1 tbsp xylitol to taste
4 tbsp lime juice
1 tbsp flaxseed oil

....

350g/12oz block tempeh, drained and
     cubed
2 tbsp tamari soy sauce
2 tbsp mirin (Japanese rice wine)
1 tbsp coconut oil
1 red pepper, cut into julienne
½ cucumber, deseeded and thinly sliced
1 red onion, finely chopped
1 carrot, cut into julienne
1 red chilli, deseeded and finely chopped
1 pak choi, shredded, or Chinese greens
Handful of fresh coriander leaves (cilantro),
     chopped

Place all the ingredients for the dressing in a food processor and blend until fairly smooth. Add a little more oil or water to thin if needed.

Place the tempeh in a shallow dish and pour over the tamari, mirin and xylitol. Allow to marinate for 30 minutes or 1 hour. Heat the coconut oil in a frying pan and sauté the tempeh in batches until golden brown. Remove from the pan and allow to cool.

Combine all the salad ingredients together in a large bowl. Add the tempeh and toss in the dressing just before serving.

Nutritional information per serving
Calories 167kcal
Protein 8.3g
Carbohydrates 8g of which sugars 7.3g
Total fat 11.4g of which saturates 4.1g

Wild Mushroom and Butterbean Soup

This soup is rich and creamy-tasting, yet without any added dairy. Mushrooms, particularly Asian varieties such as shiitake and enoki, are known for their immune-supporting properties and have been used medicinally by the Chinese for more than 6,000 years. Mushrooms are a useful source of vitamin D2 for vegans. If you have homemade chicken stock, use this for additional flavour and health benefits. Chicken stock is rich in easily digestible gelatine and is a source of essential amino acids. Adding the butterbeans provides fibre, protein and a creamy texture.

▪ SERVES 4

2 tbsp coconut oil
2 shallots, chopped
1 garlic clove, crushed
400g/14oz wild mixed mushrooms
     including shitake mushrooms
700ml/24fl oz/generous 2¾ cup
     Vegetable Stock or *Chicken Stock*
     (Chapter 1)

Heat 1 tbsp of coconut oil in large pan and sauté the shallots for 2–3 minutes until soft but not browned. Stir in the garlic and mushrooms and cook until golden for about 5 minutes. Pour in the stock and simmer for 15 minutes. Add the beans and season to taste. Blend the soup in a food processor until smooth. Season to taste and pour into a clean pan.

400g/14oz can butterbeans, drained
Freshly ground black pepper
75g/2¾oz enoki mushrooms
1 tbsp sesame seeds
Fresh parsley, chopped, to garnish

Heat the remaining coconut oil in a frying pan. Add the enoki mushrooms and sesame seeds and stir-fry for 1–2 minutes, leaving texture in the mushrooms.

Spoon the soup into bowls and scatter over the mushrooms and sesame to serve. Garnish with parsley.

Nutritional information per serving
Calories 178kcal
Protein 6.4g
Carbohydrates 14.1g of which sugars 1.5g
Total fat 10.6g of which saturates 7g

Dinner

Pomegranate Glazed Turkey with Butternut Squash and Leaf Salad

Sweet and tangy pomegranate molasses is a typical ingredient in Middle Eastern dishes. This sweet–sour marinade marries beautifully with the meaty flavour of the turkey and would be equally delicious with guinea fowl, chicken or firm fish, such as halibut. Opt for organic, free-range poultry, as it is higher in omega-3 fatty acids. Turkey is a good source of protein, B vitamins (B6, B3), selenium, choline and zinc. The butternut squash provides beta-carotene, a precursor to vitamin A.

▪ SERVES 4

Marinade
4 tbsp pomegranate molasses
2 tbsp tamari soy sauce
2 tbsp olive oil
Juice of ½ lemon
1 tsp sumac (Middle Eastern spice)

Dressing
2 tbsp pomegranate molasses
2 tbsp lemon juice
1 garlic clove, crushed
2 tbsp flaxseed oil
2 tbsp extra virgin olive oil
Freshly ground black pepper

Mix together all the marinade ingredients. Pour over the turkey and leave to marinate in the fridge for 2–3 hours or overnight.

Mix together the dressing ingredients and chill until needed.

Heat the oven to 200°C/400°F, gas mark 6.

Heat the coconut oil in a non-stick frying pan. Sauté the butternut squash for 2 minutes. Add the turkey and cook on each side for 1 minute.

Transfer the turkey and butternut squash to a roasting tray and drizzle over the remaining coconut oil. Roast in the oven for 20 minutes, or until the turkey is cooked through. (The juices will run clear when the meat is pierced in the thickest part with a skewer.) Remove from the oven and set aside. Remove the skin.

2 tbsp coconut oil

200g/7oz butternut squash, cut into cubes

4 turkey breast fillets, skin on

225g/8oz mixed leafy greens (e.g. rocket/arugula, watercress, baby spinach leaves)

Seeds of 1 pomegranate

Mix the salad leaves with the butternut squash and pomegranate seeds and toss with a little of the dressing. Place on a plate and top with the turkey. Drizzle over a little more of the dressing to serve.

Nutritional information per serving
Calories 430kcal
Protein 27g
Carbohydrates 23.5g of which sugars 17.2g
Total fat 31.4g of which saturates 4.4g

Indian Spiced Mackerel with Curried Lentils and Coriander Yoghurt Sauce

Omega-3-rich mackerel is quick and easy to cook. The lentils have been flavoured with anti-inflammatory spices, including turmeric, ginger and garlic, and a cooling yoghurt sauce, rich in probiotic bacteria. Red lentils have had their skins removed, so are lower in lectins than other pulses and beans. If lectins are a particular problem, you could serve the mackerel with *Baked Cauliflower with Curry Spices and Turmeric* instead (Chapter 3). When grilling the mackerel, be careful not to burn the skin. Once the flesh is cooked, remove the skin before eating.

▪ SERVES 4

Curried red lentils

1 tbsp coconut oil

1 onion, finely chopped

2 garlic cloves, chopped

2cm/1in piece fresh root ginger, minced

1 tsp turmeric

1 tsp garam masala

225g/8oz red lentils

600ml/21fl oz/2$^{1}/_{3}$ cups chicken or vegetable stock

Juice of ½ lemon

Freshly ground black pepper

Yoghurt sauce

200ml/7fl oz natural live yoghurt

1 tbsp fresh coriander (cilantro), chopped

1 green chilli, deseeded and finely chopped

For the lentils, heat the oil in a large pan. Add the onion, garlic, ginger, turmeric and garam masala and sauté gently for 3–4 minutes.

Add the lentils and stir to coat in the spices. Add the stock and cook covered for 40 minutes until tender. Season with lemon juice and black pepper.

For the yoghurt sauce, simply mix all the ingredients together and chill until required.

Heat the grill. Grind all the spices together to form a coarse mixture. Rub the spices all over the mackerel. Drizzle with a little olive oil.

Put the mackerel fillets on to a tray and place under the grill, skin side up, and cook for 8–10 minutes, or until the mackerel is just cooked through. Serve with the lentils and yoghurt sauce.

Spiced mackerel
1 tsp fennel seeds
1 tsp cumin seeds
½ tsp chilli powder
Pinch of cinnamon
Sea salt and freshly ground black
    pepper
4 mackerel fillets (about 115g/4oz
    each), skin on
Olive oil for drizzling

Nutritional information per serving
Calories 532kcal
Protein 38.3g
Carbohydrates 34.9g of which sugars 5.6g
Total fat 26.8g of which saturates 9.2g

Snacks and desserts

Strawberry Coconut Ice Cream

This is a creamy dairy-free ice cream, rich in vitamin C as well as immune-supporting lauric acid from the coconut oil. You can make use of frozen berries out of season. Soaking the cashew nuts before using helps to improve their digestibility and makes them easier to blend to form a creamy, smooth texture.

▪ SERVES 8

200g/7oz/1¾ cups cashew nuts
    (soaked for 1 hour, then drained)
250ml/8fl oz/1 cup water
60g/2oz organic coconut oil
150g/5oz fresh strawberries
1 tbsp xylitol (optional)
50g/1¾oz creamed coconut,
    chopped

Place the nuts and water in a blender and process for a couple of minutes until blended.

Add the rest of the ingredients and continue to blend until smooth and creamy.

Pour the mixture into an ice cream maker and churn according to the manufacturer's instructions. Alternatively, pour the mixture into a shallow freezer-proof container and freeze for 2–3 hours until firm.

Remove from the freezer 15–30 minutes before serving to allow it to soften slightly.

Nutritional information per serving
Calories 258kcal
Protein 5g
Carbohydrates 5.7g of which sugars 2.6g
Total fat 23.9g of which saturates 12.6g

Apple and Berry Spiced Compote with Crispy Almond Topping

Similar to a crumble but gluten- and grain-free, this simple dessert or breakfast dish is suitable for anyone following a 'Paleo-style' (traditional hunter-gatherer) diet. Apples are low glycemic fruits, rich in phenols and soluble fibre, especially if used unpeeled. Allow the compote to cool before adding the suggested probiotic supplements. Cinnamon may help improve insulin function and it also possesses anti-inflammatory, antimicrobial, antioxidant, anti-tumour, cholesterol-lowering and immunomodulatory effects. You can make the crumble topping in advance and store it in an airtight container for up to 1 week. The compote will keep in the fridge for 2–3 days.

- SERVES 4

130g/4½oz/1 cup almonds (skins on)
2 tbsp ground flaxseed
Pinch of mixed spice
2 tsp ground cinnamon
2 tbsp coconut oil
1 tbsp honey or maple syrup
1 tbsp vanilla extract
2 eating apples, peeled, cored and sliced
2 tbsp water or apple juice
150g/5oz mixed berries, fresh or frozen
Probiotic powder (optional – speak to your nutrition adviser to see if this is appropriate for you)

Preheat the oven to at 180°C/350°F, gas mark 4.

Place half of the almonds in a food processor or blender and grind to a fine flour. Place in a bowl with the flaxseed and 1 tsp of cinnamon and the mixed spice.

Place the remaining almonds in the food processor and break up to form coarse crumbs. Add to the bowl.

Melt the coconut oil and mix with the honey and vanilla.

Pour the coconut oil over the nuts and mix thoroughly with your hands to form a crumble mixture. Add a little apple juice if the mixture if too dry. Spread out on a baking tray and bake for 20 minutes until golden and crisp.

Place the apples in a pan and add the water or apple juice. Bring to a simmer and cook for 3–4 minutes. Add the berries and the remaining cinnamon and simmer for a couple of minutes until the fruit is soft and tender but still retains its shape. Once cool, the probiotic cultures (if using) can be added.

Sprinkle the crumble over the compote to serve.

Nutritional information per serving
Calories 326kcal
Protein 8.1g
Carbohydrates 13.6g of which sugars 11.1g
Total fat 26.8g of which saturates 8.1g

Green Olive and Shallot Tapenade

This is a delicious dip or spread, rich in healthy monounsaturated fats. Serve with vegetable sticks, crackers or rye bread, or use to fill celery stalks. This can be prepared in advance and kept in the fridge for 3–4 days. You can also serve it tossed through pasta (gluten-free if appropriate for your goals) or mixed with a little olive oil and drizzled over steamed vegetables.

▪ SERVES 8–10

1 tbsp coconut oil
2 garlic cloves, crushed
2 shallots, chopped
200g/7oz green olives, pitted
2 tbsp balsamic vinegar
Pinch of xylitol
1 tbsp fresh parsley, chopped

Heat the coconut oil in a frying pan and sauté the garlic and shallots for 2 minutes.

Place in a food processor with the remaining ingredients and pulse until chunky.

Nutritional information per tbsp

Calories 19kcal

Protein 0.2g

Carbohydrate 0.4g of which sugars 0.3g

Total fat 1.9g of which saturates 0.8g

References

1. Fasano, A. (2011) 'Zonulin and its regulation of intestinal barrier function: The biological door to inflammation, autoimmunity and cancer.' *Physiological Reviews 91*, 1, 151–75.
2. Ash, M. (2010) 'Vitamin A: The key to a tolerant immune system?' *Focus: Allergy Research News, August*. Available at www.allergyresearchgroup.com/focus/201088.htm, accessed on 25 Januaryl 2012.
3. Fasano, A. and Shea-Donohue, T. (2005) 'Mechanisms of disease: The role of intestinal barrier function in the pathogenesis of GI autoimmune diseases.' *Nature Clinical Practice Gastroenterology and Hepatology 2*, 9, 416–22.
4. Ash, M. (2010) 'Dysregulation of the Immune System: A Gastro-Centric Perspective.' In L. Nicolle and A. Woodriff Beirne (eds) *Biochemical Imbalances in Disease*. London: Singing Dragon.
5. Bengmark, S. (2006) 'Curcumin, an atoxic antioxidant and natural NFkappaB, COX2, LOX and inducible nitric oxide synthase inhibitor: A shield against acute and chronic diseases.' *Journal of Parenteral and Enteral Nutrition 30*, 1, 45–51.
6. Balagopal, P., George, D., Patton, N., Yarandi, H. *et al.* (2005) 'Lifestyle-only intervention attenuates the inflammatory state associated with obesity: A randomized controlled study in adolescents.' *Journal of Pediatrics 146*, 3, 342–8.
7. Kanterman, J., Sade-Feldman, M. and Baniyash, M. (2012) 'New insights into chronic inflammation-induced immunosuppression.' *Seminars in Cancer Biology*, Epub ahead of print.
8. Cheung, B.M. and Li, C. (2012) 'Diabetes and hypertension: Is there a common metabolic pathway?' *Current Atherosclerosis Reports*, Epub ahead of print.
9. Tilstra, J.S., Clauson, C.L., Neidernhofer, L.J. and Robbins, P.D. (2011) 'NF-κB in aging and disease.' *Aging and Disease 2*, 6, 449–65.
10. McCormick, R. (2007) 'Osteoporosis: Integrating biomarkers and other diagnostic correlates into the management of bone fragility.' *Alternative Medicine Review 12*, 2, 113–45.

11. Lietz, G., Oxley, A., Leung, W. and Hesketh, J. (2012) 'Single nucleotide polymorphisms upstream from the beta-carotene 15,15'-monoxygenase gene influence provitamin A conversion efficiency in female volunteers.' *Journal of Nutrition 142*, 1, S161–5.

12. Manicassamy, S. and Pulendran, B. (2009) 'Retionoic acid-dependent regulation of immune responses by dendritic cells and macrophages.' *Seminars in Immunology 21*, 1, 22–7.

13. Issazadeh-Navikas, S., Teimer, R. and Bockermann, R. (2011) 'Influence of dietary components on regulatory T cells.' *Molecular Medicine 18*, 1, 95–110.

14. Pino-Lagos, A., Benson, M.J. and Noelle, R.J. (2008) 'Retinoic acid in the immune system.' *Annals of the New York Academy of Sciences 1143*, 170–87.

15. Hewison, M. (2010) 'Vitamin D and the immune system: New perspectives on an old theme.' *Endocrinology and Metabolism Clinics of North America 39*, 2, 365–79.

16. Zhang, R. and Naughton, D. (2010) 'Vitamin D in health and disease: Current perspectives.' *Nutrition Journal 9*, 65.

17. Holick, M.F. (2008) 'The vitamin D deficiency pandemic and consequences for nonskeletal health: Mechanisms of action.' *Molecular Aspects of Medicine 29*, 6, 361–8.

18. Kivity, S., Agmon-Levin, N., Zisappl, M., Shapira, E.V. *et al.* (2011) 'Vitamin D and autoimmune thyroid diseases.' *Cell and Molecular Immunology 8*, 243–7.

19. Pogge, E. (2010) 'Vitamin D and Alzheimer's disease: Is there a link?' *Consultant Pharmacist 25*, 7, 440–50.

20. Yi, J., Gattoni-Celli, M., Zhu, H., Bhat, N.R. *et al.* (2011) 'Vitamin D3 enriched diet correlates with a decrease of amyloid plaques in the brain of AbetaPP transgenic mice.' *Journal of Alzheimer's Disease 25*, 2, 295–307.

21. Masoumi, A., Goldenson, B., Ghirmai, S., Avagyan, H. *et al.* (2009) '1alpha, 25-dihydroxyvitamin D3 interacts with curcuminoids to stimulate amyloid-beta clearance by macrophages of AD patients.' *Journal of Alzheimer's Disease 17*, 3, 703–17.

22. Culp, M. (2010) 'The Metabolic Syndrome Insulin Resistance, Dysglycaemia and Dyslipaemia. In Nicolle L and Woodriff Beirne (eds) *Biochemical Imbalances in Disease*. London: Singing Dragon. Page 155.

23. Esfahani, A., Wong, J.M., Mirrahimi, A., Srichaikul, K., Jenkins, D.J. and Kendall, C.W. (2009) 'The glycemic index: Physiological significance.' *Journal of the American College of Nutrition 28*, Suppl., 439–445S.

24. 'Bromelain. Monograph.' (2010) *Alternative Medicine Review 15*, 4, 361–8.

25. Johnson, J.J. (2011) 'Carnasol: A promising anti-cancer and anti-inflammatory agent.' *Cancer Letters 305*, 1, 1–7.

26. Fitzpatrick, L.R., Wang, J. and Le, T. (2001) 'Caffeic acid phenethyl ester, an inhibitor of nuclear factor-kappaB, attenuates bacterial peptidoglycan polysaccharide-induced colitis in rats.' *Journal of Pharmacology and Experimental Therapeutics 299*, 3, 915–20.

27. Kelly. G. (2011) 'Quercetin: A monograph.' *Alternative Medicine Review 16*, 2, 172–94.

28. Joseph, J.A., Shukitt-Hale, B. and Casadesus, G. (2005) 'Reversing the deleterious effects of aging on neuronal communication and behavior: Beneficial properties of fruit polyphenol compounds.' *American Journal of Clinical Nutrition 81*, 1, Suppl., 313–6S.

29. Taylor, R. (2011) 'Curcumin for IBD: A review of human studies.' *Alternative Medicine Review 16*, 2, 152–6.

30. Aggarwal, B.B. and Harikumar, K.B. (2009) 'Potential therapeutic effects of curcumin, the anti-inflammatory agent, against neurodegenerative, cardiovascular, pulmonary, metabolic, autoimmune and neoplastic diseases.' *International Journal of Biochemistry and Cell Biology 41*, 1, 40–59.

31. Collard, J. (2009) 'Histamine Intolerance.' *Allergy UK*. Available at www.allergyuk.org/fs_histamine.aspx, accessed on 7 January 2011.

32. Zhao, Y., Qin, G., Sun, Z. *et al.* (2011) 'Effects of soybean agglutinin on intestinal barrier permeability and tight junction protein expression in weaned piglets.' *International Journal of Molecular Sciences* 12, 12, 8502–12.

33. Dalla Pellagrina, C., Perbellini, O., Scupoli, M.T., *et al.* (2009) 'Effects of wheat germ agglutinin on human gastrointestinal epithelium: insights from an experimental model of immune/epithelial cell interaction.' *Toxicology and Applied Pharmacology 237*, 2, 146–53.

34. Katsuya, M., Tanaka, T. and McNeil, P. (2007) 'Lectin-based food poisoning: A new mechanism of protein toxicity.' *PLoS ONE 2*, 8, e687.

35. Cordain, L. (2006) 'Solved: The 10,000-year-old riddle of bread and milk.' *Complementary and Alternative Medicine*, July 2006.

36. Fasano, A. (2011) 'Zonulin and its regulation of intestinal barrier function: The biological door to inflammation, autoimmunity and cancer.' *Physiological Reviews 91*, 1, 151–75.

37. Sapone, A., Bai, J.C., Ciacci, C., Dolinsek, J. *et al.* (2012) 'Spectrum of gluten-related disorders: Consensus on new nomenclature and classification.' *BMC Medicine 10*, 1, 13.

38. Hafstrom, I., Ringertz, B., Spangberg, A. *et al.* (2001) 'A vegan diet free of gluten improves the signs and symptoms of rheumatoid arthritis: the effects on arthritis correlate with a reduction in antibodies to food antigens.' *Rheumatology 40*, 10, 1175–9.

39. Kjeldsen-Kragh, J. (1999) 'RA treated with vegetarian diets.' *American Journal of Clinical Nutrition 71*, 5, 1211–3.

40. Scotece, M., Conde, J., Gómez, R., López, V. *et al.* (2011) 'Beyond fat mass: Exploring the role of adipokines in rheumatic diseases.' *Scientific World Journal 11*, 1932–47.

41. Fain, J.N. (2006) 'Release of interleukins and other inflammatory cytokines by human adipose tissue is enhanced in obesity and primarily due to the nonfat cells.' *Vitamins and Hormones 74*, 443–77.

42. Desantis, A.S., Diezroux, A.V., Hajat, A., Aiello, A.E. *et al.* (2011) 'Associations of salivary cortisol levels with inflammatory markers: The Multi-Ethnic Study of Atherosclerosis.' *Psychoneuroendocrinology*, Epub ahead of print.

43. Baba, H., Ohtsuka, Y., Haruna , H., Lee, T. *et al.* (2009) 'Studies of anti-inflammatory effects of Rooibos tea in rats.' *Pediatrics International 51*, 5, 700–4.

9

Reducing Oxidative Load

Oxidation is what happens to metal when it rusts, to a sliced apple when it turns brown and to the human body when it degenerates. Specifically, oxidation is a chemical reaction in which a molecule loses an electron from one of the pairs in its outer shell. This makes the molecule unstable, a 'free radical' that sets off a chain reaction of damage to cells.

Oxidation occurs continuously within the human body, particularly during the process of cellular respiration (the metabolism of food into energy) within the mitochondria (the 'powerhouses' of the cell). A healthy body can manage a certain level of oxidative stress, through its endogenous antioxidant systems. These comprise the antioxidant (AO) enzymes (superoxide dismutase, glutathione peroxidise and catalase) and various antioxidant compounds, such as glutathione, cysteine, methionine, alpha lipoic acid, melatonin, vitamin D and CoQ10. The body can also use antioxidant substances found in food if these are sufficient in the diet.

However, in some cases the delicate balance between pro-oxidants and antioxidants in the cell is disrupted, leading to excessive oxidative stress. If this is not addressed, it can have significant health implications (see below).

Common factors involved in increased oxidative stress are:

- Endogenous oxidants:
  - poor mitochondrial function (either inherited or acquired)
  - inflammation (see Chapter 8)
  - increased metabolism, such as from high-intensity exercise
  - poor oxygen delivery to tissues from, for example, anaemia, vasoconstriction, atherosclerosis, oedema or sleep apnoea
  - poor liver detoxification systems, especially an excessively high phase 1:phase 2 ratio (see Chapter 3).

- External sources of oxidation:
    - high levels of pollution, including from smoking (active and passive) and allergens
    - dietary components, such as oxidised and *trans*-fats, processed meats and blackened foods
    - sunburn.
- Poor functioning of the endogenous AO systems (due, for example, to poor intake of nutrient cofactors) and/or low intake of dietary AOs.

Antioxidants form an extremely diverse group of compounds, first used in industrial processes (to prevent metal corrosion) and then in food preservation. Some E numbers are AOs, such as E300 (ascorbic acid) and E306 (tocopherols). AOs reduce oxidation because the electrons in their outer shell are not paired – hence, AOs are able to donate their electrons to stabilise free radicals relatively safely.

For more a more detailed discussion see Phull (2010).[1]

Some signs and symptoms of increased oxidative load

- Unexplained fatigue.
- Frequent headaches.
- Skin damage, including 'liver spots'.
- Poor cognition and memory.
- Low mood.
- Inflammatory conditions.
- Being prone to musculoskeletal injury.

Laboratory tests can be used for a wide range of pro-oxidant and AO markers, such as:

- the pro-oxidant and carcinogen p-hydroxyphenyllactate (in a urinary organic acids test)
- the DNA oxidation product 8-hydroxy-2'-deoxyguanosine (in a urinary organic acids test)
- blood levels of glutathione and other AOs, AO enzymes and lipid peroxides.

What health conditions is increased oxidative load linked to in the long term?

Excessive oxidative stress is associated with the ageing process and with many chronic diseases, including cancer, cardiovascular disease and diabetes,[2] diabetic complications,[3] Alzheimer's disease,[4] Parkinson's disease,[5] rheumatoid arthritis[6] and neurodegeneration.[7]

While it is not entirely clear whether oxidative stress is a causative factor in these diseases or a consequence of the disease process, there is some research to indicate the former. For example, there is a correlation between high plasma AO levels and lower risk of CVD and cancer.[8] There is also evidence that oxidative stress leads to insulin resistance and that increasing AO intake improves insulin sensitivity.[9]

Key nutritional interventions to consider

Overview

- Increase AO nutrients from foods (see below).

- Increase cofactors for the body to produce its own AO enzymes and compounds.

- Reduce exposure to food components that increase free radicals. These include polycyclic aromatic hydrocarbons (PAHs), nitrosamines, acrylamides and oxidised and *trans*-fats.

- Manage inflammatory processes (see Chapter 8).

- Optimise detoxification systems (see Chapter 3).

What to eat and drink

- Eat foods high in the well-established antioxidant nutrients:
  - vitamin A (the best source is organic liver but it is also present in eggs and dairy products)
  - vitamin C (bell peppers, papaya, guava, citrus, kiwi, strawberries, broccoli, Brussels sprouts, potato and other fruits and vegetables)
  - vitamin E (wheatgerm, sunflower seeds, hazelnuts, peanuts, almonds).

- Centre your diet around plant-based foods, of as wide a range of colours as possible and including the skins and outer leaves. This is the best way to ensure you are dramatically increasing your intake not only of vitamins C and E but also of the important AO phytochemicals, sometimes called plant bioactives (see Focus box 9.1 for more information).[2, 10]

- Carotenoids:
  - alpha-carotene: carrots, squash, oranges, tangerines
  - beta-carotene: orange and green leafy vegetables, tomato products, apricots, mangoes
  - lycopene: tomatoes
  - beta-cryptoxanthin: oranges
  - lutein and zeaxanthin: green leafy vegetables, especially kale and spinach.
- Flavonoids:
  - flavonols (e.g. quercetin, kaempferol, myricetin): onions, kale, broccoli, apples, tea, red wine, grapes, berries, cherries
  - anthocyanidins: dark red, blue and purple berries, sour cherries
  - flavan-3-ols:
    - catechins (e.g. epigallocatechin gallate): tea, especially green and white tea
    - pro(antho)cyanidins: apples, apricots, cherries, cocoa and dark chocolate
  - flavones: parsley, thyme, celery
  - flavanones (e.g. hesperetin, naringenin): citrus.
- Other phenolic compounds:
  - hydroxycinnamates (caffeic acid): coffee and propolis
  - ferulic acid: cereal brans
  - neochlorogenic and chlorogenic acids: prunes
  - stilbenes (resveratrol): red wine
  - vanillin, capsaicins, zingerone: vanilla, chilli, ginger.
- Phytoestrogens (isoflavones, lignans): soya, other pulses, seeds, grains, nuts.
- Plant sterols: vegetable oils, cereals, nuts, seeds, avocados.

- Glucosinolates: brassicas (Brussels sprouts, cabbage, broccoli, watercress, rocket/arugula). These are thought to be involved in reducing the damaging effects of reactive oxygen species in the development of cancer[11] (see Focus box 3.2).

- Terpenoids: herbs and spices, such as mint, sage, coriander, rosemary, ginger.

Make sure some of these plant foods are eaten raw, in order to preserve the micronutrients. However, beta-carotene and lycopene are better absorbed when the foods are cooked and eaten with fat. Glucosinolates may also be more bioavailable when the cruciferous vegetables are lightly cooked, as the raw plant contains an enzyme that can reduce the conversion of glycosinolates to their active form (isothiocyanates).[12] But note that overcooking also reduces phytochemical availability. (Foods high in AO phytochemicals are often referred to as 'high-ORAC' foods – see Focus box 9.2.)

- Eat foods containing the cofactors for the body's AO enzymes. Important cofactors are:

  - zinc (lean cuts of beef, pork, venison and lamb, crab, poultry, calf's liver, seeds, sea vegetables and wholegrains)

  - copper (organ meats, oysters, nuts and legumes)

  - selenium (Brazil nuts, meat, poultry, fish and wholegrains)

  - manganese (broccoli, orange juice, nuts, beans and wholegrains)

  - glutathione (cysteine-rich foods, such as lean meat, fish and eggs).

- Consume soluble fibre and prebiotic foods (see Chapter 2) that encourage the synthesis of n-butyrate in the colon. N-butyrate reduces the risk of colon cancer[13] and research shows that one of its beneficial roles in the human colon is that of reducing oxidative stress.[14]

What not to eat and drink

- Avoid burnt or blackened foods, from grilling, frying or griddling meats at very high temperatures or for lengthy periods of time, or from barbecuing meats. Cooking by these methods produces polycyclic aromatic hydrocarbons (PAHs).[15] PAHs increase lipid peroxidation and oxidative stress in the body.[16]

- Steer clear of processed meats, such as sausages, bacon, ham and other cured meats. The World Cancer Research Fund has linked their consumption to an increased risk of certain types of cancer.[17] Their consumption increases nitrosamines, which are linked to increased oxidative load.[18, 19]

- Don't eat processed or heated polyunsaturated fats (vegetable oils), as this causes them to oxidise (see Chapter 4).

- Avoid processed foods that contain *trans*-fats (see Chapter 4).

Lifestyle

- Reduce your stress levels, by following the guidance in Chapter 6.

- Reduce your exposure to toxins through pollution, household and personal care chemicals and smoking. For example:

  ○ switch your brands of personal care products and cosmetics to those that are chemical-free

  ○ replace your Teflon with uncoated cook- and bakeware

  ○ avoid using plastics in the microwave

  ○ ensure that containers used for food storage and smoothie shakers are free from bisphenol A (BPA)

  ○ use greaseproof paper in place of cling film or foil for wrapping food

  ○ use white vinegar and other natural household cleaning agents

  ○ take physical exercise in zones that are relatively traffic-free.

  See Focus box 10.2 for more suggestions.

- Take moderate (not excessive) exercise, as this has been shown to improve endogenous AO defence systems.[20]

Focus box 9.1   Phytochemicals
There is currently significant interest in the plant bioactives (also known as phytochemicals), many of which have potent antioxidant (AO) properties. Phytochemicals, such as carotenoids, flavonoids, glucosinolates and others, are abundantly available in fruit, vegetables, herbs, spices, edible fungi, nuts and seeds. This is because plants get energy from the sun (via photosynthesis) – hence, they need to produce chemicals to protect them from the free radicals caused by the solar radiation. See the main text for a list of the individual bioactives and the best food sources.

There is a substantial body of epidemiological, *in vitro* and animal data indicating that foods high in phytochemical antioxidants may help to reduce the risk and severity of degenerative diseases.[2, 21] For example, large cohort studies have found that people who eat more plant foods have a lower risk of cardiovascular disease,[22, 23] dementia and Alzheimer's disease[24] and some cancers;[11, 25] and many *in vitro* and animal studies have demonstrated the capacity of antioxidant nutrients to reduce the risk of oxidative damage to DNA.[26]

These types of observations have led to the suggestion that AOs may reduce the risk of chronic disease and there have followed many intervention trials of AO supplements. Surprisingly, some of the largest of these trials have concluded no significant reduction in the risk of the big killers (such as cancer and CVD) from taking AO supplements.[27, 28, 29] However, some of the studies have been criticised for their metholological shortcomings. For example, synthetic forms of micronutrients have often been used, at exceptionally high doses and sometimes in isolation from other AOs required for their recycling. (An AO will eventually turn into a pro-oxidant, as it becomes electron-depleted, but can be regenerated by other AOs.)[1] This problem is less likely to occur in foods because they contain a range of AOs that work synergistically. What we can conclude is that, rather than focus on supplements, the most important thing to get right is the diet.

In addition, phytochemicals from plant foods have other benefits, over and above their AO qualities.[30] For example, many of them help to regulate the activity of enzymes involved in inflammatory processes, cell cycle control, platelet function and other processes involved in health and disease.[10] In population studies, diets high in fruit and vegetables correlate with lower LDL-cholesterol readings,[31] which is a non-AO mechanism by which high plant food diets may reduce the risk of cardiovascular disease. Hence, the correlation between higher plant food intake and lower risk of degenerative diseases may not solely be due to an AO effect.

Phytochemicals have attracted so much scientific interest in recent years that there now exists a European-wide database on the content and biological activity of phytochemicals in commonly consumed plant foods.[2] Details of how to access the database can be found at EuroFIR (2010).[32]

It is not the phytochemicals themselves that are beneficial to us, but the metabolites that are created from them in the gastro-intestinal tract, the liver and the kidneys.[2, 10] Thus, the optimal functioning of these organ systems, including the balance of the gut microflora, is of crucial importance in extracting the full benefits from these plant foods.

In the test tube and in animal studies, the plant bioactives have powerful AO, anti-mutagenic, anti-carcinogenic and anti-hypertensive effects. While our knowledge on the extent of tissue uptake in humans still has some way to go,[10, 21] there is ample epidemiological research that associates higher plant-based diets with lower risks of chronic disease. For this reason, focusing your diet primarily on plant foods is recommended.

Focus box 9.2   ORAC

Oxygen radical absorbance capacity (ORAC) is a measure of the ability of substances to subdue oxygen free radicals in the test tube.[33]

Developed at Tufts University, Boston, for the US Department of Agriculture in the early 1990s, the scale is based on the results of animal research and studies on human blood (following participants' ingestion of the foods to be tested). It was found that foods with high ORAC scores increased the AO power of human blood and conferred some protection to middle-aged rats against long-term memory loss and damage to capillaries from oxygen.

The leaders of the Tufts research programme recommend a daily intake of 3,000–5,000 ORAC units a day, to improve plasma and tissue AO capacity.[34]

Perhaps unsurprisingly, the top-scoring foods tend to be plant foods of the like outlined in Focus box 9.1, and comprise the most deeply coloured fruits (especially berries, prunes and raisins) and vegetables (especially the dark green leaves).

Although the ORAC tool has its limitations and it has been criticised for being a test tube rather than an *in vivo* measure of AO effect, it has established itself in the consumer consciousness because it is commonly used by food and supplement manufacturers to benchmark the AO potential of their products. Be aware, however, that some of the values claimed for functional foods and food supplements have never been published in the scientific literature and are therefore difficult to evaluate.

Three-day meal plan

Dishes and snacks in italics are supported by recipes in this chapter or other chapters as indicated.

Day 1

Breakfast: Sugar-free muesli with added goji berries and mixed seeds or *Crunchy Berry Granola* (Chapter 4)

Snack: *Tangy Kale Crisps* (Chapter 7)

Lunch: *Creamy Coconut and Greens Soup*

Snack: Handful of blueberries (fresh or frozen)

Dinner: *Butternut Squash, Quinoa and Halloumi Salad with Walnut Oil Vinaigrette.* Optional dessert: *Hot Chocolate and Prune Fondant Puddings*

Day 2

Breakfast: *Green Herb Cleanser* (Chapter 3) or *Supergreens Berry Smoothie* (Chapter 3)

Snack: Handful of raw, mixed nuts

Lunch: *Lemony Prawn Salad*

Snack: *Goji and Berry Cacao Bar*

Dinner: *Mirin and Lemon Baked Salmon or Tofu* with mixed salad. Optional dessert: *Berry Mousse*

Day 3

Breakfast: *Orange Nut Shake*

Snack: Two oat cakes with almond butter

Lunch: *Crunchy Cabbage Slaw with Chilli Tahini Dressing* and a handful of tinned beans or feta cheese

Snack: *Homemade Yoghurt* (Chapter 1) with mixed berries (fresh or frozen)

Dinner: *Shredded Chicken with Tenderstem Broccoli and Sweet Soy, Ginger and Chilli Dressing* and buckwheat noodles (optional)

Drinks

- Pure, filtered water and herbal teas, especially green tea (see above). Coffee is an antioxidant-rich beverage (see Chapter 3) but we advise you to stay within your limit of caffeine tolerance, which varies considerably between individuals. If your sleep is disrupted, or if you feel 'wired' or shaky, you know you've had too much.

- Redbush and white tea.

- Freshly pressed vegetable juices (limit to one small glass a day). Unless you have gastro-intestinal dysbiosis, blood glucose and/or adrenal problems, you could drink an occasional shot of a concentrated cherry juice (available from health food stores and online), for its high levels of anthocyanin antioxidants.

Recipes

Breakfast

Orange Nut Shake

Brazil nuts, rich in the antioxidant mineral selenium, and orange, which contains vitamin C and phytochemicals, make a winning combination to support body systems in times of increased oxidative stress. This easy, dairy-free milkshake makes a simple snack or breakfast – perfect too for children or those with limited appetites. You can make up a batch and keep it in the fridge for 1–2 days.

- SERVES 2

2 oranges, peeled and deseeded
250ml/8fl oz/1 cup water or coconut water
80g/3oz Brazil nuts
1 tsp vanilla extract
30g/1oz pitted dates

Place the oranges in the blender with the water and process until smooth.

Add the remaining ingredients and continue to blend until the mixture is smooth and creamy.

Nutritional information per serving
Calories 341kcal
Protein 7.2g
Carbohydrates 21.6g of which sugars 20.3g
Total fat 25.7g of which saturates 6.5g

Lunch

Creamy Coconut and Greens Soup

This delicious soup is quick and easy to prepare and includes antioxidant-rich sweet potato, green vegetables and beans. Make use of frozen bags of edamame or broad beans, for speed.

- SERVES 4

1 tbsp coconut oil
6 spring onions (scallions), finely chopped
1 garlic clove, crushed
2 sticks celery, chopped
1 medium courgette (zucchini), cut into bite-sized chunks
300g/10½oz sweet potato, peeled cut into small cubes
Zest of 1 lemon
300ml/10½fl oz/1¼ cups vegetable stock

Heat the oil in a large pan. Add the onions, garlic and celery and fry until softened but not coloured.

Add the courgette, potatoes and lemon zest and fry for 2–3 minutes.

Add the stock and coconut milk and bring to the boil. Add the kale and beans and simmer for 15 minutes, or until the potatoes are completely cooked.

Stir in the lemon juice and season to taste.

400g/14oz can coconut milk
150g/5oz kale, chopped, thick stems
    discarded
115g/4oz edamame beans or broad
    beans
1 tbsp lemon juice
Sea salt and freshly ground black
    pepper

Nutritional information per serving
Calories 152kcal
Protein 5.4g
Carbohydrates 23g of which sugars 10.5g
Total fat 4.2g of which saturates 2.4g

Lemony Prawn Salad

This is a simple, quickly prepared, fresh-tasting salad, which combines an omega-rich lemon oil dressing with prawns, raw fennel and peppery watercress. It makes a sensational lunch option or light dinner. Toss in a handful of cherry tomatoes for additional colour. You could also accompany the salad with sourdough or gluten-free bread or baby new potatoes.

    Low in saturated fat and calories, yet rich in protein, prawns provide a healthy alternative to meat and make a quick and easy lunch option. Their amino acids help support the production of immune system compounds and the antioxidant peptide glutathione, and are also used in liver detoxification processes. Prawns are rich in selenium and also provide magnesium, zinc, copper and B vitamins. Lemon zest and watercress are high in phytochemicals and support liver detoxification.

- SERVES 4

Lemon oil dressing
Juice and zest of 1 lemon
3 tbsp flaxseed oil or walnut oil
1 tbsp extra virgin olive oil
2 tsp honey or agave nectar
Pinch of sea salt
Freshly ground black pepper

....

350g/12oz cooked king prawns
1 fennel bulb, cored and sliced thinly
    lengthways
125g/4½oz watercress, thick stalks
    removed
125g/4½oz red and yellow cherry
    tomatoes, halved

Mix together the dressing ingredients and store in the fridge for up to 3 days.

Combine the prawns, fennel, watercress and tomatoes in a large bowl. Drizzle over the dressing and mix gently just before serving.

Nutritional information per serving
Calories 235kcal
Protein 21.2g
Carbohydrates 4.5g of which sugars 4.5g
Total fat 14.7g of which saturates 1.6g

Crunchy Cabbage Slaw with Chilli Tahini Dressing

Crisp cabbage combined with fresh herbs and red onion makes a robust salad, tossed with a zesty tahini dressing. Including both red and green cabbage provides a greater variety of antioxidant and liver-supporting compounds, including polyphenols, glucosinolates and vitamin C. This salad will keep for 2–3 days in the fridge and makes a tasty and healthy accompaniment to main dishes; or, for a lunch, add some protein, such as a hard-boiled egg, mixed beans or some feta cheese. Instead of the tahini dressing, you could use the *Tofu Mayonnaise* (Chapter 1).

- SERVES 4

Dressing
2 tbsp tahini
Juice and zest of 1 lemon
2 tbsp tamari soy sauce
2 tsp chopped chilli, deseeded
1 garlic clove, crushed
2–3 tbsp water to thin as needed

125g/4½oz red cabbage
125g/4½oz green cabbage
1 red pepper, finely diced
1 small red onion, finely diced
Handful of fresh parsley, chopped
Handful of fresh mint, chopped

Place all the dressing ingredients in a blender and process until smooth. Thin with water to create a thick, pouring consistency.

Finely chop or shred the cabbage and place in a bowl with the remaining ingredients. Pour over the dressing and toss to coat completely. Chill in the fridge until needed.

Nutritional information per serving

Calories 87kcal
Protein 3.2g
Carbohydrates 7.6g of which sugars 6.5g
Total fat 4.8g of which saturates 0.7g

Dinner

Butternut Squash, Quinoa and Halloumi Salad with Walnut Oil Vinaigrette

Creamy roasted, carotenoid-rich butternut squash, drizzled with a nutty vinaigrette and accompanied with pan-fried halloumi on a bed of quinoa, creates the most delicious warm salad. Add a scattering of pumpkin seeds just before serving. If you wish to avoid frying, use crumbled feta instead of the halloumi. Try to use unfiltered olive oil, as this has a higher polyphenol content. The dressing can be prepared ahead and kept in the fridge for 2 days.

- SERVES 4–6

700g/1lb 9oz butternut squash, peeled and cut into 2cm/1in cubes
3 tbsp melted coconut oil

Walnut vinaigrette
3 tbsp sherry or balsamic vinegar
4 tbsp walnut oil
1 tbsp fresh mint, chopped
2 tbsp extra virgin olive oil
Handful of pumpkin seeds
Sea salt and freshly ground black pepper

....

150g/5oz quinoa
455ml/16fl oz/scant 2 cups vegetable stock
1 clove garlic, thinly sliced
1 red onion, finely chopped
Handful of rocket (arugula) leaves
250g/9oz halloumi cheese, cut into thin slices, or feta, crumbled
Rice flour for dusting

Preheat the oven to 200°C/400°F, gas mark 6.

Place the butternut squash on a large baking sheet. Toss with 2 tbsp of the coconut oil and season. Bake in the oven for 20 minutes until tender. Keep warm.

Meanwhile, place the quinoa in a pan with the vegetable stock and garlic. Bring to the boil, then reduce the heat to a simmer and cook with the lid on for 15 minutes. Turn off the heat and allow to stand for 5 minutes. Toss in the onion and rocket leaves.

Heat 1 tbsp of coconut oil, dust the halloumi with flour and cook it in a shallow pan until lightly golden on both sides. You may need to do this in batches. Alternatively, use crumbled feta – no need to cook.

Mix all the dressing ingredients together.

Spoon the quinoa on to a serving platter and spoon over the roasted butternut squash and halloumi or feta. Drizzle over the dressing and sprinkle with the seeds to serve.

Nutritional information per serving (6 servings)
Calories 441kcal
Protein 12.7g
Carbohydrates 25g of which sugars 8.5g
Total fat 32.2g of which saturates 12.1g

Mirin and Lemon Baked Salmon or Tofu

This is a quick and simple marinade that works well with oily fish, such as salmon or trout, and is equally delicious with tofu for a vegetarian option. You can either bake the salmon in parchment paper or cook the fillets in a baking dish, covered with the marinade. If using tofu, either place in a shallow baking dish or under the grill for a crispier texture. Serve with a mixed salad.

▪ SERVES 4

4 x 100g/3½oz organic or Alaskan salmon boneless fillets or 400g/14oz firm tofu, cut into cubes
2 tbsp lemon juice and zest
2 tbsp rice vinegar
2 tbsp mirin (Japanese rice wine)
2 garlic cloves, crushed
Handful of fresh mint leaves, chopped
Few slices of fresh lemon
Sea salt and freshly ground black pepper

Place the salmon or tofu in a shallow container. Mix together the remaining ingredients (except lemon slices) and pour over the salmon or tofu. Marinate for 1 hour.

Heat the oven to 200°C/400°F, gas mark 6.

Take four square pieces of baking parchment. Place a salmon fillet on each piece of parchment. Drizzle over the marinade and top with a few slices of lemon. Season with sea salt and black pepper. Fold up the baking parchment to form a parcel with the join at the top and the edges folded in so the juices don't spill. Don't make them too tight. Put them on a baking sheet and cook for 15–20 minutes, by which time the salmon should be cooked through. Alternatively, place the salmon in a baking dish and pour over the marinade. Top with the lemon slices and bake until tender.

Nutritional information per serving (salmon)
Calories 188kcal
Protein 20.4g
Carbohydrates 0.4g of which sugars 0.2g
Total fat 11g of which saturates 1.9g

Nutritional information per serving (tofu)
Calories 81kcal
Protein 8.3g
Carbohydrates 1g of which sugars 0.5g
Total fat 4.2g of which saturates 0.5g

Shredded Chicken with Tenderstem Broccoli and Sweet Soy, Ginger and Chilli Dressing

This is a Thai-spiced dish, bursting with fresh flavours and packed with antioxidants. Poaching the chicken keeps the meat moist and tender. Sweet-tasting tenderstem broccoli is packed full of antioxidants, including vitamin C, beta-carotene and cancer-protective glucosinolates, and provides a good source of folic acid too. Eat it on its own or with some wholemeal or buckwheat noodles.

▪ SERVES 4

4 chicken breasts

Dressing
4 tbsp tamari soy sauce
1 tbsp xylitol (optional)
2 garlic cloves, crushed
1 red chilli, deseeded and finely
   chopped
2 tsp fresh root ginger, grated
Juice of 1 lemon
1 tbsp rice vinegar

250g/9oz tenderstem broccoli,
   trimmed
½ red onion, finely chopped
1 red pepper, sliced thinly
Handful of mange tout (snow peas)
2 carrots, cut into julienne
1 tbsp sesame seeds
Trickle of sesame oil

Bring a large pan of water to the boil. Add the chicken breasts and cook for 10 minutes. Turn off the heat and leave the chicken to poach for a further 15 minutes. Remove from the pan and shred the meat, discarding the skin.

Mix all the dressing ingredients together and set aside. This will keep in the fridge for 3–4 days.

Place the broccoli in a steamer and steam for 3–4 minutes until al dente.

Place the broccoli and other ingredients in a large bowl. Pour over the dressing and mix well. Sprinkle over the sesame seeds and oil to serve.

Nutritional information per serving
Calories 254kcal
Protein 36.8g
Carbohydrates 14.2g of which sugars 13.1g
Total fat 6.6g of which saturates 1.4g

Snacks and desserts

Hot Chocolate and Prune Fondant Puddings

These gluten-free, gooey little puddings make an indulgent treat. The prunes provide soluble fibre to support digestive health and stabilise blood sugar levels. Prunes are also a good source of phytonutrients, including neochlorogenic and chlorogenic acids, which help to protect cells from free radical damage. Serve these scrummy little pots with a dollop of natural yoghurt or coconut cream.

- SERVES 4–6

150g/5oz dark chocolate or carob bars
75g/2¾oz butter or dairy-free spread
30g/1oz xylitol to taste
2 eggs, beaten
15g/½oz tapioca flour
15g/½oz rice flour
1 tsp baking powder
Pinch of salt
Pinch of ground cinnamon
50g/1¾oz pitted prunes, chopped

Preheat the oven to 180°C/350°F, gas mark 4.

Grease 4–6 small metal dariole moulds with a little butter or dairy-free spread

Place the butter and chocolate in a small pan and melt gently over a low heat. Stir well. Allow to cool slightly.

Place the remaining ingredients except the prunes in a food processor or blender, then add the chocolate mixture.

Blend until the mixture is smooth and thick. Stir in the prunes.

Divide the mixture between the dariole moulds. Then bake for 10–12 minutes until the middle is just set – you still want it to be soft and gooey inside.

Serve hot with yoghurt.

Nutritional information per serving (6 servings)
Calories 274kcal
Protein 4.1g
Carbohydrates 27.3g of which sugars 23.4g
Total fat 17.2g of which saturates 9.9g

Goji and Berry Cacao Bar

This is a raw, antioxidant-rich bar, naturally sweetened with dried fruit and frozen berries. Pecan nuts and chia seeds provide protein and essential fatty acids, while the cacao and berries provide phytonutrients. Goji berries score very highly on the ORAC scale. This makes a healthy snack, but is equally delicious as a 'breakfast-on-the-go' option.

- MAKES 12 BARS

30g/1oz goji berries
125g/4½oz/1 cup pecan nuts
125g/4½oz/1 cup pitted dates
60g/2oz/1 cup fresh or frozen
  cranberries
1 tbsp chia seeds
25g/1oz raw cacao powder

Soak the goji berries in warm water for 10 minutes, then drain.

Place the pecan nuts in a high-speed blender or food processor and process until fine.

Place the dates, goji berries and cranberries in a food processor and pulse gently to chop. Add the chia seeds, cacao powder and pecan nuts and process until the mixture forms a dough. Mix thoroughly.

Press the mixture into a 22cm/8½in traybake tin lined with baking parchment and place in the freezer for 2 hours or until firm.

Cut into 12 bars. These can be stored in the fridge for 1 week or frozen for up to 1 month.

Nutritional information per bar

Calories 123kcal

Protein 2g

Carbohydrates 10.2g of which sugars 9.2g

Total fat 8.3g of which saturates 0.9g

Berry Mousse

This dairy-free mousse is packed full of antioxidant-rich berries and it makes a tasty yet healthy dessert or sweet treat. Acai berries are rich in anthocyanins and adding acai powder is an easy way to cram in more protective antioxidants. You could also add a tablespoon of cherry concentrate juice if desired. The cashew nuts create a creamy texture and provide protein to help support blood sugar levels. For a nut-free option, replace them with Greek yoghurt or silken tofu.

▪ SERVES 4–6

125g/4½oz/1 cup cashew nuts,
  soaked for 1–2 hours then
  drained
350g/12oz strawberries
3 tbsp coconut oil, melted
2 tsp acai powder

Simply place all the ingredients in a blender or food processor and blend until smooth and creamy.

Spoon into little glasses and chill in the fridge before serving.

Nutritional information per serving (6 servings)

Calories 200kcal

Protein 4.2g

Carbohydrates 7.3g of which sugars 4.2g

Total fat 16.9g of which saturates 7.2g

References

1. Phull, S. (2010) 'Poor Energy Production and Increased Oxidative Stress'. In L. Nicolle and A. Woodriff Beirne (eds) *Biochemical Imbalances in Disease*. London: Singing Dragon.

2. Denny, A. and Butriss, J. (2007) *Plant Foods and Health*. London: British Nutrition Foundation.

3. Davi, G., Falco, A. and Patrono, C. (2005) 'Lipid peroxidation in diabetes mellitus.' *Antioxidants and Redox Signaling 7*, 1–2, 256–68.

4. Nunomura, A., Castellani, R.J., Zhu, X., Moreira, P.I., Perry, G. and Smith, M.A. (2006) 'Involvement of oxidative stress in Alzheimer's disease.' *Journal of Neuropathology and Experimental Neurology 65*, 7, 631–41.

5. Wood-Kaczamar, A., Gandhi, S. and Wood, N.W. (2006) 'Understanding the molecular causes of Parkinson's disease.' *Trends in Molecular Medicine 12*, 11, 521–8.

6. Hitchon, C.A. and El-Gabalawy, H.S. (2004) 'Oxidation in rheumatoid arthritis.' *Arthritis Research and Therapy 6*, 6, 265–78.

7. Cookson, M.R. and Shaw, P.J. (1999) 'Oxidative stress and motor neurone disease.' *Brain Pathology 9*, 1, 165–86.

8. Biesalski, H.K., Böhles, H., Esterbauer, H., Fürst, P. *et al.* (1997) 'Antioxidant vitamins in prevention.' *Clinical Nutrition 16*, 151–5.

9. Willcox , D.C., Willcox, B.J., Todoriki, H. and Suzuki, M. (2009) 'The Okinawan diet: Health implications of a low-calorie, nutrient-dense, antioxidant-rich dietary pattern low in glycemic load.' *Journal of the American College of Nutrition 28*, Suppl., 500–516S.

10. D'Archivio, M., Filesi, C., Di Benedetto, R., Giovannini, C. and Masella, R. (2007) 'Polyphenols, dietary sources and bioavailability.' *Annali dell'Istituto Superiore di Sanita 43*, 4, 348–61.

11. World Cancer Research Fund (2007) 'Food, Nutrition, Physical Activity and the Prevention of Cancer: A Global Perspective.' Available at www.dietandcancerreport.org/?p=ER, accessed on 26 April 2012.

12. Mithen, R. (2006) 'Sulphur-Containing Compounds.' In A. Crozier, M.N. Clifford and H. Ashihara (eds) *Plants' Secondary Metabolites: Occurrence, Structure and Role in the Human Diet*. Oxford: Blackwell Publishing.

13. Scharlau, D., Borowicki, A., Habermann, N., Hofmann, T. *et al.* (2009) 'Mechanisms of primary cancer prevention by butyrate and other products formed during gut flora-mediated fermentation of dietary fibre.' *Mutation Research 682*, 1, 39–53.

14. Hamer, H.M., Jonkers, D.M., Bast, A., Vanhoutvin, S.A. *et al.* (2009) 'Butyrate modulates oxidative stress in the colonic mucosa of healthy humans.' *Clinical Nutrition 28*, 1, 88–93.

15. Jedrychowski, W., Perera, F.P., Tang, D., Stigter, L. *et al.* (2012) 'Impact of barbecued meat consumed in pregnancy on birth outcomes accounting for personal prenatal exposure to airborne polycyclic aromatic hydrocarbons: Birth cohort study in Poland.' *Nutrition 28*, 4, 372–7.

16. Jeng, H.A., Pan, C.H., Diawara, N., Chang-Chien, G.P. *et al.* (2011) 'Polycyclic aromatic hydrocarbon-induced oxidative stress and lipid peroxidation in relation to immunological alteration.' *Occupational and Environmental Medicine 68*, 9, 653–8.

17. Schatzkin, A. (2007) *Animal Foods*. Available at www.dietandcancerreport.org/cancer_resource_center/downloads/speaker_slides/us/06_Schatzkin_Animal_Foods.pdf, accessed on 10 January 2012.

18. Bartsch, H., Hietanenen, E. and Malaveille, C. (1989) 'Carcinogenic nitrosamines: Free radical aspects of their action.' *Free Radical Biology and Medicine 7*, 6, 637–44.

19. Hecht, S.S. (1997) 'Approaches to cancer prevention based on an understanding of N-nitrosamine carcinogenesis.' *Proceedings of the Society for Experimental Biology and Medicine 216*, 2, 181–91.

20. Leeuwenburgh, C. and Heinecke, J.W. (2001) 'Oxidative stress and antioxidants in exercise.' *Current Medical Chemistry 8*, 7, 829–38.

21. Singh, M., Arseneault, M., Sanderson ,T., Murthy, V. and Ramassamy, C. (2008) 'Challenges for research on polyphenols from foods in Alzheimer's disease: Bioavailability, metabolism and cellular and molecular mechanisms.' *Journal of Agricultural and Food Chemistry 56*, 13, 4855–73.

22. He, F.J., Nowson, C.A. and MacGregor, G.A. (2006) 'Fruit and vegetable consumption and stroke: Meta-analysis of cohort studies.' *The Lancet 367*, 320–6.

23. Martínez-González, M.Á., de la Fuente-Arrillaga, C., López-Del-Burgo, C., Vázquez-Ruiz, Z., Benito, S. and Ruiz-Canela, M. (2011) 'Low consumption of fruit and vegetables and risk of chronic disease: A review of the epidemiological evidence and temporal trends among Spanish graduates.' *Public Health Nutrition 14*, 12, 2309–15.

24. Hughes, T.F., Andel, R. and Small, B.J. (2010) 'Midlife fruit and vegetable consumption and risk of dementia in later life in Swedish twins.' *American Journal of Geriatric Psychiatry 18*, 5, 413–20.

25. Masala, G., Assedi, M., Bendinelli, B., Ermini, I. *et al.* (2012) 'Fruit and vegetables consumption and breast cancer risk: The EPIC Italy study.' *Breast Cancer Research and Treatment 132*, 3, 1127–36.

26. Prasad, K.N. (2004) 'Multiple dietary antioxidants enhance the efficacy of standard and experimental cancer therapies and decrease their toxicity.' *Integrated Cancer Therapy 3*, 4, 310–22.

27. Omenn, G.S., Goodman, G.E., Thornquist, M.D., Balmes, J. *et al.* (1996) 'Risk factors for lung cancer and for intervention effects in CARET, the Beta-Carotene and Retinol Efficacy Trial.' *Journal of the National Cancer Institute 88*, 21, 1550–9.

28. The ATBC Cancer Prevention Study Group (1994) 'The alpha-tocopherol, beta-carotene lung cancer prevention study: Design, methods, participant characteristics and compliance.' *Annals of Epidemiology 4*, 1, 1–10.

29. Bjelakovic, G., Nikolova, D., Gluud, L.L., Simonetti, R.G. and Gluud, C. (2007) 'Mortality in randomized trials of antioxidant supplement for primary and secondary prevention: Systemic review and meta-analysis.' *Journal of the American Medical Association 297*, 8, 842–57.

30. Aolst, B. and Williamson, G. (2008) 'Nutrients and phytochemicals: From bioavailability to bioefficacy and beyond antioxidants.' *Current Opinion in Biotechnology 19*, 2, 73–82.

31. Djoussé, L., Arnett, D.K., Coon, H., Province, M.A., Moore, L.L. and Ellison, R.C. (2004) 'Fruit and vegetable consumption and LDL-cholesterol: The National Heart, Lung and Blood Institute Family Heart Study.' *American Journal of Clinical Nutrition 79*, 213–7.

32. EuroFIR (2010) 'eBASIS: BioActive Substances in Food Information System.' Available at http:// ebasis.eurofir.org/Default.asp, accessed on 8 March 2012.

33. Cao, G., Alessio, H.M. and Cutler, R.G. (1993) 'Oxygen-radical absorbance capacity assay for antioxidants.' *Free Radical Biology and Medicine 14*, 3, 303–11.

34. McBride, J. (1999) 'Can Foods Forestall Ageing?' Available at www.ars.usda.gov/is/AR/archive/ feb99/aging0299.htm, accessed on 9 January 2012.

10

Support for Balanced Brain Chemistry

How we think, feel and behave on a day-to-day basis is very much dependent on the process of 'neurotransmission'. When this process is working optimally – that is, in a way that enables us to interact positively with our environment – we are said to have well-balanced brain chemistry.

Optimal neurotransmission requires the correct and appropriate synthesis of the various brain chemicals (neurotransmitters – NTs), as well as their effective transmission along the neurons (the billions of nerve cells in the brain) and between the neurons (at the synapses). It also requires the NTs' attachment to, and activation of, the relevant receptors on the neurons' membranes and, finally, their efficient disposal, once they have fulfilled their role.

There are many types of neurotransmitters. Some of the most widely researched are as follows:

- Serotonin is often described as the 'happy' neurotransmitter. Serotonin is further metabolised to melatonin, an important antioxidant hormone that promotes sleep.

- Dopamine, adrenalin and noradrenalin (the catecholamines) have caffeine-like effects, providing drive, energy, focus and an upbeat mood. Adrenalin is the first chemical released in response to stress. Dopamine is the 'reward' neurotransmitter and is stimulated by addictive behaviours and substances.

- Glutamate is highly stimulatory.

- Gamma-aminobutyric acid (GABA) quietens brain activity, leading to a sense of calm.

- Acetylcholine aids memory, mental alertness and skeletal muscle function.

- Endorphins work like opiate drugs, relieving pain and promoting euphoria.

Some typical signs and symptoms of brain chemistry imbalances

- Addictive behaviours.

- Starch and sugar cravings; binge eating.

- Low pain threshold.

- Poor sleep.

- Inability to concentrate.

- Hyperactivity.

- Low mood.

- Irritability.

- Anxiety.

- Slow cognition, poor memory.

- Feeling of not being connected with others.

- Fatigue, apathy and lack of motivation.

These symptoms can, of course, be related to other biochemical imbalances, such as those arising from the endocrine, immune or digestive systems, so it is important to look at potential neurotransmitter imbalances in the context of the overall picture.

Chronically raised cortisol levels, for example, can contribute to the development of depression.[1, 2] Inflammation is involved in dementia and Alzheimer's disease.[3] Another example is that of oestrogen, which has a role in bolstering functional serotonin and catecholamine levels. Thus, a sharp drop in oestrogen may lead to symptoms of low serotonin and low catecholamines.[4] Conversely, chronically elevated oestrogen can lead to anxiety, hyperactivity, migraine, hypertension and other symptoms of elevated catecholamine levels.[5]

Laboratory evaluations to consider include:

- urinary levels of the precursor amino acids above

- urinary organic acids indicating serotonin (5-hydroxyindolacetate) and catecholamine (homovanillic acid, 3-methyl-4-hydroxyphenylglycol and vanilmandelic acid) status and for the functional levels of B vitamins, minerals and antioxidants

- urinary porphyrins, to test the extent to which toxic metals are affecting physiological functions

- blood levels of homocysteine, indicating methylation status (see Figure 7.1)

- red cell membrane levels/ratios of fatty acids to indicate those available for nerve cell membrane and receptor health

- serum 25-hydroxyvitamin D (see Focus box 11.2)

- inflammatory markers, such as C-reactive protein (CRP) and erythrocyte sedimentation rate (ESR).

What health conditions are brain chemistry imbalances linked to in the long term?

- Depression, which is now well-accepted as a functional deficiency of serotonin and/or noradrenalin.[4]

- Schizophrenia. Central hyperactivity of the dopaminergic system and dysfunction of the central serotonergic system are thought to be key mediating factors.[4]

- Alzheimer's disease (AD), in which there is a reduced ability to convert choline into acetylcholine within the brain.[6]

- Parkinson's disease, in which there is a destruction of the dopaminergic neurons.[7]

- Childhood behavioural problems such as attention deficit hyperactivity disorder (ADHD), which are thought to involve compromised dopaminergic and serotonergic systems.[8, 9]

- Alcoholism, under which lies compromised functioning of the dopamine, GABA and opioid systems.[10] Similar patterns have been found in drug abuse and other addictions.[11]

- Eating disorders, such as binge eating, anorexia nervosa and bulimia, which may be partly due to alterations in the dopamine, acetylcholine and opioid systems[12] and which are also associated with abnormal GABA levels.[13]

- Irritable bowel syndrome, via the gut–brain axis (see Chapter 2).

- Various syndromes of heightened pain (see Focus box 10.1).

Key nutritional interventions to consider

Aims of the dietary plan

All physiological processes are important in optimising brain chemistry. In particular, there is little value in trying to alter neurotransmitter function without addressing inflammation, blood glucose control, gastro-intestinal health, detoxification function and adrenal function. Therefore, it is important to follow the recommendations in those chapters in addition to the guidelines below.

What to eat and drink

- Focus on a low glycaemic load diet. Glucose is the primary fuel source for the brain, but supply needs to be kept balanced throughout the day. Essentially, this means building your diet around whole foods, with plenty of vegetables, pulses, nuts, seeds and their oils, lean meat, fish, eggs and poultry, some wholegrains and seasonal fruit, and reducing or removing processed foods. See Chapter 5 for a detailed discussion on this way of eating.

- Eat foods containing the raw materials for making the neurotransmitters.

  ○ To make dopamine, adrenalin and noradrenalin, you need the amino acid tyrosine or its precursor phenylalanine. These are mainly found in high-protein foods, such as eggs, soy foods, spirulina, poultry, dairy, fish and seeds (pumpkin and sesame).

  ○ Serotonin is made from the amino acid tryptophan. This is found in eggs, soy foods, spirulina, fish, cheese, pumpkin and sesame seeds, beans and pulses, game and red meat.

  Note that many other amino acids are required in the formation of NTs, such as glutamine, methionine and others. You are likely to get all you need if you eat some 'complete' protein every day (lean meat, fish, poultry, eggs, dairy, soy (tempeh, tofu or natto) or a combination of beans and grains).

  ○ Acetylcholine requires choline, found in egg yolk, fish roe, liver (and other organ meats) and lecithin granules – see our smoothie recipe below. Lack of choline intake has been found to lead to memory loss and poor skeletal muscle function.[14] Choline is also an essential component of the neuron membranes (see below).

- Take in cofactor nutrients for the enzymes that convert the raw materials into the neurotransmitters; and the enzymes that deactivate the neurotransmitters once they have fulfilled their task. A wide range of cofactors is required but in particular:

- All the B vitamins. These are found in whole foods, especially the proteins listed above, plus nuts, seeds and wholegrains.

    Vitamin B12 and folate are required for methylation. This is the biochemical process the body uses to produce not only the brain chemicals themselves but also the phospholipids, which support the neurotransmitter receptors and the myelin sheath that protects the nerve cells.[15] Green leafy vegetables are the best source of folate. (Note that some green leaves also contain oxalic acid, which can impair mineral aborption – see Chapter 3. Boiling and steaming somewhat reduce the oxalate load.) The only bioavailable source of vitamin B12 is animal protein, so vegans are recommended to test their levels in the blood.

    Vitamin B12 deficiency contributes to depression,[16] as does low folate.[17]

- Vitamin C, found in yellow pepper, papaya, guava, citrus, kiwi, strawberries, broccoli, Brussels sprouts, potato, peppers, salad greens and other fruits and vegetables.

    These vitamins are water-soluble. This means that they are excreted from the body within a few hours of absorption. Hence, they need to be eaten every day and preferably at every meal.

- Zinc is an important cofactor for serotonin and other NTs and is the most abundant trace mineral in the brain. Low levels have been associated with depression and ADHD[18] and have also been linked with low GABA levels in anorexia.[13]

    The best sources of zinc are meat, game, fish and seafood. Look to nuts, seeds and seaweeds if you are vegan.

- Iron is crucial for the structure and function of the central nervous system. Cognitive and behavioural disorders are found in children with low iron intake.[19] The most bioavailable iron is haem iron from lean red meat, especially liver and the darker meat from game, poultry and oily fish, as well as eggs. Vegetarian iron, which is less bioavailable, is found in beans, pulses, dark green leafy vegetables and dried fruit. It is better absorbed when eaten with foods rich in vitamin C, such as fruit and raw or lightly cooked vegetables. (See note on oxalic acid above.)

- Copper: good sources are meat, soy, oysters, shitake mushrooms, sesame and sunflower seeds, cashews, brazils, hazelnuts.

- Magnesium is not only a cofactor in the methyl cycle, but is also involved in nerve cell signalling at the synapse. Good sources are lightly cooked

Swiss chard and spinach, kelp, squash, pumpkin seeds, steamed broccoli, halibut and, to a lesser extent, other green vegetables, nuts and seeds.

- Get plenty of calcium, found in dairy products, green leafy vegetables, fermented soy, mung beans, almonds, Brazil nuts, flaxseeds (linseeds), sesame and chia seeds. This mineral is important for the release of NTs at the synapse, enabling the brain cells to talk to each other. A calcium-deficient diet is unlikely to directly affect brain chemistry because your brain will take calcium from your bones – but you need to eat it in order to keep your bones strong. (See note on oxalic acid on page 207.)

- Neurotransmitters released at the synapse then need to bind to receptors situated within the membrane of the target neurone. Essential polyunsaturated fats are required for the phospholipids that anchor these receptors. The phospholipids also form part of the protective myelin sheath around the neurons. Hence, a lack of essential fats is detrimental to NT receptor structure and function,[20] which, in turn, inhibits NT signalling.

  Eating oily fish, such as mackerel, herring, sardines, salmon and trout, is the easiest way to get the important omega-3 fats EPA and DHA. Flax, chia and pumpkin seeds and walnuts are good sources of other omega-3 fats for membrane health (see Chapter 4 for more information).

  A lack of essential fatty acids is implicated in many cognitive and mood disorders and improving the levels and/or ratios of omega-3 and omega-6 polyunsaturated fatty acids has frequently been found to improve symptoms.[21] There is increasing evidence, for example, that EPA may be helpful in depression.[22]

  Another fatty acid, arachidonic acid (AA), is also a crucial component of the brain but it is rarely deficient because not only is it found in meat, poultry, eggs and dairy foods, it is also produced in the body from the omega-6 fats found in seeds and seed oils.

- As in so many biochemical imbalances, eating a rainbow of deeply coloured fruits and vegetables is crucial for their supply of antioxidants. Fruits and vegetables provide vitamins C and E (especially avocados) and the phytochemicals, such as flavonoids and carotenoids, that help to protect the brain cells and neurotransmitters from free radical attack. So eat some at every meal and snack. See Chapter 9 for more information.

- Green tea has been recommended throughout this book for its antioxidant properties. Green tea also contains an amino acid called L-theanine, which has been found to increase low levels of serotonin, dopamine and GABA, enhance learning and memory and reduce anxiety.[23, 24, 25] It is also thought to modify the potentially negative effects of excessive caffeine,[26] which is possibly why most people can drink caffeinated green tea in moderation, without feeling 'wired'. A moderate intake is likely to be about two to three cups a day, although there is considerable variability in the extent to which individuals tolerate caffeine.

What **not** *to eat and drink*

- Avoid foods that cause oxidation (see Chapter 9) and/or inflammation (see Chapter 8). These chapters discuss such foods in detail but, essentially, you should reduce or avoid:

  ○ blackened or overcooked meats and fish

  ○ *trans*-, hydrogenated and oxidised fats (as discussed in Chapter 4)

  ○ a high intake of intensively farmed meat and/or dairy foods

  ○ all processed foods, especially those labelled with ingredients you don't recognise as natural

  ○ sugars, meaning added sugar, fruit juices, alcohol and white starches (white rice, pasta, breads and crackers) – see Focus box 5.3 for more on recognising sugars on food labels.

- Assess your intake of 'drugs'. Recreational drugs, nicotene, alcohol, caffeine and sugar are all highly addictive because of their ability to increase dopamine, endorphins and GABA. Sugar has been shown to be so addictive that it can surpass cocaine reward.[27]

  The problem is that, over time, heavy use of such drugs leads to a reduction in the number of dopamine, endorphin and GABA receptors in the brain. This, in turn, means that you need an increasingly higher intake of the drug, just to feel 'normal'. You're also likely to experience withdrawal symptoms if you try to take a break from your habit.

  With the exception of cigarettes and recreational drugs, most people can consume these substances occasionally, in small amounts, without detrimenal effects. Caffeine may be consumed more regularly by individuals with a higher tolerance level. (Benefits may include improved physical and mental performance[28] and a possible reduced risk of Alzheimer's disease and Parkinson's disease – see Chapter 3.) However, if you experience disrupted sleep and/or mental and physical 'crashes' 1–3 hours after consumption, your intake is likely compromising your adrenal function and brain chemistry. In such cases you should cut out all caffeinated fizzy drinks and reduce your coffee, tea and chocolate intake to a level where you are not experiencing side effects (jitters or shakes) and are not feeling dependent on them. As you may experience withdrawal symptoms, it is important to devise a reduction programme with your health adviser.

- Other problems arise with excess sugar in the diet. Hypoglycaemia, for example, disrupts brain chemistry by triggering adrenalin and noradrenalin. Excess sugar can also feed a fungal imbalance in the GI tract. A systemic overgrowth of the *Candida* yeast, which often starts in the gut, may contribute to the development of Parkinson's disease. This is because the yeast produces acetaldehyde, leading to the destruction of neurons that utilise dopamine.[29]

- Avoid any food that gives you wind or bloating or makes you feel worse than before you ate it. Common culprits are gluten grains, dairy foods and high levels of pulses and beans (including soy).

    The central nervous system (CNS) is directly connected to the gastro-intestinal (GI) tract by what is referred to as the enteric nervous system (ENS) or the gut–brain axis. Because of this link, there are correlations between bloating (and other GI symptoms) and brain chemistry problems, such as depression, anxiety and stress.[30]

    New research indicates that, in the same way that GI dysbiosis and leaky gut can contribute to allergies and autoimmune diseases (see Focus box 2.1), these factors may also promote neurological conditions, such as anxiety, depression and eating disorders.[31] In autism, up to 54 per cent of affected children have been reported to suffer from constipation, diarrhoea and bloating. It has been proposed that autism may partly be the result of GI abnormalities, such as dysbiosis, intestinal permeability and an inability to fully digest proteins from gluten grains and dairy products.[32]

    See Chapter 2 for more discussion on the gut–brain link.

Lifestyle

- Get some sunshine. Not only does it lift the spirits, and indeed full-spectrum light is a primary treatment of choice for seasonal affective disorder,[33, 34] but sunlight is the best natural source of vitamin D. Vitamin D receptors are widely distributed in the brain and low serum vitamin D levels are likely to contribute to depression,[35] cognitive impairment[36] and Alzheimer's disease.[37] See Focus box 11.2 for more information on vitamin D.

- Get eight hours of good-quality sleep a night. Research shows that sleep may be more crucial for brain function than it is for body function.[38] It is during the phases of rapid eye movement (REM) (or dreaming) sleep that memories are stored and learning is consolidated. Poor sleep causes problems with both of these functions,[39, 40] and sleep deficit may play a role in the progression of diseases such as Alzheimer's disease and ADHD.[41]

Regular, good-quality sleep is also vital for emotional health, with poor sleep resulting in irritability, short-temperedness and low mood.[42] If you have trouble sleeping, make sure your bedroom is completely dark and well-ventilated, switch off all the electrics at the plug sockets and keep the two hours prior to bedtime free of computers, television, intense exercise, caffeine and bright lighting. Relax in a warm bath with chamomile or lavender essential oils added.

- There is a great deal of evidence that regular exercise may help improve depression and mental health.[43, 44] Aerobic exercise increases the feel-good endorphins. The most effective exercise for mood disorders is that done outside in natural light. Aim for 30 minutes daily of an exercise that you enjoy, such as a brisk walk with a friend.

- Make time to engage in other types of activity that make you feel good (to raise your endorphins). This might be a particular type of social interaction, or it might be yoga, touching and petting animals, playing games with your children, taking an aromatherapy bath, listening to or playing music, or singing – what do *you* love to do?

- Reduce your exposure to toxic metals, especially mercury, cadmium, lead and aluminium. These may inhibit neurotransmitter function by competing with the cofactor minerals listed above.[4]

  Aluminium and mercury have been linked with the development of Alzheimer's disease and multiple sclerosis, respectively.[4, 45] Anxiety and depression were included in mercury and lead toxicity symptoms experienced by individuals exposed to the air at Ground Zero following the 11 September attacks on the World Trade Centre.[46]

  See Focus box 10.2 for some tips on reducing toxin exposure. If you are particularly concerned about previous exposure, undertake a urinary porphyrin test (see above).

- Improve your ability to cope with stress, by either removing the stressor, walking away from the stressor or changing the way you feel and think about the stressor. Mood swings, poor memory and cognition, apathy, anxiety and depression are all associated with imbalances in the stress hormones. Much is written about this in Chapter 6 – so please refer to the recommendations therein.

- Keep your brain active as you get older. You can do this by reading books and newspapers, learning new skills, doing crosswords and puzzles and regularly engaging in stimulating social interaction. Making good use of your brain may help to reduce age-related cognitive decline.[47]

Focus box 10.1   Supporting the brain can help control pain

Recent work in the area of mindfulness meditation has demonstrated the power of the mind to control pain.[48] There is increasing evidence that what goes on in the brain (the balance of the neurotransmitters) has more of an influence on pain perception than does the extent of the tissue damage at the site of the pain.

For example, in a large database of osteoarthritis patients, researchers found very little correlation between the level of pain experienced and the extent of tissue damage seen on MRI scans. Instead, they found that the patients who had lower levels of dopamine, adrenalin and noradrenalin (due to a genetic variation) had three times the risk of hip pain than the patients not of this genotype.[49] The genetic variation meant that a key enzyme that breaks down these catecholamines was up-regulated – thus, lower catecholamines led to increased pain sensitivity. (Indeed, tricyclic and SNRI antidepressants (which keep catecholamines in circulation) are used in many musculoskeletal pain disorders with some success.)

Serotonin also has a role in pain perception. Both migraine and fibromyalgia are associated with low levels of this neurotransmitter. Increasing serotonin levels (through conventional medication and/or food supplements) has been found to reduce fibromyalgia pain[50, 51, 52] and the number and severity of migraine attacks.[53, 54]

Both these examples show that identifying and intervening in brain chemistry can directly alter pain perception. Rebalancing neurotransmitters can also improve mood, sleep and the ability to cope with stress, all of which can independently aid our ability to manage pain.

Focus box 10.2   Environmental toxins – some tips for reducing your exposure

Food and drink

- Don't cook at high temperatures.

- Don't heat polyunsaturated oils.

- Avoid processed foods, especially those with added colourings, sweeteners and flavourings.

- Switch to as much organic produce as possible. In particular, use organic dairy products (milk, cheese, yoghurt, ice cream, etc.), meats (grass-fed) and eggs. Wash all fruits and vegetables before eating.

- Avoid eating the larger oily fish (e.g. swordfish, tuna, marlin and shark), as they are higher in mercury and chemical pollutants.

- Water can contain many toxins and in general it is better to filter tap water with a multi-stage carbon filter or reverse osmosis filter.

- Minimise your intake of bottled water in soft plastic containers, as chemicals from the plastics often leach into the water. Mineral waters in glass bottles are generally safe, unless the quality of the source is uncertain.

- Avoid sipping your takeaway hot drink through the plastic lid.

- Similarly, avoid using plastics in the microwave and make sure that containers used for food storage and smoothie shakers are free from bisphenol A (BPA).

- Replace any Teflon cook- and bakeware with uncoated glass, clay, stone or enamel versions.

- Minimise the use of cling wraps and aluminium foil. Replace them with paper wraps, such as baking parchment.

Your environment

- Avoid using pesticides or herbicides in your home or garden.

- When choosing hair care and skin care products, look for those without added alcohol, sodium lauryl sulfate, paraben, phthalate or other petrochemicals.

- Avoid aluminium-containing antiperspirants and antacids.

- Minimise the amount of standard carpeting in your home, as this is usually treated with chemicals. Use natural carpets or hardwoods instead.

- Consider whether you need to waterproof and flameproof your furniture coverings and clothes.

- Use paints labelled low- or no-VOC. Paints and finishes release low-level toxic emissions into the air for years after application. The source of these toxins is a variety of volatile organic compounds (VOCs), which may have short- and long-term adverse health effects.

- Take steps to control the levels of dust, bacteria and moulds in your home. Make use of house plants. Consider using an air filter and/or ioniser to reduce the debris in the air.

- Purchase natural cleaning products. Spirit vinegar and bicarbonate of soda are good-value options.

- Minimise your exposure to low-level electromagnetic fields, by restricting your mobile phone use and limiting the amount of electrical equipment in the bedroom.

- Avoid spending long periods of time in heavy traffic, and if you are exercising out of doors stick to traffic-free zones.

- Don't smoke (and avoid passive smoking). It can be difficult to give up the habit because nicotine is so highly addictive. Some people find hypnotherapy and/or psychotherapy helpful.

Three-day meal plan

Dishes and snacks in italics are supported by recipes in this chapter or other chapters as indicated.

Day 1

Breakfast: *Banana Cherry Brain-Food Smoothie*

Snack: *Homemade Sauerkraut* (Chapter 1) with carrot sticks

Lunch: *Warm Red Mullet Salad Niçoise*

Snack: *Hemp Seed and Walnut Dip* with celery sticks

Dinner: *Chicken Lettuce Wraps*

Day 2

Breakfast: *Seeded Protein Bars*

Snack: *Homemade Yoghurt* (Chapter 1)

Lunch: *Nutrient-Packed Salad* (Chapter 1), topped with a poached egg

Snack: *Coconut Blueberry Crumble*

Dinner: *Tomato Rice Soup with Turkey Meatballs* and steamed broccoli

Day 3

Breakfast: *Buckwheat and Amaranth Apple Porridge*, topped with some mixed seeds and a little milk or almond milk

Snack: A small handful of fresh coconut chunks

Lunch: *Baby Beets with Asparagus, Pickled Walnuts and Goat's Cheese*

Snack: *Ginger Roasted Pineapple* and a handful of nuts

Dinner: *Braised Venison or Lamb Casserole* with wilted shredded greens

Drinks

- Herbal teas: relaxing teas include valerian, hop, passion flower, oat flower, marshmallow root, chamomile, lemon balm and kava; stimulating teas include ginger, green, ginseng, liquorice, tulsi, gingko, Schisandra and Ashwagandha.

Recipes

Breakfast

Banana Cherry Brain-Food Smoothie

Yoghurt is a useful source of protein, containing all the essential amino acids, including tryptophan and the tyrosine precursor phenylalanine. Bananas are an additional source of tryptophan, while the Montmorency cherry juice provides melatonin. Adding a spoonful of lecithin granules is an easy way to increase your intake of choline – the precursor to acetylcholine. Bursting with antioxidants, healthy fats and protein, this makes a healthy snack or quick breakfast option.

- SERVES 4

50g/1¾oz whey protein or hemp protein powder, berry or vanilla flavour (additive-free)
2 tbsp ground flaxseed
1 tbsp lecithin granules
280g/10oz/2 cups frozen pitted cherries
2 tbsp Montmorency cherry juice concentrate (available from health food stores and online)
2 ripe bananas, chopped
Handful ice
250ml/8fl oz/1 cup natural yoghurt or soy yoghurt
250ml/8fl oz/1 cup milk or vanilla almond milk (no added sugar)

Place all the ingredients in a high-speed blender and process until smooth and creamy.

Add a little more milk or water to thin as needed.

Nutritional information per serving
Calories 260kcal
Protein 10.3g
Carbohydrates 38.9g of which sugars 27.3g
Total fat 7.1g of which saturates 1.5g

Seeded Protein Bars

Similar to flapjacks, these bars are bound together with dates and nut butter rather than sugars or syrups. The protein powder provides the complete complement of essential amino acids, while the psyllium, chia and oats contain solube fibre and slow-releasing carbohydrate. These nutrients also make the bars useful as a post-exercise snack.

- MAKES 15 BARS

225g/8oz pitted chopped dates
Juice and zest of 3 lemons
115g/4oz nut butter (e.g. almond, cashew or tahini)
60g/2oz coconut oil, melted
150g/5oz/1½ cups gluten-free oats or millet flakes
150g/5oz/1½ cups buckwheat flakes
50g/1¾oz protein powder, plain or vanilla flavour (additive-free)
30g/1oz/scant ¼ cup pumpkin seeds
30g/1oz/scant ¼ cup desiccated coconut
1 tbsp psyllium husks (optional)
30g/1oz/scant ¼ cup sunflower seeds
2 tbsp ground chia seeds or flaxseed
½ tsp bicarbonate of soda

Preheat the oven to 190°C/370°F, gas mark 5. Grease and line a 20 x 30cm/8 x 12in traybake tin with baking parchment.

Place the dates, lemon juice and zest, nut butter and coconut oil in a food processer and blend to create a thick paste.

Place all the dry ingredients in a large bowl and mix together. Pour over the date paste and mix thoroughly (it may be easier to do this with your hands). Spoon the mixture into the tin and press down firmly, smoothing the surface.

Place the mixture in the oven and bake for 20–25 minutes until the top is golden. Remove the tray from the oven. Leave to cool and then cut into 15 bars.

Store in the fridge in an airtight container or freeze for up to 1 month.

Nutritional information per bar
Calories 275kcal
Protein 6.6g
Carbohydrates 24.8g of which sugars 10.8g
Total fat 16.5g of which saturates 7.4g

Buckwheat and Amaranth Apple Porridge

This is a warming, gluten-free breakfast option, rich in amino acids and fibre. Top with fresh berries, dried fruit or a handful of nuts and seeds and pour over a little milk or almond milk to serve. If amaranth is difficult to find, substitute with quinoa grains. If time is short in the mornings, you can prepare this porridge the night before, then add a little hot water or milk and reheat it when required.

▪ SERVES 4

75g/2¾oz buckwheat groats
50g/1¾oz amaranth or quinoa
Juice and zest of ½ lemon
1 tsp ground cinnamon
125ml/4fl oz/½ cup apple juice
200ml/7fl oz water
30g/1oz cashew nuts
30g/1oz dried apricots
150ml/5fl oz/scant ⅔ cup almond milk or milk alternative (optional)

Toast the buckwheat in a pan, stirring over a medium heat for 2–3 minutes until fragrant. Add the amaranth or quinoa and continue stirring until lightly toasted.

Add the lemon juice, zest, ground cinnamon, juice and water to the grains. Bring to a boil. Reduce the heat to a very low simmer and cover. Cook for about 20 minutes, or until most the liquid is absorbed and the grains are soft.

Blend together the cashew nuts, apricots and almond milk to form a thick sauce.

Stir the sauce into the porridge to create a creamy texture. Serve with additional almond milk if desired.

> **Nutritional information per serving**
>
> **Calories 191kcal**
> **Protein 5.8g**
> **Carbohydrates 29.9g of which sugars 6.3g**
> **Total fat 5.4g of which saturates 0.9g**

Lunch

Warm Red Mullet Salad Niçoise

A variation on a classic salad, this is high in protein from the eggs and fish. Red mullet can be obtained from sustainable sources and it contains some omega-3 fats to support neuronal membranes. If unavailable, salmon would make a good alternative.

▪ SERVES 4

4 new potatoes
4 organic or free-range eggs
100g/3½oz green beans, trimmed

Dressing
1 tsp Dijon mustard
Pinch of xylitol (optional)
3 tbsp walnut oil
2 tbsp lemon juice
3 tbsp extra virgin olive oil
Sea salt and freshly ground black
    pepper

1 tbsp coconut oil
4 red mullet fillets, skin on
1 tbsp salted butter or ghee
2 little gem lettuces, leaves
    separated
16 black olives, pitted
150g/5oz cherry tomatoes, halved
1 tbsp capers
2 avocados
Juice of ½ lemon

Cook the potatoes in boiling water for 15–20 minutes until tender. Drain, then halve.

Boil the eggs for 6–7 minutes, then drain and place in ice cold water. Once cool, shell.

Cook the beans in boiling water for 2 minutes. Drain, then refresh under cold water.

Mix the dressing ingredients together. Season to taste.

Heat the coconut oil in a frying pan and pan-fry the mullet fillets skin side down for 5 minutes. Add the butter or ghee and turn the fillets over. Cook for a further minute, then remove the pan from the heat.

Place the potatoes, green beans, lettuce, olives, cherry tomatoes and capers in a bowl and toss together. Slice the avocado and drizzle with a little lemon juice and add to the salad. Cut the eggs in half and place on top of the salad. Drizzle over the some of the dressing.

Divide the salad between four plates and top each one with a mullet fillet.

> **Nutritional information per serving**
>
> **Calories 475kcal**
> **Protein 26.7g**
> **Carbohydrates 5.3g of which sugars 2.7g**
> **Total fat 38.6g of which saturates 8.6g**

Baby Beets with Asparagus, Pickled Walnuts and Goat's Cheese

This is a simple, refreshing salad, rich in folate and B vitamins for cognitive function, and antioxidants to protect cells from free radical damage. Goat's cheese is a useful source of protein and the amino acid tryptophan, which the body converts into our 'feel good' neurotransmitter serotonin. This salad is quick and easy to prepare and the inclusion of walnuts and walnut oil adds valuable omega-3 essential fats too.

▪ SERVES 4

12 raw baby beetroots
1 tsp caraway seeds
3 tbsp olive oil or coconut oil,
   melted
1 tbsp apple cider vinegar
250g/9oz asparagus spears

Dressing
1 tbsp apple cider vinegar
3 tbsp walnut oil
Sea salt and freshly ground black
   pepper

Large handful of lamb's lettuce and
   watercress leaves
150g/5oz goat's cheese, broken into
   small chunks
2 pickled walnuts, chopped into
   small pieces

For the roasted beetroots, preheat the oven to 200°C/400°F, gas mark 6.

Place a large sheet of baking parchment on top of a large sheet of foil. Place the beetroots on to the baking parchment. Sprinkle over the caraway seeds and drizzle over the olive oil (or melted coconut oil) and vinegar. Wrap the beetroots up in the parchment and foil to form a parcel and roast in the oven for 45–60 minutes, or until tender.

While warm, peel the beetroots and cut into wedges or slices.

Steam the asparagus for 5 minutes or until just tender.

Make up the dressing by whisking the vinegar and oil together with a little sea salt and freshly ground black pepper to taste.

To serve, arrange the lamb's lettuce and watercress on plates and top with the beetroot and asparagus. Scatter the goat's cheese and pickled walnuts over the top. Drizzle over the dressing just before serving.

Nutritional information per serving
Calories 364kcal
Protein 12.7g
Carbohydrates 9.1g of which sugars 8.7g
Total fat 30.8g of which saturates 9.1g

Dinner

Chicken Lettuce Wraps

This is a simple, healthy dish using large lettuce leaves as wraps. It is perfect as a lighter meal for lunch or dinner. For a vegetarian option, use firm tofu cut into slices.

▪ SERVES 4

Marinade
4 tbsp lime juice (about 2 limes)
2 tbsp fish sauce
1 tsp xylitol or ¼ tsp stevia
1 red chilli, seeded and thinly sliced
2 tbsp mint leaves, chopped
4 spring onions (scallions), chopped

....

2 chicken breasts, skinless and
    boneless
8 large romaine lettuce leaves
1 carrot, cut into julienne
Handful of beansprouts
Strips of red pepper

Mix together the lime juice, fish sauce, xylitol or stevia, chilli, mint and spring onions for the marinade.

Place the chicken breasts in a pan and cover with water. Bring to the boil, then simmer for 15 minutes. Take off the heat and leave to cool in the water for a further 5 minutes. Remove from the pan and slice thinly, then add to the marinade. Leave to marinate for 15 minutes before using.

Fill the lettuce leaves with the chicken and vegetables and wrap around the filling to serve.

Nutritional information per serving
Calories 101kcal
Protein 19g
Carbohydrates 3g of which sugars 2.6g
Total fat 1.5g of which saturates 0.4g

Tomato Rice Soup with Turkey Meatballs

This is a speedy meal-in-a-bowl lunch or dinner option. Turkey is high in protein and a good source of tryptophan. It also contains selenium, zinc and vitamins B3 and B6. Brown rice provides tryptophan, selenium and magnesium – all important nutrients for neurotransmitter function.

▪ SERVES 4

1 tbsp coconut oil
1 onion, chopped
75g/2¾oz brown rice
½ tsp chilli powder
1 red pepper, diced
450g/1lb tomatoes, quartered
400g/14oz can chopped tomatoes
1 litre/2 pints/4 cups organic chicken
    stock
400g/14oz turkey mince
Pinch of paprika
Sea salt and freshly ground black
    pepper

Heat the coconut oil in a large saucepan. Add the onion and rice and cook for 2–3 minutes. Add the chilli powder and stir in the pepper and fresh tomatoes. Cook over a low heat until softened. Add the can of chopped tomatoes and 500ml chicken stock. Bring to the boil, then lower the heat and simmer for 20 minutes until the rice is tender.

Place the remaining stock in a pan and bring it to a gentle simmer. Season the mince with paprika, sea salt and pepper. Shape into walnut-size balls and drop them into the stock. Poach for 10 minutes, until cooked through.

Remove the meatballs with a slotted spoon and divide between bowls. Add a little of the reserved stock to thin the soup if needed. Spoon over the soup to serve.

Nutritional information per serving
Calories 321kcal
Protein 32.6g
Carbohydrates 24.3g of which sugars 9.4g
Total fat 10.5g of which saturates 4.2g

Braised Venison or Lamb Casserole

This is a tasty, tender one-pot dish, which can be cooked the day before, ready for reheating when needed. Venison is a rich source of protein, tryptophan, B vitamins, iron, zinc and selenium, yet is low in saturated fat. Being a lean meat, it can dry out quickly, but marinating and slow cooking keeps it moist. Although higher in fat, lamb is a good alternative if venison is not readily available. Serve with leafy green vegetables, such as shredded greens, kale or broccoli.

- SERVES 6

700g/1lb 9oz venison shoulder or lamb, cut into bite-sized chunks
400ml/14fl oz/scant 1⅔ cups red wine
3 sprigs fresh thyme
4 garlic cloves, peeled
2 fresh bay leaves
1 tsp juniper berries, crushed
2 tbsp coconut oil
2 onions, chopped
2 carrots, sliced
2 celery stalks, chopped
2 plum tomatoes, skinned and chopped
200ml/7fl oz/generous ¾ cup beef stock
3 tbsp tomato purée
16 black pitted olives

Mix the venison, red wine, thyme, garlic, bay leaves and juniper berries in a bowl until well combined. Cover with cling film and leave in the fridge to marinate overnight.

Remove the meat from the fridge and leave to come to room temperature. Drain the venison, reserving the liquid, herbs and garlic.

Preheat the oven to 150°C/300°F, gas mark 2.

Heat the coconut oil in a large casserole and fry the venison shoulder, turning frequently, until browned all over. Remove from the pan and set aside.

Add the chopped onion, carrot, celery and reserved garlic and herbs to the pan and cook for 5 minutes, or until caramelised.

Add the tomatoes, reserved marinade, beef stock, tomato purée and olives and bring the mixture to the boil. Cook for 5 minutes to reduce the volume of the liquid. Place the venison into the pan, cover with the lid and cook in the oven for 2½ hours until the meat is very tender.

Nutritional information per serving (venison)

Calories 221kcal
Protein 27.1g
Carbohydrates 4.4g of which sugars 3.9g
Total fat 5.7g of which saturates 3.7g

Snacks and desserts

Hemp Seed and Walnut Dip

This creamy dip is a delicious alternative to hummus, especially spread on celery or other vegetable sticks. It can also be used as a sandwich filler or topping on oat cakes and flaxseed crackers. Hemp and walnut are both good sources of omega-3 fats, important for neurotransmitter function.

- SERVES 8

150g/5oz raw shelled hemp seeds
3 tbsp walnut butter
Juice of ½ lemon
1 clove garlic, crushed
Pinch of sea salt
Freshly ground black pepper
2–3 tbsp walnut oil

Place all the ingredients in a food processor and blend to form a smooth, creamy dip.

Add a little more oil if necessary to achieve the desired consistency. Season with sea salt and black pepper to taste.

Nutritional information per tbsp

Calories 111kcal
Protein 4.9g
Carbohydrates 1.4g of which sugars 0.1g
Total fat 9.8g of which saturates 0.8g

Coconut Blueberry Crumble

This is an easy-to-assemble crumble dish, high in protein and packed with antioxidants. Instead of blueberries, you could use mixed berries or bags of frozen fruit, defrosted. While this dish can be baked in the oven like a traditional crumble, it is equally delicious served raw.

▪ SERVES 6

115g/4oz/scant 1½ cups shredded
   coconut
115g/4oz/scant ¾ cups pecan nuts
60g/2oz/½ cup dates
400g/14oz fresh blueberries
1 tsp ground cinnamon
2 tbsp red grape juice

Make the crumble topping. Place the coconut, nuts and dates in a food processor and process to make coarse crumbs.

Spoon the blueberries, cinnamon and grape juice into a baking dish. Top with the crumble topping.

If baking the crumble, place in a preheated oven at 190°C/375°F, gas mark 5, and bake for 20 minutes until lightly golden.

Nutritional information per serving

Calories 287kcal
Protein 3.5g
Carbohydrates 11g of which sugars 11g
Total fat 25.5g of which saturates 11.3g

Ginger Roasted Pineapple

An easy-to-prepare dessert or snack, this is equally as delicious as part of a breakfast option. Ginger is a wonderfully warming spice. Serve with *Homemade Yoghurt* (dairy or soy) (Chapter 1) if desired.

▪ SERVES 4

15g/½oz butter or coconut oil
350g/12oz fresh pineapple chunks
2 pieces of stem ginger, chopped
2 tbsp ginger syrup from jar
1–2 tbsp lime juice to taste

Heat a frying pan. Melt the butter or coconut oil in the pan and, when beginning to foam, add the pineapple pieces. Sauté for a couple of minutes, then add the ginger and syrup. Increase the heat slightly and add the lime juice. Allow the mixture to bubble for 1 minute until syrupy. Spoon into bowls and serve warm.

Nutritional information per serving

Calories 87kcal
Protein 0.5g
Carbohydrates 14.8g of which sugars 14.7g
Total fat 3.3g of which saturates 2g

References

1. Swaab, D.F., Bao, A.M. and Lucassen, P.J. (2005) 'The stress system in the human brain in depression and neurodegeneration.' *Aging Research Reviews 4*, 2, 141–94.

2. McEwan, B.S. (2006) 'Protective and damaging effects of stress mediators: Central role of the brain.' *Dialogues in Clinical Neuroscience 8*, 4, 367–81.

3. Tilstra, J.S., Clauson , C.L., Neidernhofer , L.J. and Robbins, P.D. (2011) 'NF-kB in aging and disease.' *Aging and Disease 2*, 6, 449–65.

4. Puri, B. and Lynam, H. (2010) 'Dysregulated Neurotransmitter Function.' In L. Nicolle and A. Woodriff Beirne (eds) *Biochemical Imbalances in Disease*. London: Singing Dragon.

5. Neil, K. (2010) 'Sex Hormone Imbalances.' In L. Nicolle and A. Woodriff Beirne (eds) *Biochemical Imbalances in Disease*. London: Singing Dragon. Page 245.

6. Higgins, J.P. and Flicker, L. (2001) 'Lecithin for dementia and cognitive impairment.' *Cochrane Database of Systematic Reviews 2003*, 3, CD001015.

7. Epp, L.M. and Mravec, B. (2006) 'Chronic polysystemic candidiasis as a possible contributor to onset of idiopathic Parkinson's disease.' *Bratislava Medical Journal 107*, 6–7, 227–30.

8. Stark, R., Bauer, E., Merz, C.J., Zimmermann, M. *et al.* (2010) 'ADHD related behaviours are associated with brain activation in the reward system.' *Neuropsychologia 49*, 3, 426–34.

9. Ribasés, M., Ramos-Quiroga, J.A., Hervás A., Bosch, R. *et al.* (2009) 'Exploration of 19 serotoninergic candidate genes in adults and children with attention-deficit/hyperactivity disorder identifies association for 5HT2A, DDC and MAOB.' *Molecular Psychiatry 14*, 1, 71–85.

10. Ray, L.A., Courtney, K.E., Bujarski, S. and Squeglia, L.M. (2012) 'Pharmacogenetics of alcoholism: A clinical neuroscience perspective.' *Pharmacogenomics 13*, 2, 129–32.

11. Wise, R.A. (1996) 'Neurobiology of addiction.' *Current Opinion in Neurobiology 6*, 2, 243–51.

12. Avena, N.M. and Bocarsly, M.E. (2011) 'Dysregylation of brain reward systems in eating disorders: Neurochemical information from animal models of binge eating, bulimia nervosa and anorexia nervosa.' *Neuroparmacology*, Epub ahead of print.

13. Birmingham, C.L. and Gritzner, S. (2006) 'How does zinc supplementation benefit anorexia nervosa?' *Eating and Weight Disorders 11*, 4, e109–11.

14. Buchman, A.L. (2009) 'The addition of choline to parenteral nutrition.' *Gastroenterology 137*, 5, Suppl., S119–28.

15. Karakula, H., Opolska, A., Kowal, A., Domański, M., Plotka, A. and Perzyński, J. (2009) 'Does diet affect our mood? The significance of folic acid and homocysteine.' *Polski Merkuriusz Lekarski 26*, 152, 136–41.

16. Tiemeier, H., van Tuijl, H.R., Hofman, A., Meijer, J., Kiliaan, A.J. and Breteler, M.M. (2002) 'Vitamin B12, folate and homocysteine in depression: The Rotterdam Study.' *American Journal of Psychiatry 159*, 12, 2099–101.

17. About-Saleh, M.T. and Coppen, A. (2006) 'Folic acid and the treatment of depression.' *Journal of Psychosomatic Research 61*, 3, 285–7.

18. Cyhlarova, E. and Hart, G. (2011) 'Nutrition and mental health.' *Nutrition Practitioner 12*, 1,4–16.

19. Harris, R.J. (2004) 'Nutrition in the 21st century: What is going wrong?' *Archives of Disease in Childhood 89*, 2, 154–8.

20. Witt, M.R. and Nielson, M. (1994) 'Characterization of the influence of unsaturated free fatty acids on brain GABA/benzodiazepine receptor binding in vitro.' *Journal of Neurochemistry 62*, 4, 1432–9.

21. Hanciles, S. and Pimlott, Z. (2010) 'PUFAs in the Brain.' In L. Nicolle and A. Woodriff Beirne (eds) *Biochemical Imbalances in Disease*. London: Singing Dragon.

22. Martins, J.G. (2009) 'EPA but not DHA appears to be responsible for the efficacy of omega-3 long chain polyunsaturated fatty acid supplementation in depression: Evidence from a meta-analysis of randomized controlled trials.' *Journal of the American College of Nutrition 28*, 5, 525–42.

23. Nathan, P.J., Lu, K., Gray, M. and Oliver, C. (2006) 'The neuropharmacology of L-theanine: A possible neuroprotective and cognitive enhancing agent.' *Journal of Herbal Pharmacatherapy 6*, 2, 21–30.

24. Higashiyama, A., Htay, H.H., Ozeki, M., Juneja, L.R. and Kapoor, M.P. (2011) 'Effects of L-theanine on attention and reaction time response.' *Journal of Functional Foods,* Epub ahead of print.

25. Park, S.K., Jung, I.C., Lee, W.K., Lee, Y.S. *et al.* (2011) 'A combination of green tea extract and L-theanine improves memory and attention in subjects with mild cognitive impairment: A double-blind placebo-controlled study.' *Journal of Medicinal Food 14*, 4, 334–43.

26. Kelly, S.P., Ramirez, G.M., Montesi, J.L. and Foxe, J.J. (2008) 'L-theanine and caffeine in combination affect human cognition as evidence by oscillatory alpha-band activity and attention task performance.' *Journal of Nutrition 138*, 1572–7S.

27. Lenoir, M., Serre, F., Cantin, L. and Ahmed, S.H. (2007) 'Intense sweetness surpasses cocaine reward.' *PLoS ONE 2*, 8, e698.

28. Lara, D.R. (2010) 'Caffeine, mental health and psychiatric disorders.' *Journal of Alzheimer's Disease 20*, Suppl. 1, S239–48.

29. Epp, L.M. and Mravec, B. (2006) 'Chronic polysystemic candidiasis as a possible contributor to onset of idiopathic Parkinson's disease.' *Bratislava Medical Journal 107*, 6–7, 227–30.

30. Yoon, S., Grundmann, O. and Koepp, L. (2011) 'Management of IBS in adults: Conventional and complementary/alternative approaches.' *Alternative Medicine Review 16*, 2, 134–51.

31. Fetissov, S.O. and Dechelotte, P. (2011) 'The new link between gut-brain axis and neuropsychiatric disorders.' *Current Opinion in Clinical Nutrition and Metabolic Care 14*, 5, 447–82.

32. Catell, J. (2011) 'Autism: The gut-brain connection.' *The Nutrition Practitioner 12*, 1, 22–30.

33. Westrin, A. and Lam, R.W. (2007) 'SAD: A clinical update.' *Annals of Clinical Psychiatry 19*, 4, 239–46.

34. Miller, A.L. (2005) 'Epidemiology, etiology and natural treatment of SAD.' *Alternative Medicine Review 10*, 1, 5–13.

35. Ganji ,V., Milone, C., Cody, M.M., McCarty, F. and Wang, Y.T. (2010) 'Serum vitamin D concentrations are related to depression in young adult US population: The Third National Health and Nutrition Examination Survey.' *International Archives of Medicine 3*, 29.

36. Zhang, R. and Naughton, D. (2010) 'Vitamin D in health and disease: Current perspectives.' *Nutrition Journal 9*, 65.

37. Pogge, E. (2010) 'Vitamin D and Alzheimer's disease: Is there a link?' *Consultant Pharmacist 25*, 7, 440–50.

38. Savage, V.M. and West, G.B. (2007) 'A quantitative, theoretical framework for understanding mammalian sleep.' *Proceedings of the National Academy of Sciences 104*, 3, 1051–6.

39. Machi, M.S., Staum, M., Callaway, C.W., Moore, C. *et al.* (2012) 'The relationship between shift work, sleep and cognition in career emergency physicians.' *Academic Emergency Medicine 19*, 1, 85–91.

40. Carskadon, M.A. (2011) 'Sleep's effects on cognition and learning in adolescence.' *Progress in Brain Research 190*, 137–43.

41. Wang, G., Grone, B., Colas, D., Appelbaum, L. and Mourrain, P. (2011) 'Synaptic plasticity in sleep: Learning, homeostasis and disease.' *Trends in Neuroscience 34*, 9, 452–63.

42. Harvard Medical School (2006) 'Importance of Sleep: Six Reasons Not to Scrimp on Sleep.' Harvard Health Publications. Available at www.health.harvard.edu/healthbeat/co_reg.php, accessed on 2 February 2012.

43. Kirby, S. (2005) 'The positive effect of exercise as a therapy for clinical depression.' *Nursing Times 101*, 13, 28–9.

44. Blumenthal, J., Babyak, M.A., Doraiswamy, P.M., Watkins, L. *et al.* (2007) 'Exercise and pharmacotherapy in the treatment of major depressive disorder.' *Psychosomatic Medicine 69*, 7, 587–96.

45. Attar, A.M., Kharkhaneh, A., Etemadifar, M., Keyhanian, K., Davoudi, V. and Saadatnia, M. (2011) 'Serum mercury level and multiple sclerosis.' *Biological Trace Element Research 146*, 2, 150–3.

46. Kokayi, K., Altman, C.H., Calelly, R.W. and Harrison, A. (2006) 'Findings of and treatment for high levels of mercury and lead toxicity in Ground Zero rescue and recovery workers and lower Manhattan residents.' *Explore 2*, 5, 400–7.

47. Mahncke, H.W., Bronstone, A. and Merzenich, M.M. (2006) 'Brain plasticity and functional losses in the aged: Scientific bases for a novel intervention.' *Progress in Brain Research 157*, 81–109.

48. BBC News (2012) 'Scans "show mindfulness meditation brain boost".' Available at www.bbc.co.uk/news/health-16406814, accessed on 2 February 2012.

49. Clauw, D.J. and Witter, J. (2009) 'Pain and rheumatology: Thinking outside the joint.' *Arthritis and Rheumatism 60*, 2, 321–4.

50. Caruso, I., Sarzi Puttini, P., Cazzola, M. and Azzolini, V. (1990) 'Double-blind study of 5HTP versus placebo in the treatment of primary fibromyalgia syndrome.' *Journal of International Medical Research 18*, 3, 201–9.

51. Sarzi Puttini, P. and Caruso, I. (1992) 'Primary fibromyalgia syndrome and 5HTP: A 90-day open study.' *Journal of International Medical Research 20*, 2, 182–9.

52. Juhl, J.H. (1998) 'Fibromyalgia and the serotonin pathway.' *Alternative Medicine Review 3*, 5, 367–75.

53. Yoon, M.S., Savidou, I., Diener, H.C. and Limmroth, V. (2005) 'Evidence-based medicine in migraine prevention.' *Expert Review of Neurotherapeutics 5*, 3, 333–41.

54. Titus, F., Dávalos, A., Alom, J. and Codina, A. (1986) '5HTP versus methysergide in the prophylaxix of migraine: Randomized clinical trial.' *European Neurology 25*, 5, 327–9.

11

Healthy Ageing

This chapter brings together the concepts introduced in the preceding sections, and complements them with a look at current research into the theory of healthy ageing.

Fundamentally, we age because the DNA, lipids and proteins in our cells accumulate damage. Yet, longevity and state of health in the later years are extremely variable between populations and are therefore thought to be modifiable.

Current research on ageing

Epigenetic changes in ageing

The rate at which you age is very much determined by the epigenetic changes you accumulate throughout your life, as a result of your environmental experiences, including your diet and lifestyle.

Epigenetic changes are heritable changes in gene *expression* that are not caused by changes to the DNA *sequence*. (They are heritable in that the changes that occur during your life can be passed on to your offspring.)

Research has focused on epigenetic changes to the biochemical processes of:

- DNA methylation (see Chapter 3 and Figure 7.1 for more on methylation)

- methylation and acetylation of the histones – the little sphere-like proteins around which DNA can wind for compaction. (For a more detailed discussion of the process of histone acetylation, see the free access paper Li, Daniel and Tollefsbol (2011).[1])

Aberrant alterations in the function of these processes occur more frequently the older we get, and are key drivers in age-related disorders. For example, ageing tends to cause a reduction in global DNA methylation *and* an increase in the methylation of certain regions of specific genes. DNA hypermethylation and histone hypoacetylation tend to silence genes, while DNA hypomethylation and acetylated histones promote gene transcription (activation). Thus, a tumour suppressor gene that is hypermethylated may become silenced, increasing the risk of cancer.[2]

Epigenetic changes affect a great many genes, including those involved in telomerase activity. This brings us to a related focus of study in ageing, that of telomere dynamics (telomere length and attrition rate).

Telomeres – the limiting factor to a healthy old age

Telomeres are regions of DNA that protect the ends of chromosomes from damage. Over time, with each DNA replication, the telomeres become shorter. Telomeres that become too short trigger the cell to stop replicating – the cell ceases to function and dies. This is a key part of the ageing process. To counter the shortening process, the body uses the enzyme telomerase to elongate the telomeres.

Thus, the shorter the telomere, the greater the age of the cell, and it is thought that telomere erosion is a driver of age-associated organ decline[3] and the development of many degenerative diseases.[4]

Data from animal studies indicates that increasing telomerase may slow the ageing process.[3] Conversely, telomerase inhibition is being researched as a possible therapy for cancer, since this arrests cell cycling.[5] Such a dichotomy makes this a particularly complex and challenging area of research.

Telomere length varies greatly between individuals of the same chronological age. This is partly due to genetics, but is also influenced by diet and lifestyle (see below).

SIRT-1 – a longevity gene?

A key gene receiving research focus in ageing is that of SIRT-1. SIRT-1 is one of seven 'silent information regulator' genes (also known as 'sirtuins'), which are implicated in longevity. Activation of SIRT-1 has been found to increase lifespan in animal studies.[6] This is partly because it regulates epigenetic changes (see above), in particular, histone acetylation.[1]

Some key biochemical processes involved

Inextricably involved in these drivers of the ageing process are other biochemical processes, of the like that we have discussed in the preceding chapters. Problems with these will contribute to cellular damage, eventually leading to tissue and organ dysfunction, otherwise known as premature ageing. Here are just some examples:

- Oxidative stress is associated with telomere erosion[7] and is well documented to contribute to ageing and age-related chronic diseases.[8] In particular, oxidation of mitochondrial DNA causes defects in the process of metabolising macronutrients into energy. This leads to electron leakage, which speeds up the ageing process.[9, 10] Long-lived individuals (centenarians) tend to have lower levels of oxidation.[11] See Chapter 9 for more on oxidation.

- Excess insulin (from insulin resistance) is associated with accelerated shortening of telomeres,[12] whereas human longevity is associated with insulin sensitivity.[13] See Chapter 5.

- Hyperglycaemia causes glucose to combine with proteins in the body, leading to the production of advanced glycation end products (AGEs). These cause tissue damage and are implicated in many diseases of ageing.[14] Such damage can also be caused by AGEs found in cigarettes and the diet (discussed below). See Chapter 5.

- Poor adrenal function, whether the adrenals are hyperactive or in a state of exhaustion, is linked to poor resistance against age-related degeneration. What's more, population studies show that optimal levels of the adrenal hormone DHEA are associated with increased longevity and fewer age-related diseases;[15] and it has been suggested that some of the manifestations of ageing may be caused by DHEA deficiency.[16] See Chapter 6.

- Increased inflammation appears to be part of the ageing process[17] and a strong body of evidence points to chronic inflammation being the driving force behind most of the today's degenerative diseases. The development of such diseases now seems to be a relatively 'normal' part of the ageing process, and is the key barrier to achieving maximum lifespan. Moreover, all the physiological processes outlined here eventually lead to inflammation. See Chapter 8 for a fuller discussion.

Epigenetic changes and changes to these biochemical processes are thought to be reversible. Hence, there is potential to consider diet and lifestyle as interventions in delaying the effects of ageing. Although much of the research is preliminary, positive dietary changes generally carry no health risk and are thus recommended here.

Key nutritional interventions to consider

Overall strategy

- Follow the general healthy eating guidelines in Chapter 1.

- Identify any potential biochemical imbalances affecting you, and follow the diet and lifestyle guidelines in the relevant chapters.

- Consider implementing the additional diet and lifestyle interventions (below) that are of particular current scientific interest in the ageing process.

What to eat and drink

- Populations that have been studied for their longevity and slow rates of ageing, such as that of Okinawa in Japan, tend to eat diets that have a low glycaemic load, are heavy in fruit and vegetables, have a healthy fat profile (higher in monounsaturated fats and omega-3 polyunsaturates and lower in saturated and *trans*-fats), include fish and legumes and are lower in meat, dairy, refined grains, sugar and calories.[15] Other diets associated with a reduction in degenerative disease risk, such as the traditional Mediterranean diet and the DASH (dietary approaches to stop hypertension) diet, also share these characteristics. For more information on the characteristics of populations where people live measurably longer lives, see Buettner (2008).[18]

- Make root vegetables your main source of starch. The staple carbohydrate in the Okinawan diet is the sweet potato, which is lower in calories, of a lower GL and higher in antioxidants (especially carotenoids) than white potatoes and many grains.

- Other Okinawan staples that have 'superfood' properties include the following:

  - Soy foods. Eat miso, tamari soy sauce, tofu, tempeh and natto. See our recipe for *Natto Fried Rice* below.

  - Bitter melon. Use in salads and stir-fries and see our recipe for *Stir-Fried Bitter Melon with Egg* (Chapter 5).

  - Shiitake mushrooms. See our recipe for *Wild Mushroom and Butterbean Soup* (Chapter 8). They are packed with micronutrients and are a source of vitamin D for vegans (see Focus box 11.2).

  - Burdock root. This is best used as a tea.

○ Seaweeds, such as kombu, hijuki and wakame. See our recipe for *Sea Vegetable Salad with Japanese Dressing* (Chapter 6).

○ Phytochemical-rich herbs and spices, such as turmeric and fennel.

- In animal studies the phytochemical resveratrol has been shown to extend lifespan and reduce the damaging metabolic effects of obesity, by activating the SIRT-1 gene. Clinical trials are now being undertaken.[6, 19]

  The best sources of resveratrol are grapes (in the skins) and red wine. Alcohol intake should, of course, be limited. The lifestyle habits of some high-longevity populations include red wine in moderation and normally with a high plant-based meal. We therefore suggest a maximum of one 125ml/4fl oz glass of dark red wine (pinot noir and Sardinian cannonau wines are higher in resveratrol) on a maximum of five days a week, with a meal. However, this is not recommended for individuals who are at risk of developing an alcohol addiction, nor for individuals with a higher than average risk of cancer – these people should avoid alcohol as much as possible.[20]

- Incorporate the particular phytochemicals that are currently being trialled for their potential to modify aberrant epigenetic changes that exacerbate the effects of ageing.[19] These are as follows:

  ○ Sulforaphane, which is converted from glucosinolates, found in broccoli (especially broccoli sprouts), cauliflower, kale and other cruciferous vegetables. See Focus box 3.2 for more information on glucosinolates. Chapter 3 includes various recipes for cruciferous vegetables.

  ○ Epigallocatechin gallate, from green tea.

  ○ Genistein, which is an isoflavone found in soy foods (see above).

- The fermented soy food natto is not only high in genistein but is also the best food source of vitamin K2. Vitamin K is important for the prevention of age-related degeneration from calcium mishandling (see Focus box 11.1). Good food sources for vitamin K1 are green leaves, broccoli, Brussels sprouts and plant oils, such as rapeseed and olive oils. Natto contains the highest levels of vitamin K2, as seen, although there is also some in liver and fermented cheeses, such as Gorgonzola, Roquefort, Parmesan, semi-hard Munster, curd cheese, Swiss Emmental cheese and Norwegian Jarlsberg. Note that it is best to eat cheese only occasionally, due to its high content of (saturated and arachidonic) animal fat. See our recipe below for *Emmental-Stuffed Aubergine*.

- Eat foods, including some raw, that help to inhibit glycation and the production of AGEs (see above). These are the flavonoids quercetin (found in onions and apples), rutin (buckwheat is a good source – see our recipe below for *Buckwheat and Almond Bread*), epigallocatechin gallate (green tea again), kaempferol (onions, leeks, citrus fruits, grapes and many other fruits and vegetables) and proanthocyanidins (deeply coloured berries).[21, 22, 23]

- Regularly eating an array of brightly and deeply coloured fruits and vegetables may also help to boost your antioxidant capacity (see Focus boxes 9.1 and 9.2). A reduction in oxidative stress is thought to be one of the mechanisms by which the practice of calorie restriction (see below) may increase the length and quality of life.[24] Include raw foods daily, such as mixed salad, raw marinated vegetables and vegetable sticks.

- Include foods that contain nutrients to support methylation. These nutrients are methyl donors, such as methionine and vitamin B12 (from eggs, poultry, fish, soy products and lean, organic or wild meat), betaine (seafood and spinach) and folate (leafy greens).

  Inadequate dietary folate and ageing synergistically disturb the normal process of methylation, leading to high homocysteine levels and increasing cancer risk.[25] Vitamin B6 (found in wholegrains) is also important for the metabolism of homocysteine. See Chapters 3 and 7 for more on methylation.

- Eat foods rich in vitamin D (see Focus box 11.2): oily fish, shellfish, egg yolk, mushrooms and fortified foods (these vary between countries).

- As we age, it is important to ensure we get a good source of highly bioavailable protein every day. This is particularly important in preserving muscle mass. Proteins that have the highest 'biological value' are those found in dairy products and egg whites. (These are proteins that contain all the essential amino acids and which are more easily digested, absorbed and utilised by the body.) Some people don't tolerate dairy products well. If you are one of them, you could try lactose-free dairy or aim to eat 1–2 eggs a day (eggs do not raise blood levels of cholesterol). Wild fish and organic poultry are also good sources of protein. You could also add a high-quality protein powder to smoothies, soups and/or baked products that are not ordinarily protein-rich. See Focus box 11.3 for more information on protein powders.

What not to eat and drink

- Do not eat too much. Excessive weight gain is associated with insulin resistance and inflammation. What's more, according to evidence from animal studies, the practice of calorie restriction (CR) is the most well-established environmental manipulation for extending lifespan.[24] CR has been shown to regulate the epigenetic pathways discussed above, which in turn increases telomerase activity[1] and SIRT-1 expression. The 'healthy ageing' consequences include enhanced cholesterol metabolism, improved insulin sensitivity and reduced glucose levels, improved mitochondrial numbers and function and reduced fat storage.[6, 19, 26] Interestingly, human populations with higher proportions of centenarians tend to have a lower caloric intake.[14, 15]

The ideal calorie intake varies between individuals, according to biochemistry and levels of physical activity. In general, try to take in less than the government's recommended 'average' allowance of 2,000 calories per day for women and 2,500 caloires per day for men. Your diet should be nutrient-dense, rather than energy-dense. It should also be satisfying and you should not deprive yourself of food if you are genuinely hungry.

The practice of intermittent fasting (IF) (where food is only available on alternate days) has also been associated with increased lifespan in animals, as well as with cardio- and neuro-protection and increased resistance to cancer.[27] However, we are not advocating this practice here, due to the potential negative consequences for some individuals, including those with poor glucose control. If you are interested in the practice of IF for health, discuss this with your healthcare practitioner.

- Minimise your intake of sugar, as high blood glucose promotes glycation (see above). See Focus box 5.3 for a list of terms used to denote sugar on food labels. In particular, try not to eat too much fructose because, although it does not adversely affect blood glucose regulation in the short term, it strongly promotes the formation of AGE products.[28] Although most of the negative effects come from eating processed foods, rather than fruits, it would be wise to consume only 2–3 pieces of fruit a day, with a preference for the fruits lower in fructose where possible, such as berries.

- You should also look to reduce intake of AGEs from food. These are found in protein- and fat-rich foods that have been heated to high temperatures to enhance flavour, colour and aroma (a process technically known as the Maillard reaction). The highest food sources are caramelised toppings, pan-fried meats, poultry and cheeses and baked milks, such as custard.[14, 29] We recommend avoiding all processed foods. Another way to reduce AGEs in foods is to cook at lower temperatures, use moist heat rather than dry heat, use shorter cooking times, avoid browning and add acidic ingredients, such as lemon juice or vinegar.

- Aside from the AGE foods, you should also avoid *trans*-fats and any blackened foods, including vegetables, as they increase oxidative load (see Chapter 9).

Lifestyle

- Do not smoke. Tobacco contains AGEs[14] and it down-regulates SIRT-1 expression.[6]

- Pay attention to the overall balance of your life. Aim, on a daily basis, to be:

  - mentally and creatively stimulated but not 'stressed out'

  - connected to people/feeling that you belong to a community: sharing experiences, challenges, hopes and fears

  - experiencing joy and laughter (depression has been associated with accelerated ageing)[30]

  - physically active

  - spending time outside in the daylight and, preferably, the sunlight

  - relaxing, resting, breathing and sleeping well.

- Each of these areas is discussed in the preceding chapters.

Focus box 11.1   Are you gamma-carboxylating?

The biochemical process of gamma-carboxylation is vital for health in the later years. It's a process that activates certain proteins in the body, so that they can attract and hold on to calcium. This is crucial for blood coagulation and also for preserving the health of our bones and our arteries as we get older.

The problem is that many people are not getting enough of the dietary cofactor needed for optimal gamma-carboxylation, and thus for the proteins to bind calcium effectively. The cofactor in question is vitamin K, both K1 and K2.

So, vitamin K is necessary for gamma-carboxylation. But how exactly does this help us keep healthy as we age?

First and foremost, plasma-clotting factors need to be carboxylated in order to start the coagulation cascade; and a lack of vitamin K leads to a tendency towards excessive bleeding.

Second, vitamin K works in bone tissue. It carboxylates (activates) the protein osteocalcin, so that it can hang on to calcium and consolidate it within the bone.[31] People with better vitamin K status (K1 and K2) appear to have fewer fractures;[31, 32, 33] and increasing vitamin K intake improves the amount of osteocalcin that is carboxylated, as well as improving markers of bone health.[31, 34–39] (Note that some of the trials have used doses far above what could realistically be obtained from the diet. These tend to be the trials of a type of K2 called MK-4.[38, 39] The studies of K1 and another type of K2 called MK-7 include those with more reasonable doses.)[40]

A third role of gamma-carboxylation, and thus of vitamin K, is to activate a protein called matrix Gla protein (MGP). When MGP binds calcium, it inhibits calcification of blood vessels, cartilage and other soft tissue.[41] Vascular calcification is a particular problem in ageing because it hardens any pre-existing plaque, reducing blood vessel elasticity and increasing the risk of heart attack and stroke. A direct relationship has been found between the levels of coronary artery calcium and the number of years of life lost, leading some researchers to use coronary calcification as a predictor of an individual's biological age.[42]

Population studies indicate a link between higher dietary intake of vitamin K2 and lower rates of arterial calcification[31] and cardiovascular disease (CVD).[43, 44] Controlled trials show that vitamin K1 may also be helpful.[41, 45]

A possible widespread insufficiency of the vitamin K cofactor

Most people typically get enough vitamin K from the diet for blood clotting purposes. But many experts now believe that a *sub*-clinical deficiency could be widespread and could be contributing to osteoporosis, atherosclerosis and other age-related diseases.[31, 46–48]

This is because proteins in bone and arterial tissue need far higher vitamin K levels for full carboxylation than do blood clotting proteins.[46, 48] The activation of osteocalcin, for example, requires vitamin K at levels ten times that required for blood clotting.[38]

How do you know if you are fully carboxylating?

In the medical setting, an abnormally long prothrombin time is used to identify outright vitamin K deficiencies. However, a more sensitive indicator of functional vitamin K insufficiency is that of serum undercarboxylated osteocalcin (ucOC)[31, 49] and this is now available to healthcare practitioners.

A diet rich in vitamin K should include sources of both K1 (green leafy vegetables and plant oils) and K2 (natto and fermented cheeses) – see the main text for more detailed information on food sources. Lower rates of hip fracture among elderly women are found in eastern Japan, where natto is most widely eaten.[47]

It's also important to be aware that blood-thinning medications, such as warfarin, are vitamin-K antagonists and that vascular calcification is a known side effect of these drugs.[31, 50] Naturally, if you are looking to increase your vitamin K intake and are taking one of these medications, you should consult your doctor.

Focus box 11.2   Vitamin D – crucial for healthy ageing

Vitamin D is well known for its importance in skeletal health. But large-scale population studies also link vitamin D deficiency with many degenerative diseases of ageing.

Vitamin D's wide-ranging roles include controlling calcium metabolism (with vitamin K), regulating cell proliferation and differentiation, promoting immune tolerance (see Chapter 8 and also Focus box 2.1), producing antibiotic substances to control microbes and aiding insulin secretion. It's hardly surprising, then, that vitamin D insufficiency has been implicated in osteoporosis,[51] muscle weakness and falls,[51] upper respiratory tract infections and other infectious immune disorders,[52–54] psoriasis, rheumatoid arthritis and other inflammatory autoimmune conditions,[51, 53] cancer,[51, 53–57] cognitive decline,[51, 58] mood disorders[59] and cardiovascular disease.[51]

The main source of vitamin D is sunlight. But many people in the UK do not get enough year-round sun to synthesise optimal vitamin D levels. This is because it is only available in the summer and its synthesis is significantly diminished under cloud cover, clothing and sunscreen. Even in the summer, it is estimated that 45 per cent of the English population have vitamin D levels of less than 40nmol/L (deficient) and that 75 per cent fail to reach the 'optimal' level of 75nmol/L.[60, 61]

This situation is causing such concern to some experts that they are calling for vitamin D deficiency to be classified as a major 'lifestyle' risk, like smoking, alcohol, obesity and being sedentary.[60, 61]

The best dietary source of vitamin D3 is cod liver oil (at approximately 1,350 IU per tbsp), followed by oily fish (447 IU and 388 IU for 3oz cooked salmon and mackerel respectively).[62] There is also a little in egg yolk, tinned tuna and fortified foods, such as margarine. So try to eat eggs and oily fish regularly. Some mushrooms contain D2 (the precursor to D3), which is the main dietary source for vegans.

It is also important to expose your skin to sunlight, in the middle of the day, every day from April to September, without sunscreen. Start with 2–3 minutes only and build up gradually to a maximum of 30 minutes, taking care not to burn. Seven major UK health charities, including Cancer Research UK and Diabetes UK, have now developed a new joint position statement on vitamin D and sun exposure: 'Enjoying the sun safely, while taking care not to burn, can help to provide the benefits of vitamin D without unduly raising the risk of skin cancer.'

How do you know if you are getting enough vitamin D? We recommend that you run a blood test for serum 25-hydroxyvitamin D (25(OH)D3). The average serum level is estimated to be 54nmol/L (Haggenau 2009) but many experts say that the minimum level to aim for is 75nmol.[60, 61] Some experts even believe that we should be looking to reach levels as high as 100–150nmol/L if we want to reduce the risk of chronic diseases.[63, 56, 64] Their argument is that the existing laboratory reference ranges for serum 25(OH)D are too low, as they are set at the level observed in people who are considered 'normal' only because they do not have rickets, and that the prevention of longer-latency diseases requires far higher serum levels.

Although there is still disagreement about desirable levels of vitamin D and its effects on human health, it has been claimed that 'increasing serum levels at the population level appears to be the most cost-effective way to reduce [chronic] disease rates'.[55] Thus, anyone hoping for a healthy old age should make a start by getting themselves tested.

Focus box 11.3   Protein powders

The use of protein powders is a convenient way to increase your intake of high-quality, easily digestible protein, particularly on those occasions where time does not allow for a sit-down meal. They are also used for sports training and recovery, post-surgical recovery and during periods of appetite loss, such as post-illness or during chemotherapy.

Protein powders vary tremendously in terms of their constituents and their quality, so we have provided a summary of some of the most popular types available.

Whey protein

Whey is often thought of as the premier protein powder of choice. It contains an array of proteins: beta-lactoglobulin, alpha-lactalbumin and serum albumin. The amino acid profile and other components present are similar to those found in human breast milk.

Whey is easily digested by the body. It is rich in sulphur amino acids for the synthesis of glutathione, which is important for antioxidant and detoxification processes. Whey protein has also been shown to enhance healthy bone metabolism[65] and improve markers of cardiovascular health, such as blood pressure and the inflammatory marker C-reactive protein.[66] Whey contains high levels of branch-chain amino acids (BCAAs), useful for preventing muscle catabolism during exercise, and glutamine, important fuel for muscle synthesis.[67]

Processing methods vary — microfiltration and ion exchange are used to separate the fat and lactose from the protein. We recommend 'cold-processing' because heat treatments can degrade the protein and also damage immune-supportive micronutrients. In addition, some people find the 'hydrolysed' form of whey easier to digest. Organic powders are also available.

Whey powders often combine isolate and concentrate forms of the protein. Although the isolate form may be of a higher biological value (i.e. it may be better absorbed and utilised), it tends to lack the active components that the concentrate form contains. These include the immunoglobulins IgG1, IgG2, secretory IgA and IgM.

Casein protein powder is not recommended as it is often highly processed and not easily absorbed. Whole casein, such as in raw milk and aged cheese, is better absorbed and can be used to yield a steady, long-lasting anabolic effect on your muscles. (This is not appropriate if you are milk sensitive, however.) For the best anabolic effects it is suggested you choose quality whey protein for muscle nourishment and post-exercise recovery, while at night you eat a casein-rich food, to keep your muscles in a sustained anabolic mode during the sleeping hours.

Soya

Soya protein is often chosen by those who are sensitive to milk products. Soya protein has also been demonstrated to help lower cholesterol levels,[68] hence it may be an appropriate choice for cardiovascular health. It is rich in arginine and glutamine, which are key fuel sources during exercise. Arginine is also important for blood vessel dilation and glutamine is important for gut, immune and detoxification support. Soya digests more slowly than whey, giving a prolonged release of amino acids, although the biological value is lower compared to animal proteins. It may also provide additional health benefits associated with phytoestrogens.

Egg

Although less popular than whey, egg protein has an excellent amino acid profile and a high biological value, making it a good choice for muscle building. It is a slower releasing protein than whey and may therefore be useful during the day to help stabilise blood sugar levels.

Other options

Hemp protein, pea, rice and blended sprouted seed protein powders are also available and are popular vegan choices.

Pea protein is easily digestible and contains high levels of lysine, BCAAs (to help maintain muscle tissue during exercise), glutamine (aiding muscle recovery) and arginine (to help with muscle metabolism and energy). It is slow-digesting and may therefore promote satiety. Preliminary research indicates it may have a potential role in supporting kidney function.[69]

Hemp protein is also easy to digest, comprising around 65 per cent globulin edestin and 35 per cent albumin protein, more than any other plant. It is also a source of fibre and beneficial omega-3, 6 and 9 fatty acids. It contains some vitamins and minerals, including iron.

Rice protein is a useful source for those with allergies to dairy, egg or soy. It is commonly mixed with other protein powders and/or vitamins and minerals.

All protein powders should, of course, be considered as a supplement to, rather than a replacement for, a healthy diet. It is important to check labels. Your product should be low-glycaemic, low-carbohydrate and should not contain any artificial sweeteners, sugar alcohols, glycerine, sugar, artificial flavourings or fillers. It should also be certified free of genetically modified organisim (GMO) ingredients. Some powders contain supplementary nutrients, such as green algae, fibre, probiotics, vitamins, minerals and antioxidants.

Three-day meal plan

Dishes and snacks in italics are supported by recipes in this chapter or other chapters as indicated.

Day 1

Breakfast: *Berry Protein Shake*

Snack: *Avocado Spiced Hummus* with carrot sticks

Lunch: *Braised Cabbage in Red Wine.* Optional dessert: *Soaked Prunes with Orange and Ginger*

Snack: *Raspberry Buckwheat Slice*

Dinner: *Slow-Roasted Lemon-Spiced Lamb with Garlicky Wilted Kale*

Day 2

....

Breakfast: *Green Herb Cleanser* (Chapter 3)

Snack: *Buckwheat and Almond Bread* with almond or hemp seed butter (available from health food shops)

Lunch: *Emmental-Stuffed Aubergine* with a salad of green leaves

Snack: *Yoghurt and Berry Parfait*

Dinner: *Chicken and Okra Tomato Curry* with a salad of green leaves

Day 3

....

Breakfast: *Black and Green Smoothie*

Snack: Handful of mixed seeds

Lunch: *Lettuce Waldorf Wraps*

Snack: *Mango Green Pudding*

Dinner: *Natto Fried Rice* with steamed greens

Drinks

....

- Choose from fresh, unfiltered water, herbal teas (ashwaghanda, green tea, white tea, redbush tea), *Alkaline Detox Broth* (Chapter 3), which can be sipped throughout the day, and/or miso soup.

Recipes

Breakfast

Berry Protein Shake

This is a tangy and creamy milkshake. The addition of hemp seeds adds omega-3 fats and protein to the drink, but for additional protein consider adding a scoop of protein powder. Soaking the nuts helps to make them more digestible and easier to blend.

- SERVES 4

30g/1oz/¼ cup almonds, soaked for at least 1 hour

30g/1oz/¼ cup cashew nuts, soaked for at least 1 hour

1 tbsp hemp seeds, soaked

900ml/32fl oz/3½ cups water or coconut water

300g/10½oz mixed berries (use a bag of frozen berries if desired)

1–2 tbsp xylitol or pinch of stevia to taste if needed

Place the nuts, seeds and water in a blender and process until smooth and creamy. Pour through a sieve to create a smoother texture if desired.

Place back in the blender with the berries and xylitol and blend again until smooth.

Nutritional information per serving

Calories 151kcal

Protein 6.1g

Carbohydrates 5.9g of which sugars 4g

Total fat 11.5g of which saturates 1.5g

Black and Green Smoothie

This is an antioxidant-rich smoothie packed with sweet berries and mineral-rich greens. Adding hemp protein provides valuable amino acids, fibre and essential fats.

▪ SERVES 1

250ml/8fl oz coconut water or water
4 tbsp blueberries (ideally frozen)
4 tbsp strawberries (ideally frozen)
4 tbsp raspberries (ideally frozen)
1 small banana
Handful of kale leaves
30g//1oz/1 scoop hemp protein powder

Simply place all the ingredients in a processor and blend until smooth.

Nutritional information per serving

Calories 217kcal

Protein 17.2g

Carbohydrates 26.9g of which sugars 21.3g

Total fat 4.3g of which saturates 0.2g

Lunch

Braised Red Cabbage in Red Wine

Rich in antioxidants, this combination of red wine, apples and cabbage creates a vibrant accompaniment to meat or fish, but could equally well form a light lunch if you add a little protein, such as tofu, nuts or beans. It is also delicious served cold and will keep in the fridge for 2–3 days. Red cabbage is a good source of vitamins K1 and C, folate and carotenoids and is particularly high in polyphenols.

▪ SERVES 4–6

2 tbsp coconut oil
1 red onion, finely sliced
2 dessert apples, peeled, cored and
  sliced
1kg/2lb 3oz red cabbage, finely
  sliced
75g/2¾oz raisins
100ml/3½fl oz/scant ½ cup sherry
  vinegar
100ml/3½fl oz/scant ½ cup red wine
Sea salt and freshly ground black
  pepper

Melt the coconut oil in a large casserole dish over a medium heat and sauté the onion for 2–3 minutes until softened. Stir in the apple and cabbage and cook for 5 minutes.

Add the raisins, sherry vinegar and red wine.

Cover with a lid, then cook for 1 hour, until all the vegetables are just tender. Season to taste.

Nutritional information per serving (4 servings)
Calories 188kcal
Protein 3.6g
Carbohydrates 25.7g of which sugars 25g
Total fat 5.4g of which saturates 3.9g

Emmental-Stuffed Aubergine

Swiss Emmental cheese is fermented by *proprioni* bacteria, producing a type of vitamin K2 called MK-9(H4). Aged cheeses, such as Emmental and Gouda, provide friendly bacteria and, like other cheeses, are rich in protein, vitamin A and calcium. However, as cheese is relatively high in saturated fat, it should only be consumed in moderation. Instead of Emmental, you could also use Jarlsberg, Gouda or Munster. This is a delicious vegetarian meal which can be prepared in advance and heated when needed. Serve with a leafy green salad.

▪ SERVES 4

2 large aubergines (eggplants)
30ml/2 tbsp lemon juice
Sea salt and freshly ground black
  pepper
2 tsp coconut oil
1 shallot, finely chopped
½ courgette (zucchini), finely
  chopped
4 sun-dried tomatoes in oil, drained
30g/1oz black pitted olives, chopped
1 tbsp fresh mint
1 tbsp pine nuts
90g/3¼oz Emmental cheese, grated

Preheat the oven to 190°C/375°F, gas mark 5. Cut the aubergines in half lengthways and score the cut sides. Place scored side up on a baking sheet. Rub in the lemon juice and sprinkle with a little sea salt. Bake in the oven for 20 minutes until soft.

Allow to cool slightly, then scoop the flesh out of the aubergines without damaging the skin and chop finely.

Heat the oil in a frying pan and sauté the shallot and courgette for 5 minutes until soft. Add the aubergine flesh and mix thoroughly.

Drain and chop the tomatoes; chop the olives and mint. Place in a bowl with the remaining ingredients and season to taste.

Spoon the filling into the aubergines and return to the oven for 10 minutes until the cheese has melted.

Nutritional information per serving
Calories 189kcal
Protein 8.5g
Carbohydrates 3.1g of which sugars 2.7g
Total fat 15.9g of which saturates 6.4g

Lettuce Waldorf Wraps

This low-carb vegan wrap is made using large green leaves, such as romaine, collard greens, or cabbage. Quick and easy to assemble, these make a perfect light lunch or healthy snack. Packed with flavonoids and other antioxidants, and omega-3 fats, this is a delicious recipe for healthy ageing. Instead of the lettuce leaves, you could use sheets of nori seaweed. The nut dressing is also delicious drizzled over steamed vegetables or spread on crackers.

▪ SERVES 4

Nut dressing
125g/4½oz/1 cup cashew nuts
2 tbsp lemon juice
1 tbsp nutritional yeast flakes
Pinch of garlic salt
5 tbsp water

....

1 green apple, finely chopped
3 sticks celery, chopped
4 tbsp walnut pieces
4 tbsp dried unsweetened
    cranberries
8 large romaine lettuce leaves or
    collard or spring greens

To make the nut dressing, simply place all the ingredients in a high-speed blender and blend until smooth, adding enough water to produce a thick creamy dressing.

Place all the filling ingredients in a bowl and toss in about 3 tbsp of the dressing to coat.

If using collard leaves or cabbage, cut the leaves away from the thick centre of the stem and roll each leaf gently with a rolling pin to make them more pliable. Romaine leaves do not require rolling. Spoon a little of the filling across the shorter width of each leaf. Roll up into a wrap and serve with the dressing on the side.

Nutritional information per serving
Calories 192kcal
Protein 4.1g
Carbohydrates 12g of which sugars 11.1g
Total fat 14.2g of which saturates 1.9g

Dinner

Slow-Roasted Lemon-Spiced Lamb with Garlicky Wilted Kale

This meltingly tender lamb dish is satisfyingly rich and virtually cooks itself. The mild spices provide additional flavour as it cooks and combines well with the wilted kale. Accompany with *Cauliflower Tahini Mash* (Chapter 3). Any leftovers can be used for lunch the following day.

▪ SERVES 6–8

1.5kg/3lb shoulder of lamb
1 tsp coriander seeds
1 tbsp thyme, chopped
1 tsp black peppercorns
2 star anise, roughly crushed
2 lemons, zest only
2 tbsp olive oil

Preheat the oven to 160°C/300°F, gas mark 2, and place the lamb into a roasting tray. Score the skin with a very sharp knife.

Crush the coriander seeds, thyme, peppercorns and star anise in a pestle and mortar. Mix the spices with the lemon zest and the oil. Rub the mixture into the shoulder, massaging into the meat. Ideally, leave to marinate at room temperature for 30–60 minutes.

300ml/10½fl oz/scant 1¼ cups lamb stock

200ml/7fl oz/generous ¾ cup red wine

2 tsp coconut oil

1 garlic clove, crushed

400g/14oz kale, shredded

Pour the stock and red wine into the roasting tray. Place the lamb into the oven to cook for 4–5 hours or until the meat falls away from the bone, basting occasionally with the juices from the pan. Remove from the oven and lift out the lamb. Allow it to rest in a warm place, covered, for 15 minutes.

Skim the fat from the cooking juices left in the bottom of the roasting tray. Place the tray over the hob and add a little more stock or boiling water to create a thin gravy.

Heat the coconut oil in a frying pan. Add the garlic and shredded kale to the pan and stir-fry for about 2 minutes until the kale is looking cooked. Add a splash of water if the pan is too dry. Slice the lamb and serve with the gravy and kale.

> **Nutritional information per serving (6 servings)**
> **Calories 358kcal**
> **Protein 36.5g**
> **Carbohydrates 1.1g of which sugars 0.9g**
> **Total fat 20.8g of which saturates 8.8g**

Chicken and Okra Tomato Curry

This nutritious curry contains okra, also known as ladies' fingers, which is particularly rich in soluble fibre (pectin and gums) for digestive function and healthy cholesterol levels. Okra is a good source of beta-carotene, vitamins B6 and C, iron and calcium. It also contains glutathione, a powerful antioxidant that supports detoxification. The tomatoes and sweet potato provide antioxidant carotenoids, including lycopene. Accompany with a green leafy salad.

▪ SERVES 4

1 tbsp coconut oil

1 tsp yellow mustard seeds

4 boneless, skinless chicken thighs, cut into small strips

1 sweet potato, peeled and chopped into cubes

1 red onion, finely chopped

2 garlic cloves, crushed

2cm/1in piece of ginger, finely grated

1 green chilli, seeded and finely chopped

Heat the coconut oil in a large frying pan. Add the mustard seeds and fry until they pop. Add the chicken pieces and cook for 2–3 minutes, or until browned all over.

Stir in the sweet potato, onion, garlic, spices and sea salt and sauté for 1–2 minutes. Add the rest of the ingredients and bring the mixture to a simmer. Cook for 20 minutes until the chicken is cooked through. Add a little water or stock if the mixture becomes too dry.

½ tsp ground cumin
½ tsp ground coriander
1 tsp ground turmeric
½ tsp sea salt
350g/12oz okra, trimmed, sliced
    diagonally into 2cm/1in pieces
400g/14oz tinned tomatoes

Nutritional information per serving

Calories 224kcal
Protein 20.8g
Carbohydrates 15.7g of which sugars 8.9g
Total fat 9.2g of which saturates 3.8g

Natto Fried Rice

Natto is a traditional Japanese dish made from soybeans fermented with *Bacillus subtilis*. The fermentation process makes the beans easier to digest and enables us to better absorb the nutrients. Natto has a stringy consistency and a strong smell and it can be an acquired taste. Eaten as a breakfast staple in Japan for over 1,000 years, natto is a great source of protein and is particularly rich in vitamin K2 (see text). If you are new to using natto, this is a good recipe to get you started and works well as a light lunch. Accompany with steamed greens or a leafy green salad.

▪ SERVES 4

150g/5oz brown basmati rice
1 tbsp coconut oil
4 spring onions (scallions), finely
    chopped
1 leek, finely sliced
115g/4oz/2 packets of natto (available
    from online Japanese food suppliers)
2 organic eggs, beaten
Freshly ground black pepper
1 tbsp tamari soy sauce

Place the rice in a pan and cook in simmering water until cooked and tender, about 20 minutes.

Heat the coconut oil in a wok or large frying pan. Sauté the spring onions and leek for 2–3 minutes until softened.

Beat the natto in a bowl with the eggs until thoroughly combined.

Add the egg and natto to the pan, stirring so that it does not burn. As it begins to set, add the cooked rice and stir well for 3–4 minutes until warmed through and lightly golden. Season with black pepper and tamari.

Nutritional information per serving

Calories 264kcal
Protein 11.6g
Carbohydrates 34.1g of which sugars 1.9g
Total fat 9.4g of which saturates 3.6g

Snacks and desserts

Avocado Spiced Hummus

This is a great alternative to standard hummus, packed with healthy monounsaturated fats, B vitamins, folate, vitamin K and soluble fibre. Nutritional yeast flakes are optional but do provide additional B vitamins to the dish.

- SERVES 4–6

1 ripe avocado, cut in half, skin and stone removed
400g/14oz can chickpeas, drained and rinsed
2 garlic cloves, crushed
Juice and zest of 1 lemon
½ tsp ground cumin
1 tsp nutritional yeast flakes (optional)
½ tsp smoked paprika
Sea salt to taste

Place all the ingredients into a food processor and blend until smooth.

Spoon into a bowl and cover with cling film. Chill in the fridge until needed.

Nutritional information per tbsp

Calories 21kcal
Protein 0.9g
Carbohydrates 1.7g of which sugars 0.1g
Total fat 1.2g of which saturates 0.2g

Soaked Prunes with Orange and Ginger

Prunes are particularly high on the ORAC scale (see Focus box 9.2), containing phytonutrients important in protecting cells from free radical damage. This is a simple dessert or snack which you can prepare ahead, leaving the prunes to soak in the juice. Serve with a handful of nuts or natural yoghurt.

- SERVES 4

200ml/7fl oz/generous ¾ cup freshly squeezed orange juice
½ tsp cinnamon
½ tsp grated fresh ginger
1 tbsp xylitol (optional)
20 pitted prunes

Place the orange juice, spices and xylitol in a small saucepan and bring to the boil. Add the prunes and simmer on a very low heat for 5 minutes.

Allow the mixture to cool.

Nutritional information per serving

Calories 68kcal
Protein 1g
Carbohydrates 16.8g of which sugars 16.8g
Total fat 0.2g of which saturates 0g

Raspberry Buckwheat Slice

Satisfy those sweet cravings with this fruity, moist bar filled with fresh berries. The use of dried fruit means there is no need to include added sugars, making this a healthier option than most other cereal bars. Buckwheat flakes and nuts provide slow-releasing carbohydrate and protein. Cashew nuts are rich in copper and iron to help support red blood cell synthesis, essential for maintaining energy and cognitive function.

- MAKES 12 SLICES

200g/7oz raspberries
150g/5oz/1¼ cups cashew nuts
225g/8oz/2¼ cups buckwheat flakes
125g/4½oz dates, chopped, or raisins
1 tbsp vanilla extract
125g/4½oz coconut oil or butter, melted

Preheat the oven to 190°C/375°F, gas mark 5.

Mash the raspberries with a fork in a bowl and set aside.

Process the nuts in a food processor to form a fine flour. Add the buckwheat flakes and process again to break them down. Place in a large bowl.

Place the dates or raisins, vanilla and butter in a food processor and blend to form a paste. Add to the dry ingredients and mix well with your hands to form a crumbly dough.

Place half of the mixture into a greased and lined 20cm/8in square shallow baking tin. Press the mixture down well with the back of a metal spoon.

Spread the mashed raspberries over the nut base, then top with the remaining nut mixture, pressing down lightly.

Bake in the oven for 25–30 minutes until golden brown. Allow to cool, then cut into 12 slices.

Nutritional information per slice
Calories 250kcal
Protein 4.9g
Carbohydrates 21.1g of which sugars 8.1g
Total fat 16.2g of which saturates 6.6g

Buckwheat and Almond Bread

This is a dark, slightly sweet-tasting gluten-free bread, with a delicious nutty flavour. The seeds add a wonderful crunch. Buckwheat is a good source of the antioxidant flavonoid rutin, which helps to extend the protective effects of vitamin C. It also contains soluble fibre and lignans. If you need to avoid dairy, use coconut oil or a dairy-free spread.

- MAKES 1LB LOAF, ABOUT 12 SLICES

115g/4oz/scant ¾ cup rice flour
100g/3½oz/heaped ½ cup potato flour
85g/3¼oz/scant ⅔ cup buckwheat flour
50g/1¾oz ground almonds
1 tsp gluten-free baking powder
1 tsp xanthan gum
1 tsp molasses
1 tbsp easy-blend dried yeast
50g/1¾oz dairy-free spread, coconut oil or unsalted butter, cut into small pieces
30g/1oz/¼ cup mixed seeds (e.g. sesame, sunflower, flaxseed)
½ tsp sea salt or seagreens
400ml/14fl oz warm water

Sift the flours into a large mixing bowl and stir in the ground almonds, baking powder, xanthan gum, molasses and yeast.

Rub in the dairy-free spread, oil or butter until the mixture resembles breadcrumbs. Mix in the seeds and season with sea salt or seagreens.

Pour in the warm water and beat to form a batter.

Cover with cling film and leave to rise for 1 hour.

Preheat the oven to 200°C/400°F, gas mark 6.

Grease a 450g/1lb loaf tin. Spoon the dough into the tin and allow it to rise again for 20 minutes.

Bake for 45–50 minutes until it is golden brown and cooked through.

Transfer to a cooling rack and allow to cool before cutting and serving.

Nutritional information per slice

Calories 161kcal
Protein 4.2g
Carbohydrates 19.2g of which sugars 0.9g
Total fat 7.3g of which saturates 2.6g

Yoghurt and Berry Parfait

Using a variety of berries, cherries and red grapes in this dish provides plenty of antioxidants. If you cannot tolerate dairy, use plain soy yoghurt or serve with a nut cream instead. This is a simple layered dish, ideal for breakfast, snacks or a healthy dessert.

▪ SERVES 4

115g/4oz fresh strawberries
75g/2¾oz toasted flaked almonds
400g/14oz low-fat live Greek yoghurt or soy yoghurt
400g/14oz mixed berries, cherries and red grapes, fruits sliced if large

Place the strawberries in a blender and process to form a smooth sauce.

Sprinkle a few almonds in the base of four glasses. Spoon in a little yoghurt, then top with berries. Drizzle over a little sauce then repeat the layering, ending with fruit, the sauce and a scattering of almonds.

Place in the fridge until ready to eat.

Nutritional information per serving

Calories 226kcal
Protein 9.9g
Carbohydrates 20.3g of which sugars 20.3g
Total fat 11.6g of which saturates 1.5g

Mango Green Pudding

This dessert is simple and speedy to make and is a good way to cram more greens into your diet. To increase the protein content, you could add a scoop of protein powder. Instead of flaxseed, you could add a teaspoon of psyllium husks to create a thicker pudding. Allow the pudding to chill for 15 minutes to help it thicken slightly.

- SERVES 4

2 ripe mangos
2 large handfuls of spinach leaves
1 tbsp ground flaxseed
Coconut water to blend if needed

Simply place all the ingredients in a food processor or blender and process until smooth. Add a little coconut water if needed to help it blend together.

Spoon into bowls to serve.

Nutritional information per serving

Calories 72kcal
Protein 2.3g
Carbohydrates 11.5g of which sugars 10.5g
Total fat 2g of which saturates 0.3g

References

1. Li, Y., Daniel, M. and Tollefsbol, T.O. (2011) 'Epigenetic regulation of caloric restriction in aging.' *BMC Medicine 9*, 98.

2. Lu, Q., Qui, X. and Hu, N. (2006) 'Epigenetics, disease and therapeutic interventions.' *Ageing Research Reviews 5*, 4, 449–67.

3. Jaskelioff, M., Muller, F. and Paik, J. (2010) 'Telomerase reactivation reverses tissue degradation in aged telomerase-deficient mice.' *Nature 469*, 102–6.

4. Bendix, L. and Kolvraa, S. (2010) 'The role of telomeres in aging-related disease.' *Ugeskrift for Laeger 172*, 40, 2752–5.

5. Shawi, M. and Autexier, C. (2008) 'Telomerase, senescence and ageing.' *Mechanisms of Ageing and Development 129*, 1–2, 3–10.

6. Kelly, G. (2010) 'A review of the sirtuin system, its clinical implication and the potential role of dietary activators like resveratrol: Part 1.' *Alternative Medicine Review 15*, 3, 245–63.

7. Demissie, S., Levy, D. and Benjamin, E.J. (2006) 'Insulin resistance, oxidative stress, hypertension and leukocyte telomere length in men from the Framingham heart study.' *Aging Cell 5*, 4, 325–30.

8. Malinin, N.L., West, X.Z. and Byzova, T.V. (2011) 'Oxidation as "the stress of life".' *Aging 3*, 9, 906–10.

9. Greaves, L.C., Reeve, A.K., Taylor, R.W. and Turnbull, D.M. (2012) 'Mitochondrial DNA and disease.' *Journal of Pathology 226*, 2, 274–86.

10. Kidd, P. (2005) 'Neurodegeneration from mitochondrial deficiency.' *Alternative Medicine Review 10*, 4, 268–93.

11. Barbieri, M., Rizzo, M.R., Manzella, D., Grella, R. *et al.* (2003) 'Glucose regulation and oxidative stress in healthy centenarians.' *Experimental Gerontology 38*, 1–2, 137–43.

12. Demissie, S., Levy, D. and Benjamin, E.J. (2006) 'Insulin resistance, oxidative stress, hypertension and leukocyte telomere length in men from the Framingham heart study.' *Aging Cell 5*, 4, 325–30.

13. Barbieri, M., Boccardi, V. and Papa, M. (2009) 'Metabolic journey to healthy longevity.' *Hormone Research 71*, Suppl. 1, 24–7.

14. Luenvano-Contreras, C. and Chaman-Novadofski, K. (2010) 'Dietary advanced glycation end products and aging.' *Nutrients 2*, 12, 1247–65.

15. Willcox, D.C., Willcox, B.J., Todoriki, H. and Suzuki, M. (2009) 'The Okinawan diet: Health implications of a low-calorie, nutrient-dense, antioxidant-rich dietary pattern low in glycemic load.' *Journal of the American College of Nutrition 28*, Suppl., 500–516S.

16. Gaby, A. (1996) 'Dehydroepiandrosterone: Biological effects and clinical significance.' *Alternative Medicine Review 1*, 2, 60–69.

17. Tilstra, J.S., Clauson, C.L., Neidernhofer, L.J. and Robbins, P.D. (2011) 'NF–kB in aging and disease.' *Aging and Disease 2*, 6, 449–65.

18. Buettner, D. (2008) *Blue Zones: Lessons for Living Longer from the People Who've Lived the Longest.* Washington, DS: National Geographic.

19. Kelly, G. (2010) 'A review of the sirtuin system, its clinical implication and the potential role of dietary activators like resveratrol: Part 2.' *Alternative Medicine Review 15*, 4, 313–28.

20. World Cancer Research Fund (2007) 'Food, Nutrition, Physical Activity and the Prevention of Cancer: A Global Perspective.' Available at www.dietandcancerreport.org/?p=ER, accessed on 26 April 2012.

21. Asgary, S., Naderi ,G., Sarrafzadegan, N., Ghassemi, N. *et al.* (1999) 'Antioxidant effect of flavonoids on hemoglobin glycosylation.' *Pharmaceutica Acta Helvetica 73*, 5, 223–6.

22. Urios, P., Grigorova-Borsos, A.M. and Sternberg, M. (2007) 'Flavonoids inhibit the formation of the cross-linking AGE pentosidine in collagen incubated with glucose, according to their structure.' *European Journal of Nutrition 46*, 3, 139–46.

23. Wolfram, S. (2007) 'Effects of green tea and EGCG on cardiovascular and metabolic health.' *Journal of the American College of Nutrition 26*, 4, 373–88S.

24. Speakman, J.R. and Mitchell, S.E. (2011) 'Caloric restriction.' *Molecular Aspects of Medicine 32*, 3, 159–221.

25. Choi, S.W. and Friso, S. (2005) 'Interactions between folate and arginine for carcinogenesis.' *Clinical Chemistry and Laboratory Medicine 43*, 10, 1151–7.

26. Elliot, P. and Jirousek, M. (2008) 'Sirtuins: Novel targets for metabolic disease.' *Current Opinion in Investigational Drugs 9*, 4, 371–8.

27. Froy, O. and Miskin, R. (2010) 'Effect of feeding regimens on circadian rhythms: Implications for aging and longevity.' *Aging 2*, 1, 7–27.

28. Gaby, R. (2005) 'Adverse effects of dietary fructose.' *Alternative Medicine Review 10*, 4, 294–306.

29. Uribarri, J., Woodruff , S., Goodman, S., Cai, W. *et al.* (2010) 'Advanced glycation end products in foods and a practical guide to their reduction in the diet.' *Journal of the American Dietetic Association 110*, 6, 911–16.e12.

30. Wolkowitz , O., Reus, V. and Mellon, S. (2011) 'Of sound mind and body: Depression, disease and accelerated ageing.' *Dialogues in Clinical Neuroscience 13*, 25–39.

31. Kidd, P. (2010) 'Vitamins D and K as pleiotropic nutrients: Clinical importance for the skeletal and cardiovascular systems and preliminary evidence for synergy.' *Alternative Medicine Review 15*, 3, 199–222.

32. Kaneki, M., Hodges, S.J., Hosoi, T., Fujiwara, S. *et al.* (2001) 'Japanese fermented soybean food as the major determinant of the large geographic difference in circulating levels of vitamin K2: Possible implications for hip-fracture risk.' *Nutrition 17*, 4, 315–21.

33. Booth, S.L. (2009) 'Roles for vitamin K beyond coagulation.' *Annual Review of Nutrition 29*, 89–110.

34. Katsuyama, H., Ideguchi, S., Fukunaga, M., Fukunaga, T. *et al.* (2004) 'Promotion of bone formation by fermented soybean (Natto) intake in premenopausal women.' *Journal of Nutritional Science and Vitaminology 50*, 2, 114–20.

35. Forli, L., Bollerslev, J., Simonsen, S., Isaksen, G.A. *et al.* (2010) 'Dietary vitamin K2 supplement improves bone status after lung and heart transplantation.' *Transplantation 89*, 4, 458–64.

36. Takemura, H. (2006) 'Prevention of osteoporosis by foods and dietary supplements. "Kinnotsubu honegenki": A fermented soybean (natto) with reinforced vitamin K2 (menaquinone-7).' *Clinical Calcium 16*, 10, 1715–22.

37. Cheung, A.M., Tile, L., Lee, Y., Tomlinson, G. *et al.* (2008) 'Vitamin K supplementation in postmenopausal women with osteopenia (ECKO trial): A randomized controlled trial.' *PLoS Medicine 5*, 1, e196.

38. Plaza, S.M. and Lamson, D.W. (2005) 'Vitamin K2 in bone metabolism and osteoporosis.' *Alternative Medicine Review 10*, 1, 24–35.

39. Cockayne, S., Adamson, J., Lanham-New, S., Shearer, M.J., Gilbody, S. and Torgerson, D.J. (2006) 'Vitamin K and the prevention of fractures: A systematic review and meta-analysis of randomized controlled trials.' *Archives of Internal Medicine 166*, 12, 1256–61.

40. Brugè, F., Bacchetti, T., Principi, F., Littarru, G.P. and Tiano, L. (2011) 'Olive oil supplemented with menaquinone-7 significantly affects osteocalcin carboxylation.' *British Journal of Nutrition 106*, 1058–62.

41. Braam, L.A., Hoeks, A.P., Brouns, E., Hamulyák, K., Gerichhausen, M.J. and Vermeer, C. (2004) 'Beneficial effects of vitamins D and K on the elastic properties of the vessel wall in postmenopausal women: A follow-up study.' *Thrombosis and Haemostasis 91*, 2, 373–80.

42. Shaw, L.J., Raggi, P., Berman, D.S., Callister, T.Q. *et al.* (2006) 'Coronary artery calcium as a measure of biologic age.' *Atherosclerosis 188*, 1, 112–9.

43. Geleijnse, J.M., Vermeer, C., Grobbee, D.E., Schurgers, L.J. *et al.* (2004) 'Dietary intake of menaquinone is associated with a reduced risk of coronary heart disease: The Rotterdam Study.' *Journal of Nutrition 134*, 11, 3100–5.

44. Gast, G.C., de Roos, N.M., Sluijs, I., Bots, M.L. *et al.* (2009) 'A high menaquinone intake reduces the incidence of coronary heart disease.' *Nutrition, Metabolism, and Cardiovascular Diseases 19*, 7, 504–10.

45. Shea, M.K., O'Donnell, C.J., Hoffmann, U., Dallal, G.E. *et al.* (2009) 'Vitamin K supplementation and progression of coronary artery calcium in older men and women.' *American Journal of Clinical Nutrition 89*, 1799–807.

46. McCann, J. and Ames, B. (2009) 'Vitamin K, an example of triage theory: Is micro-nutrient inadequacy linked to diseases of ageing?' *American Journal of Clinical Nutrition 90*, 889–907.

47. Stevenson, M., Lloyd-Jones, M. and Pappaioannu, D. (2009) 'Vitamin K to prevent fractures in older women: Systematic review and economic evaluation.' *Health Technology Assessment 13*, 45.

48. Vermeer, C. and Theuwissen, E. (2011) 'Vitamin K, osteoporosis and degenerative diseases of ageing.' *Menopause International 17*, 1, 19–23.

49. McCormick, R. (2007) 'Osteoporosis: Integrating biomarkers and other diagnostic correlates into the management of bone fragility.' *Alternative Medicine Review 12*, 2, 113–45.

50. Crowther, M.A., Ageno, W., Garcia, D., Wang, L. *et al.* (2009) 'Oral vitamin K versus placebo to correct excessive anticoagulation in patients receiving warfarin: A randomized trial.' *Annals of Internal Medicine 150*, 5, 293–300.

51. Zhang, R. and Naughton, D. (2010) 'Vitamin D in health and disease: Current perspectives.' *Nutrition Journal 9*, 65.

52. White, J.H. (2008) 'Vitamin D signaling, infectious diseases, and regulation of innate immunity.' *Infection and Immunity 76*, 9, 3837–43.

53. Hewison, M. (2010) 'Vitamin D and the immune system: New perspectives on an old theme.' *Endocrinology and Metabolism Clinics of North America 39*, 2, 365–79.

54. Sabetta, J.R., DePetrillo, P., Cipriani, R.J., Smardin, J. and Landry, M.L. (2010) 'Serum 25(OH)D and the incidence of acute viral respiratory tract infection in the healthy adults.' *PLoS One 5*, 6, e11088.

55. Grant, B. (2011) 'The Impact of Improving Vitamin D Levels – Health and Financial Outcomes.' Sunlight, Nutrition and Health Research Centre. Presented at the Vitamin D Experts' Forum, London, April 2011.

56. Baggerly, C. and Garland, C. (2011) 'Vitamin D and Breast Cancer Prevention.' Presentation at the Vitamin D Experts' Forum, London, April 2011.

57. Holick, M.F. (2008) 'Vitamin D and sunlight: Strategies for cancer prevention and other health benefits.' *Clinical Journal of the American Society of Nephrology 3*, 5, 1548–54.

58. Pogge, E. (2010) 'Vitamin D and Alzheimer's disease: Is there a link?' *Consultant Pharmacist 25*, 7, 440–50.

59. Murphy, P.K. and Wagner, C.L. (2008) 'Vitamin D and mood disorders among women: An integrative review.' *Journal of Midwifery and Women's Health 53*, 5, 440–6.

60. Gillie, O. (2006) 'A new government policy is needed for sunlight and vitamin D.' *British Journal of Dermatology 154*, 1052–61.

61. Gillie, O. (2011) Sunlight Robbery: The Failure of UK Policy on Vitamin D: In Search of Evidence-Based Public Health Policy.' Presented at the Vitamin D Experts' Forum, London, April 2011.

62. Office of Dietary Supplements (ODS) (2011) *Dietary Supplement Fact Sheet: Vitamin D.* National Institutes of Health. Available from http://ods.od.nih.gov/factsheets/vitamind/, accessed on 1 June 2011.

63. Heaney, R.P. and Holick, M.F. (2011) 'Why the IOM recommendations for vitamin D are deficient.' *Journal of Bone and Mineral Research 26*, 3, 455–7.

64. Zitterman, A. (2003) 'Vitamin D in preventive medicine: Are we ignoring the evidence?' *British Journal of Nutrition 89*, 552–72.

65. Hoffman, J. and Falvo, M. (2004) 'Protein – which is best?' *Journal of Sports Science and Medicine 3*, 118–130.

66. Pins, J.J. and Keenan, J.M. (2006) 'Effects of whey peptides on cardiovascular disease risk factors.' *Journal of Clinical Hypertension 8*, 11, 775–82.

67. Cribb, P., Williams, A. and Carey, M. (2002) 'The effect of whey isolate on strength, body composition and plasma glutamine.' *Medical Science in Sports and Exercise 34*, 5, S299.

68. Anderson. J.W., Johnstone, B.M. and Cook-Newell, M.E. (1995) 'Meta-analysis of the effects of soy protein intake on serum lipids.' *New England Journal of Medicine 333*, 276–82.

69. Aluko, R. (2009) 'Proteins from garden pea may help fight high blood pressure, kidney disease.' *Science Daily*, 22 March 2009. Available at www.sciencedaily.com/releases/2009/03/090322154407.htm, accessed on 26 April 2012.

Index